Textbook of Pediatric Otorhinolaryngology—
Head and Neck Surgery

VOLUME II
HEAD AND NECK

Textbook of Pediatric Otorhinolaryngology— Head and Neck Surgery

VOLUME II
Head and Neck

Edited by

Chris De Souza, M.S., D.O.R.L., D.N.B., F.A.C.S.

Consulting ENT Surgeon
The Holy Family Hospital
The Holy Spirit Hospital
The Lilavati Hospital
Bombay, India

Visiting Assistant Professor
The State University of New York

James Stankiewicz, M.D.

Professor and Vice Chairman
Department of Otolaryngology—Head and Neck Surgery
Loyola University Chicago Medical Center
Maywood, Illinois

Phillip K. Pellitteri, D.O.

Associate, Section of Otolaryngology/Head and Neck Surgery
Vice Chairman, Division of Surgery
Penn State Geisinger Medical Center
Penn State Geisinger Health System

Associate Professor of Clinical Surgery
Penn State College of Medicine
Hershey, Pennsylvania

SINGULAR PUBLISHING GROUP, INC.
SAN DIEGO · LONDON

Notice: The indications, procedures, drug dosages, and diagnosis and remediation protocols in this book have been recommended in the clinical literature and conform to the practices of the general medical and health services communities. All procedures put forth in this book should be performed only by trained, licensed practitioners. The diagnostic and remediation protocols and the medications described do not necessarily have specific approval by the Food And Drug Administration for use in the disorders and/or diseases and dosages for which they are recommended. Because standards of practice and usage change, it is the responsibility of practitioners to keep abreast of revised recommendations, dosages, and procedures.

Singular Publishing Group, Inc.
401 West "A" Street, Suite 325
San Diego, California 92101-7904

Singular Publishing Ltd.
19 Compton Terrace
London, N1 2UN, UK

Singular Publishing Group, Inc., publishes textbooks, clinical manuals, clinical reference books, journals, videos, and multimedia materials on speech-language pathology, audiology, otorhinolaryngology, special education, early childhood, aging, occupational therapy, physical therapy, rehabilitation, counseling, mental health, and voice. For your convenience, our entire catalog can be accessed on our website at **http://www.singpub.com.** Our mission to provide you with materials to meet the daily challenges of the ever-changing health care/educational environment will remain on course if we are in touch with you. In that spirit, we welcome your feedback on our products. Please telephone (**1-800-521-8545**), fax (**1-800-774-8398**), or e-mail (**singpub@mail.cerfnet.com**) your comments and requests to us.

© 1999 by Singular Publishing Group, Inc.

Typeset in 10/12 Palatino by So Cal Graphics
Printed in the United States by BookCrafters

All rights, including that of translation, reserved. No part of this publication may be reproduced, stored in a retrieval system, or transmitted in any form or by any means, electronic, mechanical, recording, or otherwise, without the prior written permission of the publisher.

Library of Congress Cataloging-in-Publication Data

Textbook of pediatric otorhinolaryngology : head and neck surgery /
   editors, Chris de Souza, James Stankiewicz, Phillip K. Pellitteri.
      p. cm.
   Includes bibliographical references and index.
   ISBN 1–50593–958–1 (set : hardcover)
   1. Pediatric otolaryngology. 2. Head—Surgery. 3. Neck—Surgery.
I. De Souza, Chris. II. Stankiewicz, James A. III. Pellitteri,
Phillip K.
   [DNLM: 1. Otorhinolaryngologic Diseases—in infancy & childhood
2. Head—surgery. 3. Neck—surgery.   WV 140T355 1998]
RF47.C4T49 1998
618.92'09751—dc21
DNLM/DLC
for Library of Congress   98–8530
                                                                     CIP

Contents

Foreword

The field of pediatric otorhinolaryngology has undergone tremendous growth and clinical refinement during the past 25 years. There have been a large number of advances, including development of more effective techniques for laryngotracheal reconstruction, improvement in the methods for managing congenital laryngeal abnormalities, perfection of the instrumentation for bronchoesophagology and sinus surgery, and introduction of rigid fixation for maxillofacial trauma and craniofacial reconstruction. In otology, we have seen the success of cochlear implantation, the evolution of clinical practice guidelines for otitis media, and significant advances in pediatric audiology and immittance testing.

Research in pediatric otorhinolaryngology has flourished and has led to the better understanding of numerous congenital and acquired problems of infants and children, including genetic hearing loss and various craniofacial syndromes. The research studies in laboratories around the world have been supplemented by numerous practice-based studies, including the recent focus on clinical outcomes and patient satisfaction.

Educational programs for physicians who desire to specialize in this field also have undergone considerable changes. A number of outstanding fellowships have been created. There is a trend for these programs to last 2 years, rather than 1 year, as was previously the case. In addition, we have seen a substantive increase in publications and other continuing medical education programs.

We are indeed fortunate that Drs. Christopher de Souza, James Stankiewicz, and Phillip K. Pellitteri have expended the enormous effort necessary to produce this book. They have not only shared their own considerable experience, but have also recruited an outstanding international faculty of contributors. The entire editorial panel is composed of clinicians who have dealt with both children and adults and therefore have the unique perspective of studying diseases at all ages. Each author brings a special flavor to this well-organized book, both in presenting his or her unique experience and in challenging the reader to compare that experience with his or her own.

It is my hope that this book will receive the wide distribution and thoughtful acceptance that it merits. There is no doubt that patient care around the world will be enhanced by careful consideration of the principles presented by the editors and contributors. The children and families entrusted to our care are indeed special. The opportunity to help them deal with disease, disability, and disfigurement is one of our greatest privileges. The sharing of our clinical experiences is one of our primary responsibilities. This book gives superb evidence of the dedication and commitment to that high purpose.

Frank E. Lucente, M.D., F.A.C.S.
Professor and Chairman
Department of Otolaryngology
College of Medicine
State University of New York
Health Science Center at Brooklyn

Preface to Volume II

It is with a sense of great pride and accomplishment that we, the editors, offer this initial edition of the *Textbook of Pediatric Otorhinolaryngology—Head and Neck Surgery*. This work was developed and produced in an effort to provide a practical, comprehensive reference for physicians and surgeons who deal with disorders of the head and neck in children.

The text's intended audience is broad, including physicians and surgeons in training, both graduate and undergraduate, as well as those currently in practice in both the private and academic sectors. The text is comprised of contributions dealing with a comprehensive array of pediatric head and neck problems written by an international panel of authorities with acknowledged expertise in their respective disciplines. The focus of the text is to provide a practical contemporary approach to the management of a wide variety of head and neck disorders encountered in children. In doing so, the book offers perspectives on embryologic development and anatomy, epidemiology and pathophysiology, evaluation and diagnostic protocols, and therapeutics, both medical and surgical, for various disorders attributable to congenital, inflammatory, neoplastic, and traumatic etiologies.

It is our hope that this text will serve as a practical contemporary guide and reference for all students and practitioners who wish to expand their knowledge base and practice expertise in the field of pediatric head and neck disease.

Contributors to Volume II

Philip Abraham, M.D., D.N.B. (GE), F.I.C.P.
Professor and Chairman
Department of Gastroenterology
King Edward Memorial Hospital and
Seth G.S. Medical College
Parel, Mumbai, India

Prashant Bhandarkar, M.D., D.N.B., DM (Gastro)
Lecturer in Gastroenterology
Department of Gastroenterology
Seth G. S. Medical College and KEM Hospital
Parel, Mumbai, India

Shobna J. Bhatia, M.D., D.N.B. (GE)
Associate Professor and Head,
Department of Gastroenterology
TN Medical College and BYL NAIR Charitable Hospital
Mumbai, India

Thomas J. Bitterly, M.D., F.A.C.S
Section Head
Plastic and Reconstructive Surgery
Penn State Geisinger Medical Center
Danville, Pennsylvania

David H. Darrow, M.D., D.D.S.
Department of Otolaryngology—Head and Neck
Surgery
Eastern Virginia Medical School
Norfolk , Virginia

Craig S. Derkay, M.D., F.A.A.P., F.A.C.S.
Associate Professor
Department of Otolaryngology—Head and Neck
Surgery
Eastern Virginia Medical School
Norfolk, Virginia

Joseph G. DeSantis, M.D., F.A.C.S.
Associate
Section of Plastic and Reconstructive Surgery
Penn State Geisinger Medical Center
Danville, Pennsylvania

Chris de Souza, M.S., D.O.R.L, D.N.B., F.A.C.S.
Consulting ENT Surgeon
The Holy Family Hospital
The Holy Spirit Hospital
The Lilavati Hospital
Bombay, India
Visiting Assistant Professor
The State University of New York

William S. Gibson Jr., M.D.
Associate
Section of Otolaryngology—Head and Neck Surgery
Penn State Geisinger Medical Center
Danville, Pennsylvania

Clinical Associate Professor
Department of Otolaryngology/Head and Neck Surgery
Thomas Jefferson University School of Medicine
Philadelphia, Pennsylvania

Thomas L. Kennedy, M.D., F.A.C.S.
Associate
Section of Otolaryngology/Head and Neck Surgery
Penn State Geisinger Medical Center
Danville, Pennsylvania

Clinical Associate Professor
Department of Otolaryngology/Head and Neck Surgery
Thomas Jefferson University School of Medicine
Philadelphia, Pennsylvania

Michael E. Lessin, B.S.D., D.D.S.
Section Head, Dental Medicine and Oral and
Maxillofacial Surgery
Penn State Geisinger Medical Center
Danville, Pennsylvania

Clinical Associate Professor
Oral & Maxillofacial Surgery
West Virginia Health Sciences Center
Morgantown, West Virginia
Medical College of Pennsylvania—Hahnemann University
Philadelphia, Pennsylvania

Brad Millman, M.D.
Associate
Section of Otolaryngology/Head and Neck Surgery
Penn State Geisinger Medical Center

Danville, Pennsylvania
Clinical Assistant Professor
Department of Otolaryngology/Head & Neck Surgery
Thomas Jefferson University School of Medicine
Philadelphia, Pennsylvania

Cheri Ann Nathan, M.D.
Assistant Professor
Department of Otolaryngology/Head and Neck Surgery
Louisiana State University Medical Center
Shreveport, Louisiana

Phillip K. Pellitteri, D.O.
Associate, Section of Otolaryngology/Head and Neck
Surgery
Vice Chairman, Division of Surgery
Penn State Geisinger Medical Center
Penn State Geisinger Health System
Danville, Pennsylvania

Associate Professor of Clinical Surgery
Penn State College of Medicine
Hershey, Pennsylvania

Jan Schwartz, M.D.
Associate, Section of Anesthesiology
Penn State Geisinger Medical Center
Penn State Geisinger Health System
Danville, Pennsylvania

Fred Stucker, M.D., F.A.C.S.
Professor and Chairman
Department of Otolaryngology/Head and Neck Surgery
Louisiana State University Medical Center
Shreveport, Louisiana

George Tenedios, M.D.
Associate, Section of Anesthesiology
Penn State Geisinger Medical Center
Penn State Geisinger Health System
Danville, Pennsylvania

S. P. Wagh, M.S., D.O.R.L.
Professor and Chairman
Department of Otolaryngology
RN Cooper Hospital
Bombay, India

Edward Wood, M.D.
Associate, Section of Otolaryngology/Head and Neck
Surgery
Penn State Geisinger Medical Center
Danville, Pennsylvania

Clinical Assistant Professor
Department of Otolaryngology/Head and Neck Surgery
Thomas Jefferson University School of Medicine
Philadelphia, Pennsylvania

Robert F. Yellon, M.D.
Department of Pediatric Otolaryngology
Children's Hospital of Pittsburgh
Pittsburgh, Pennsylvania

Gregory C. Zwack, M.D.
Resident, Department of Otolaryngology–Head and
Neck Surgery
Eastern Virginia Medical School
Norfolk, Virginia

Dedication

This book is dedicated to Dr. Michael Glasscock, Dr. Michael Paparella, and the late Dr. Joe V. Desa. All of them are internationally well known, respected, admired, and liked by their colleagues. I have been fortunate enough to have been taught by all three of them. I dedicate this book to them with great affection, respect, and admiration.

Chris de Souza
Bombay, India

1

Congenital and Developmental Airway Problems in Children

William S. Gibson, Jr., M.D.

This chapter will attempt to cover the more common congenital and developmental airway problems in children. The subject matter covered will deal with lesions affecting airway obstruction, beginning at the nose and progressing through the respiratory system into the tracheobronchial tree. The discussion will include lesions of the nose, nasopharynx, oral cavity, hypopharynx, larynx, and tracheobronchial tree. Following a brief synopsis of the embryology of the nose and nasopharynx, discussion of the embryologic significance of abnormalities will be included where this information may provide insight.

EMBRYOLOGY OF THE NOSE AND NASOPHARYNX

Any variation of normal embryologic development results in pathologic changes, and an understanding of the embryology of the nose and face is therefore important. The dominating feature at 3 to 4 weeks in the development of the nose is the prominent frontonasal process. The earliest beginning of the nose is represented by thickening of the ectoderm of the lateral surfaces of the head and, as the ectoderm thickens, a pit develops and deepens giving a lateral and medial nasal process which communicates with the mouth. By the 8th week a nasal bridge and tip are developing. During this time the olfactory sensory system is developing and the convergency of digestive, olfactory, and

respiratory elements are complex; therefore, the possibility of anomalous development is significant. Failure of fusion of the two medial nasal processes will create defects of the columella, philtrum, and upper lip. At 24 weeks the nostrils are open. Although complete atresia of the external nares is rare, stenosis of the nasal passageway may occur. Other congenital defects of the nose are a result of the interruption of any of a number of sequences of differentiation and reacting of these morphogenically and/or gene-controlled activities.

Nose

Severe craniofacial malformations may occur that cover a spectrum of dysmorphisms. These may include absence of the nose, a single nostril, and duplication of nasal remnants. Other more common syndromic diagnoses will include trisomy 21 and 13. It is important to note that, because infants are obligate nose breathers, immediate recognition and airway bypass must be accomplished. The minor obstruction usually related to Down syndrome may be secondary to an increase in generalized adipose tissue deposits in the nasal passageway or nasopharynx. Stenosis of the nasal pyriform aperture may be congenital and due to overgrowth of the nasal process of the maxilla. Axial computed tomography (CT) will confirm the diagnosis. A sublabial approach has provided an appropriate method of repair (Brown, Myer, & Manning, 1989; Ey, Han, Towbin, & Jaun, 1988).

1

A soft intranasal mass occurring along the inferior aspect of the newborn nose may be a lacrimal cyst produced by failure of the lacrimal duct to open at its position in the inferior meatus. This may be unilateral or bilateral and requires only an opening in the cyst for adequate drainage. This lesion is usually associated with excessive tearing noted on the side of involvement and, because of the continuous flow of the lacrimal fluid into the nose after repair, the cyst rarely re-forms.

Glial tissue occurring outside the cranium may appear as an intranasal mass (Figure 1–1). There may be a fibrous stalk connecting the lesion with the intracranial origin but rarely does a cerebrospinal fluid leak occur. External gliomas may occur near the root of the nose or just lateral to it (Figure 1-2). Pulsations or transillumination may suggest an encephalocele. Diagnosis requires a CT scan to determine any bony defects but magnetic resonance imaging (MRI) is important if any intracranial connection is suspected (Harley, 1991; Lusk & Lee, 1986). Management should include neurosurgical consultation, and if an intracranial connection is suggested, a combined approach is indicated. An isolated glial mass in the nose has been safely removed by intranasal techniques (Strauss, Callicott, & Hargett, 1966).

Choanal atresia occurs in about 1 in 5,000 to 1 in 8,000 live births and is felt to have a female to male ratio of 2:1. This lesion may occur bilaterally or unilaterally with a ratio of 1:2. It may be isolated but may, in as much as 40% of cases, occur as part of other midface anomalies such as Charge association or Treacher Collins syndrome. At least three theories suggesting an etiology have been proposed and, in 1982, a fourth theory was suggested (Hengerer & Strome, 1982). The most commonly accepted theory is persistence of the buccopharyngeal membrane. A persistence of the nasobuccal membrane and an abnormal location of mesoderm-forming adhesions in the choanal region represent two other ideas. The misdirection of mesodermal elements secondary to other local factors completes the list of proposed theories.

Bilateral atresia presents as an airway emergency in the newborn. The characteristic "snorting" with obvious failure to move air is noticed and this is improved when the child takes a gulp or gasp of air. Since newborn infants are obligate nose breathers and have a strong suck reflex, Dr. Francis McGovern created a unique use for the baby nipple to use in the newborn (McGovern, 1961) (Figure 1–3). This technique uses a baby nipple with the end cut off to allow sucking

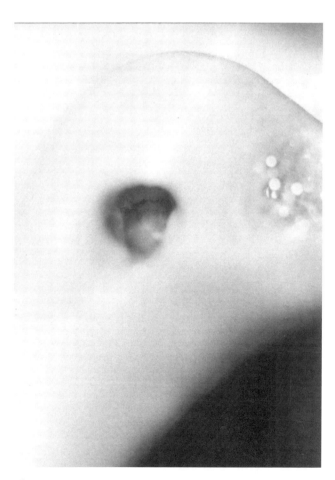

Figure 1–1. Nasal glioma—intranasal.

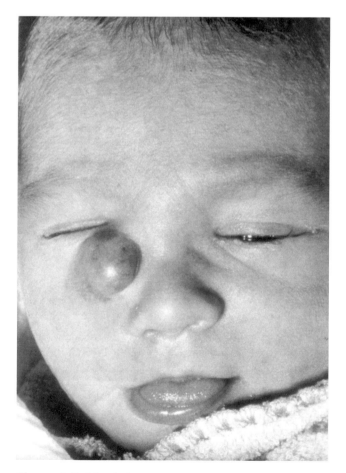

Figure 1–2. Nasal glioma presenting outside of nose.

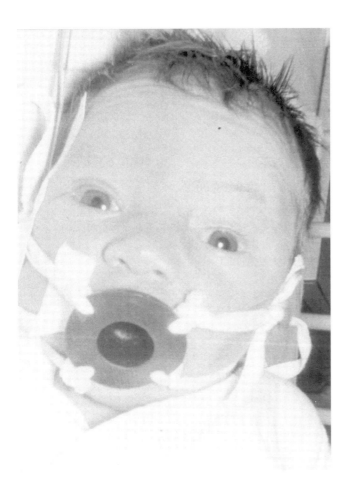

Figure 1–3. McGovern nipple.

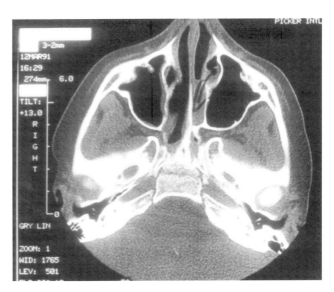

Figure 1–4. Axial CT showing unilateral choanal atresia.

return it to its normal position in the midline may prevent future cosmetic and physiologic problems.

With the exception of neural masses mentioned earlier, primary tumors within the nose per se are rare. Hemangiomas may present as nasal tumors but are generally on the external nose, although intranasal extension may be seen (Figure 1–5).

Nasopharynx

Obstruction to air flow through the nasopharyngeal area is most often related to hypertrophy of adenoidal tissue. The adenoid is a superior component of Waldeyer's ring of lymphoid tissue. It is at the midline and may hypertrophy to the extent of obstructing the posterior nasal choanae. The tissue is cystic and is microscopically identical to palatine tonsils except that the adenoid has a respiratory epithelial covering. The adenoid tissue usually atrophies at puberty but some adults may show a significant response to bacterial or viral illnesses with infectious mononucleosis being a particular example.

A child's sleep pattern may be disturbed because of airway obstruction. Symptoms include restlessness, unusual movement positions, irregular snoring, and often frank apnea (more than 10 seconds cessation of breathing). As a result of this pattern, the child may experience daytime somnolence. Weider noted that 75% of children with enuresis ceased bed wetting following relief of their severe upper airway obstruction (Weider, Sateia, & West, 1991). Coates noted that children frequently gained weight or grew in height following relief of their airway obstruction. He suggested that since some of Human Growth Hormone is secreted during nonrapid eye movement (REM) (stages 3 and

of air and therefore eliminating the need for nasal breathing. This will suffice until a more definitive measure is planned. The diagnosis is usually made by inability to pass a rubber catheter through the nasal passageway with confirmation of the anatomic configuration defined by axial CT (Crockett, Healy, McGill, & Friedman, 1987) (Figure 1–4). Definitive management may include CO_2 laser (Healy, McGill, Jako, Strong, & Vaughan, 1978), puncturing or drilling the atretic plate, or transpalatal repair (Owens, 1965). The latter technique has allegedly carried a higher incidence of subsequent palatal defects. All procedures require some form of stenting, usually an endotracheal tube secured for 4 to 6 weeks (Gleeson & Hibbert, 1985). The use of an operating microscope and endoscopic sinus surgery instruments, along with a drill or laser, has proven to work well for this repair.

Acquired nasal lesions may cause airway obstruction. The nasal septum may be displaced from the maxillary crest at birth. Some feel this is related to birth canal trauma, but Hartikainen-Sorri felt the problem originated during intrauterine life (Hartikainen-Sorri, Sorri Voinio-Mattila, & Ojala, 1983). Early manipulation using a Freer elevator to lift the displaced septum and

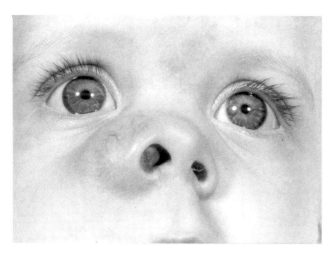

Figure 1–5. Nasal hemangioma occluding right nasal passageway.

4) sleep, and that since the children with severe upper airway obstruction rarely get into non-REM sleep, the hormone secretions may be only 60% of normal. The mean level of Human Growth Hormone postoperatively returned to a level comparable to the control group without obstructive sleep problems in Coates' trial (H.L. Coates, personal communication, 1991).

Nasopharyngeal stenosis is relatively uncommon and is currently related to poor surgical techniques. Excessive curetting or injury to the nasopharyngeal surface of the soft palate may result in a cicatricial banding of the nasopharynx. Other causes may be caustic or thermal burns, and less common now, syphilis. Indirect examination with a mirror or with the flexible nasopharyngoscope will show a narrowing of the space between the palate and the posterior pharyngeal wall. Surgical correction may be difficult; however, Cotton utilized a laterally based pharyngeal flap and was successful in relieving airway obstruction in all seven cases reported (Cotton, 1985).

Tumors of the nasopharynx are uncommon and a differential would include encephaloceles, gliomas, dermoids, hemangiomas, and neurofibromas. A rare case of an adult teratoma in a newborn was described by Raines and Yarington (1964).

Oral Cavity

Airway obstruction in the oral cavity arises because of limited space in the posterior and inferior mouth. This position is mainly compromised by the tongue position. The tongue may be too large secondary to a disease process such as Beckwith-Wiedemann syndrome or relatively large because of a small mandible as in the Pierre-Robin sequence. The tongue is usually sucked downward and posteriorly during inspiration and blocks the airway. Often jaw thrusting or

placing the child in a face-down position will help to relieve this obstruction and avoid surgical intervention.

Macroglossia related to Beckwith-Wiedmann syndrome may cause severe airway obstruction in early childhood and may require a tracheotomy. However, children older than 1 year will usually have relief of obstructive symptoms by having a tonsillectomy and adenoidectomy (Rimmel, Shapiro, Shoemaker, & Kenna, 1995).

Lymphatic malformations have been referred to as lymphangiomas and usually become manifest with the first 2 years of life. Enlargement is usually in the anterior two-thirds of the tongue and may increase in size following an infection of the upper airway (Vogel, Mulliken, & Kaban, 1986). Tongue reduction has been mainly done for orthodontic, psychologic, or cosmetic factors and should be customized in each case to provide reduction in the desired areas (Morgan, Friedman, Duncan, & Sulek, 1996).

Ectopic thyroid tissue may be present in the tongue base just behind the foramen caecum. This represents a failure of the developing thyroid to descend and in many cases will be the only functioning thyroid tissue. This must be considered if surgical or chemical ablation is necessary and appropriate thyroid replacement will be needed.

Larynx

Congenital problems of the larynx may be related to embryologic development. The lower respiratory system develops from a ventral outpouching called the tracheobronchial groove. This begins in about the 4th week. The lining epithelium arises from this foregut diverticulum. The embryo at 5 to 6 mm shows a prominence, which will become the epiglottis, and an eminence between the third and fourth arch. A slit that opens the primitive pharynx between the lateral folds of the 4th and 5th arches will become the laryngeal glottis. Failure to open at this time manifests as an atretic glottis and webbing represents incomplete opening of this slit. The lateral bands are known as arytenoid swellings; they will grow upward toward the tongue base and meet the inferior and lateral epiglottis. Failure of these lateral arches to fuse will result in posterior clefting of the larynx. The process is nearly complete in the 40 mm embryo at about the 8th to 9th week of development.

Laryngomalacia is the most common cause of stridor in the newborn and early childhood and the specific etiology remains unknown. A generalized state of localized hypotonia has been suggested (Belmont & Grundfast, 1984). This weakness manifests itself by an infolding of supraglottic tissue (epiglottic and aryepiglottic folds) on inspiration thus producing a ball-valve-like action and occluding the airway. The voice remains normal. The presence of gastroesophageal reflux in 50% of one series suggests a possible relationship (Polonovski, Contencin, Francois, Viala, & Narcy, 1990). The finding that antireflux treatment offers some improvement further suggests an association. Tracheotomy is rarely necessary while surgery on the redundant fold may be required in 5–10% of cases (Mancuso, Choi, Zalzal, & Grundfast, 1996). Regardless, it appears that the clinical problem resolves by 2 years of age.

Laryngeal cysts may be present at birth and consequently will immediately manifest themselves. Inspiratory stridor with a grunting expiratory phase as well as a muffled voice are the usual presenting symptoms. A laryngeal exam will reveal a smooth cystic mass generally arising in the supraglottic area from the medial aspect of the aryepiglottic fold and ventricle. A bronchoscope will easily pass through the airway and the obstruction will be immediately relieved. Aspiration of the cyst helps to identify the problem, but will also give immediate, although temporary, relief. Definitive surgery includes direct CO_2 laser ablation of the lesion or an uncapping of the apparent sac. Desanto (1974) classified these as saccular, ductal, and thyroid cartilage foramina.

A newborn with complete glottic atresia will not be able to breathe. There must be an alert and aggressive obstetrician or pediatrician in the delivery room who can do a forced intubation or stab tracheotomy to open the child's airway.

Severe stridor with a relatively normal voice may suggest bilateral vocal cord paralysis. Congenital bilateral paralysis may be associated with congenital, neurologic, or laryngeal anomalies or acquired lesions such as Arnold-Chiari malformation, hydrocephalus, and meningomyelocele (Holinger, Holinger, & Holinger, 1976). Relief of intracranial pressure by shunting may correct the problem in the latter group. Tracheotomy may be required with subsequent laser arytenoidectomy for airway improvement allowing tracheal decannulation. Unilateral paralysis is usually associated with trauma and, because of the long intrathoracic course, the left recurrent nerve is most often injured. Stridor may be severe and the voice may be hoarse (Grundfast & Harley, 1989).

Clefting of the larynx occurs because of a premature rest of the caudal-cranial fusion of the developing tracheoesophageal septum. A complete septum, including fusion of the cricoid cartilage, is in place by the 6th to 7th week of embryologic development. Classification includes: Evans type 1, which is a cleft limited to the inner arytenoid area; Evans type 2, extending through the posterior lamina of the cricoid cartilage; and Evans type 3, extending distally as a cleft of the tracheoesophageal membrane (Evans, 1985). Airway obstruction may be related to choking because of aspiration or edema of the mucosal folds around the cricoid cleft

(Prescott, 1995). Conservative management may suffice for Evans type 1 clefts. Prescott (1995) suggests a posterior cartilage graft for Evans type 2 and the findings of Evans type 3 cleft suggest that emergency measures be taken (Cotton & Schreiber, 1981).

Infantile subglottic hemangiomas can be a cause of stridor and severe airway obstruction. This lesion typically manifests itself before 6 months of age and may be misdiagnosed as croup, laryngomalacia, or tracheomalacia. Because of the response of hemangioma to steroid therapy, this misdiagnosis may be carried further. The diagnosis is made by direct laryngoscopy and bronchoscopy (Figure 1–6). Since most hemangiomas will involute with time, small lesions may be conservatively watched; often the lesion obstructs the airway to a critical point. Treatment options to be considered include: tracheotomy, cryotherapy, radiotherapy, steroids, and laser surgery (Mulder & Vandenbroch, 1989). Three cases were reviewed where the lesion was removed through a cricotracheotomy incision (Figure 1–7). This technique has been used by Evans (Evans & Todd, 1974) and two cases were subsequently reported by Seid, Pransky, and Kearns (1991). Each mode of therapy has its drawbacks, however. The open technique is very promising; the author has performed two cases with this technique and considers it the treatment of choice for larger lesions (Figure 1–8). Smaller lesions may be controlled with a CO_2 laser.

Both congenital and acquired subglottic stenosis in the pediatric age group pose problems in management. Cotton and Myer (1984) suggest that a newborn larynx should admit a 3-mm bronchoscope through the subglottic area and further suggest the diagnosis is only made by rigid bronchoscopic examination. The inci-

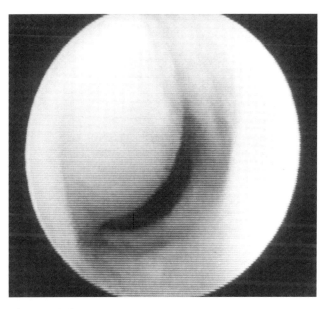

Figure 1–6. Subglottic hemangioma obstructing at least 80% of airway.

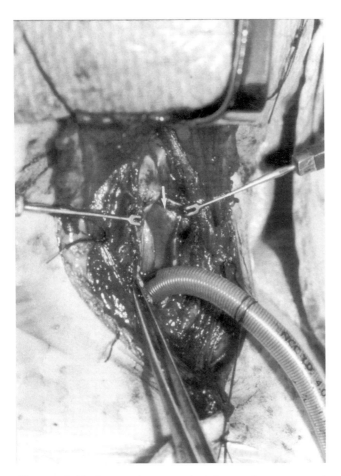

Figure 1–7. Cricotracheotomy incision and exposure of subglottic hemangioma.

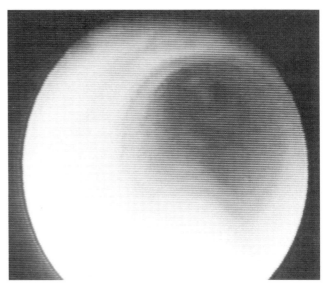

Figure 1–8. Bronchoscopic view of trachea 3 weeks after cricotracheotomy and removal of hemangioma.

dence of congenital stenosis is smaller than the incidence of acquired stenosis and therefore poses less of a problem for correction. Whereas most congenital lesions have been handled by conservative means, the open technique utilizing costal or auricular cartilage or laryngotracheoplasty must be employed in the case of an acquired stenosis. The incidence of acquired subglottic stenosis in neonates following prolonged intubation currently seems to be about 4–8% and is less than reported in the early 1980s. This decrease seems to be directly related to strict rules and management of the intubated neonate. The smallest diameter tube allowing airway support is used and firm stabilization of the tube to decrease "wearing" motion in the trachea is important. The degree of obstruction has been classified by Cotton (1984) as grade 1 through grade 4. Grade 1 is less than 70% obstruction, grade 2 is 70–80%, grade 3 is more than 90% but a lumen is still present, and grade 4 is complete obstruction. Laryngotracheal reconstruction methods include anterior cartilage grafting, posterior cartilage graft, anteroposterior cartilage graft, posterior cricoidotomy, and anterior castellation (Cotton, Gray, & Miller, 1989). Gastroesophageal reflux may inhibit proper healing and most surgeons now aggressively treat for reflex during the pre- and postoperative

period (Cotton, Myer, & O'Connor, 1995). A review of 203 patients showed an overall success rate of 92% with decannulation being the endpoint of success (Cotton, 1984).

Improved intensive care management has permitted many of these less severe forms to be corrected in a one-stage manner. This utilizes a period of postoperative intubation that allows epithelialization around the endotracheal tube. The success of this method depends upon the quality of nursing staff, anesthesiologist, and intensivist, along with an adequate intensive care facility (Cotton et al., 1989).

Human papilloma virus (types 6 and 11) is the etiologic agent for recurring respiratory papillomatosis. This histologically benign disease may be solitary or multiple and seems to have a predilection for certain anatomic areas, namely where ciliated and squamous epithelium are juxtaposed (Kashima, Mounts, Levanthal, & Rhuban, 1993). The term "juvenile laryngeal papillomatosis" suggests that this lesion has a predilection for young people and anatomically occurs in the larynx. That this same virus is found in genital and cervical warts suggests a possible relationship in children with laryngeal papillomatosis. This relationship has not been established. Airway obstruction is caused by growth of papillomas in the glottic region and for a period may be insidious such that the only symptom is hoarseness. Treatment is medical, immunological, or surgical, or some combination of these. Although there is no cure, the CO_2 laser seems to be used for control of growth. Abramson has shown success in photocoagulation therapy utilizing dihematoporphyrin ether (Abramson, et al., 1992). The use of interferon has had varying success and a position paper by Healy suggests that the long-term benefits may be limited; in some cases, a progression of the disease occurs (Healy et al., 1988).

Tracheal Lesions

Lesions causing airway obstruction in the tracheo-bronchial tree may be intrinsic or extrinsic. Tracheomalacia or bronchomalacia causes obstruction secondary to softening of the tracheal rings. Because of this softness, intrathoracic pressure during forced expiration causes a collapsing of the anterior posterior diameter of the airway. At bronchoscopy with the child spontaneously ventilating, the airway may appear more oval than round and narrowing will be noted during the expiratory phase. The collapsed area may be segmental or cover the entire length of the trachea. A 40–80% collapse is defined as partial while a greater than 80% collapse is severe (Grenholz, Karrer, & Lilly, 1986). The localizer segmental tracheomalacia is usually related to extrinsic vascular compression by the anominate artery or aortic arch (Mair & Parsons, 1992; Triglia, Guis, & Louis-Borrione, 1994). Diagnosis may be suggested by rigid bronchoscopy, although MRI, angiography, and echography have been used. Suspension of the offending vessel to the undersurface of the sternum or division of the offending paired arch may correct this vascular compression.

Tracheostenosis may be segmental or may involve any length of the tracheobronchial tree. This entity may be due to complete tracheal rings and the airway compromise is usually manifest by the 1st year of life. Diagnosis is best made by bronchoscopy and often uses only the telescope to determine the length and severity of the narrowed segment. Short segments of 102 cm may be primarily resected (Weber, Eigen, Scott, Krishna, & Grosfeld, 1982) while a tracheoplasty using rib cartilage or pericardial graft has been advocated (Andrews, Cotton, Bailey, Myer, & Vester, 1994). These procedures are done with the child on cardiopulmonary bypass and in conjunction with a cardiothoracic surgeon.

References

Abramson, A. L., Shikowitz, M. J., Mullooly, V. M., Steinberg, B. M., Amella, C. A., & Rothstein, H. R. (1992). Clinical effects of photodynamic therapy on recurrent laryngeal papillomas. *Archives of Otolaryngology—Head and Neck Surgery, 118*, 25–29.

Andrews, T. M., Cotton, R. T., Bailey, W. W., Myer, C. M., & Vester, S. R. (1994). Tracheoplasty for congenital complete tracheal rings. *Archives of Otolaryngology—Head and Neck Surgery, 120*, 1363–1369.

Belmont, J. R., & Grundfast, K. (1984). Congenital laryngeal stridor (laryngomalacia): Etiologic factors and associated disorders. *Annals of Otology, Rhinology and Laryngology, 93*, 430–437.

Brown, O. E., Myer, C. M., & Manning, S. C. (1989). Congenital nasal pyriform aperture stenosis. *Laryngoscope, 99*, 86–91.

Cohen, S. R., Geller, K. A., Seltzer, S., & Thompson, J. W. (1980). Papilloma of the larynx and tracheobronchial tree in children. A retrospective study. *Annals of Otology, Rhinology and Laryngology, 89*, 497–503.

Cotton, R. T. (1984). Pediatric laryngeal stenosis. *Journal of Pediatric Surgery, 19*, 699–704.

Cotton, R. T. (1985). Nasopharyngeal stenosis. *Archives of Otolaryngology, 111*, 146–148.

Cotton, R. T., Gray, S. D., & Miller, R. P. (1989). Update of the Cincinnati experience in pediatric laryngotracheal reconstruction. *Laryngoscope, 99*, 1111–1116.

Cotton, R. T., & Myer, C. M. (1984). Contemporary surgical management of laryngeal stenosis in children. *American Journal of Otolaryngology, 5*, 360–368.

Cotton, R. T., Myer, C. M., O'Connor, D. M., & Smith, M. E. (1985). Pediatric laryngotracheal reconstruction with cartilage grafts and endotracheal tube stenting: A single-stage approach. *Laryngoscope, 105*, 818–821.

Cotton, R. T., & Schreiber, J. T. (1981). Management of laryngotracheoesophageal cleft. *Annals of Otology, Rhinology and Laryngology, 90*, 401–405.

Crockett, D. M., Healy, G. B., McGill, T. J., & Friedman, E. M. (1987). Computed tomography in the evaluation of choanal atresia in infants and children. *Laryngoscope, 97*, 174–183.

Desanto, L. W. (1974). Laryngocele, laryngeal mucocele, large saccules and laryngeal saccular cyst—a developmental spectrum. *Laryngoscope, 84*, 1291–1296.

Evans, J. N. G. (1985). Management of cleft larynx and tracheoesophageal clefts. *Annals of Otology, Rhinology and Laryngology, 94*, 627–630.

Evans, J. N., & Todd, G. B. (1974). Laryngotracheoplasty. *Journal of Laryngology and Otology, 88*, 589–597.

Ey, E. H., Han, B. K., Towbin, R. B., & Jaun, W. K. (1988). Bony inlet stenosis as a cause of nasal airway obstruction. *Radiology, 168*, 477–479.

Greenholtz, S. K., Karrer, F. M., & Lilly, J. R. (1986). Contemporary surgery of tracheomalacia. *Journal of Pediatric Surgery, 21*, 511–514.

Gleeson, M. J., & Hibbert, J. (1985). A stent for the corrective management of bilateral choanal atresia. *Laryngoscope, 95*, 1409–1410.

Grundfast, K. M., & Harley, E. (1989). Vocal cord paralysis. *Otolaryngologic Clinics of North America, 22*, 569–597.

Harley, E. H. (1991). Pediatric congenital nasal masses. *Ear, Nose, and Throat Journal, 70*, 28–32.

Hartikainen-Sorri, H. L., Sorri, M., Voinio-Mattila, J., & Ojala, K. (1983). Aetiology and detection of congenital nasal deformities. *International Journal of Pediatric Otorhinolaryngology, 6*, 81–89.

Healy, G. B., Gelber, R. D., Trowbridge, A. L., Grundfast, K. M., Ruben, R. J., & Price, K. N. (1988). Treatment of recurring respiratory papillomatosis with human leukocyte Interferon. *New England Journal of Medicine, 319*, 401–407.

Healy, G. B., McGill, T., Jako, G. J., Strong, M. S., & Vaughan, C. W. (1978). Management of choanal atresia with the carbon dioxide laser. *Annals of Otology, Rhinology and Laryngology, 87*, 658–662.

Holinger, L. D., Holinger, P. C., & Holinger, P. H. (1976). Etiology of bilateral abductor vocal cord paralysis. *Annals of Otology, Rhinology and Laryngology, 85*, 428–436.

Hengerer, A. S., & Strome, M. (1982). Choanal atresia: A new embryologic theory and its influence on surgical management. *Laryngoscope, 92*, 913–921.

Kashima, H., Mounts, P., Leventhal, B., & Rhuban, R. H. (1993). Sites of predilection in recurrent respiratory papillomatosis. *Annals of Otology, Rhinology and Laryngology, 102*, 580–583.

Lusk, R. P., & Lee, P. C. (1986). Magnetic resonance imaging of congenital midline nasal masses. *Journal of Otolaryngology—Head and Neck Surgery, 95*, 303–305.

Mair, E. A., & Parsons, D. S. (1992). Pediatric tracheobronchial malacia and major airway collapse. *Annals of Otology, Rhinology and Laryngology, 101*, 300–309.

Mancuso, R. F., Choi, S. S., Zalzal, G. H., & Grundfast, K. M. (1996). Laryngomalacia—the search for the second lesion. *Archives of Otolaryngology—Head and Neck Surgery, 122*, 302–306.

McGovern, F. H. (1961). Bilateral choanal atresia in the newborn—a new method of medical management. *Laryngoscope, 71*, 480–483.

Morgan, W. E., Friedman, E. M., Duncan, N. O., & Sulek, M. (1996). Surgical management of macroglossia in children. *Archives of Otolaryngology—Head and Neck Surgery, 122*, 326–329.

Moss, R. B., & King, V. V. (1985). The management of sinusitis and cystic fibrosis by endoscopic surgery and serial antimicrobial lavage. *Archives of Otolaryngology—Head and Neck Surgery, 121,* 566–572.

Mulder, J. J. S., & Vandenbrock, P. (1989). Surgical treatment of infantile subglottic hemangioma. *International Journal of Pediatric Otorhinolaryngology, 17,* 51–63.

Owens, H. (1965). Observations in treating 25 cases of choanal atresia by the transpalatine approach. *Laryngoscope, 75*(1), 84–104.

Podoshin, L., Gertner, R., Fradis, M., & Berger, A. (1991). Incidence and treatment of deviation of nasal septum in newborns. *Ear, Nose, and Throat Journal, 70,* 485–487.

Polonovski, J. M., Contencin, P., Francois, M., Viala, P., & Narcy, P. (1990). Aryepiglottic fold excision for the treatment of severe laryngomalacia. *Annals of Otology, Rhinology and Laryngology, 99,* 625–627.

Prescott, C. A. J. (1995). Cleft larynx: Repair with a posterior cartilage graft. *International Journal of Pediatric Otorhinolaryngology, 31,* 91–94.

Raines, D., & Yarington, C. T. (1984). Adult nasopharyngeasl teratoma in the newborn. *Annals of Otology, Rhinology, and Laryngology, 73,* 957–962.

Rimell, F. L., Shapiro, A. M., Shoemaker, D. L., & Kenna, M. A. (1995). Head and neck manifestations of Beckwith-Weidemann syndrome. *Otolaryngology—Head and Neck Surgery, 113,* 262–265.

Seid, A. V., Pransky, S. M., & Kearns, D. V. (1991). Open surgical approach to subglottic hemangioma. *International Journal of Pediatric Otorhinolaryngology, 22,* 85–90.

Strauss, R. B., Callicott, J. H., & Hargett, I. R. Intranasal neuroglial heterotopia—so called nasal glioma. *American Journal of Diseases of Children, 111,* 317–320.

Triglia, J. M., Guis, J. M., & Louis-Borrione, C. (1994). Tracheomalacia caused by arterial compression in esophageal atresia. *Annals of Otology, Rhinology and Laryngology, 103,* 516–521.

Vogel, J. E., Mulliken, J. V., & Kaban, L. V. (1986). Macroglossia: A review of the condition and a new classification. *Plastic and Reconstructive Surgery, 78,* 715–723.

Weber, T. R., Eigen, H., Scott, P. H., Krishna, G., & Grosfeld, J. L. (1982). Resection of congenital tracheostenosis involving the carina. *Journal of Thoracic and Cardiovascular Surgery, 84,* 200–203.

Weider, D. J., Sateia, M. J., & West, R. P. (1991). Nocturnal enuresis in children with upper airway obstruction. *Otolaryngology—Head and Neck Surgery, 105,* 427–432.

2

Cleft Lip and Palate

Brad Millman, M.D.

Clefts of the palate and lip are the most commonly reported congenital facial malformations (McCarthy, Cutting, & Hogan, 1990). Reports of stomal cleft deformities date back several thousand years to ancient civilizations such as the Greeks, Romans, and Incans. Clefting of the lip or palate may occur as an isolated event or in combinations.

To understand the embryologic etiology of the cleft lip and palate one must first review the normal development of the oral and nasal cavities. The primary palate is located anterior to the incisive foramen and develops into the alveolar arch, upper lip, and anterior portion of the hard palate. Cleft lip is caused by the failure of the primary palate to fuse in the midline, specifically, by the failure of the medial nasal process to meet the lateral nasal and maxillary nasal processes during formation of the embryo. The cleft palate is formed by a defect in migration and fusion of the secondary palate in the midline. The secondary palate is formed by the medial movement of the maxillary palatal shelves, which fuse in the midline, later forming the central and posterior hard palate and soft palate (Siebert & Bumsted, 1993).

It is estimated that a cleft anomaly occurs in one out of every 680 births. Approximately 20% are isolated cleft lips, 45% are clefts of the lip and palate, and 35% are clefts of the palate only (Drillen, Ingram, & Wilkerson, 1966). The incidence of isolated cleft palate is not increased when a parent has cleft lip and/or palate. Conversely, studies of families with cleft lip alone or with cleft palate alone had an increased risk of cleft lip and palate (Fraser, 1970; McCarthy, 1990).

The etiology of oral clefting is unknown, but genetic factors may play a role in some cases. Transmission via male sex-linked recessive genes is not uncommon,

but spontaneous malformations due to environmental factors are also suspected. Some of these suspected environmental factors include: viral infections, vitamin deficiencies, anti-metabolite actions, and intrauterine posture of the fetus.

There are many classifications of cleft lip and palate malformations. Davis and Ritchie classified these malformations into three groups including clefts of the lips, palate, and combinations respectively (Davis & Ritchie, 1922). In 1967 the International Confederation for Plastic and Reconstructive Surgery classified these anomalies based on embryological development. Group one consisted of clefts involving the anterior (primary) palate. This was further divided into clefts of the lip and alveolus. Group two consisted of clefts involving the anterior and posterior (primary and secondary) palate. This group was further divided into clefts of the lip, alveolus, hard palate, and soft palate. The third group consisted of clefts involving only the posterior (secondary) palate and was divided into hard and/or soft palate defects. Total and partial cleft could be added for further subdivisions within each group. There is also a classification for the rare cases of clefting of the face such as median, transverse, vertical, and several other very rare cleft malformations (McCarthy et al., 1990).

Clefting may also be a part of a syndrome. It is estimated that 14% of individuals with cleft lip alone or with cleft palate alone are associated with a syndrome (Johnston, Bronsky, & Millicovsky, 1990). The cleft lip and palate patients associated with a syndrome are usually trisomic, have multiple organ system malformations, and commonly die before the age of 3 (Ross & Johnston, 1972). Although no classification is uniformly accepted, the classification system developed in the early 1960s describes a useful and commonly accepted system (University of Iowa Cleft Palate Team, unpublished data, 1962) (Figure 2–1).

Over the past century, medical and surgical treatment of cleft lip and palate has advanced greatly. The development of a team approach specifically treating the psychosocial aspects, feeding and speech aspects, otologic concerns, and improved aesthetic procedures allows these children to lead healthy normal lives.

The child with cleft lip and/or palate faces feeding challenges. This may be to varying degrees, but is worse immediately after birth. In children with cleft

palate, the lack of tissue closing off the oral cavity reduces the "sucking" ability of the infant. The oral bolus enters the nasal cavity, increasing the possibility of aspiration and choking events. Feeding generally is less efficient and is greatly prolonged. In one study, 72% of cleft palate infants experienced moderate to severe feeding problems (Zickenfoose, 1957).

There are devices to help overcome the infants' feeding difficulties. Compressible plastic bottles with soft rubber crisscrossed nipples are commercially available or may be modified from the normal bottles. This type of nipple requires less of a vacuum needed for

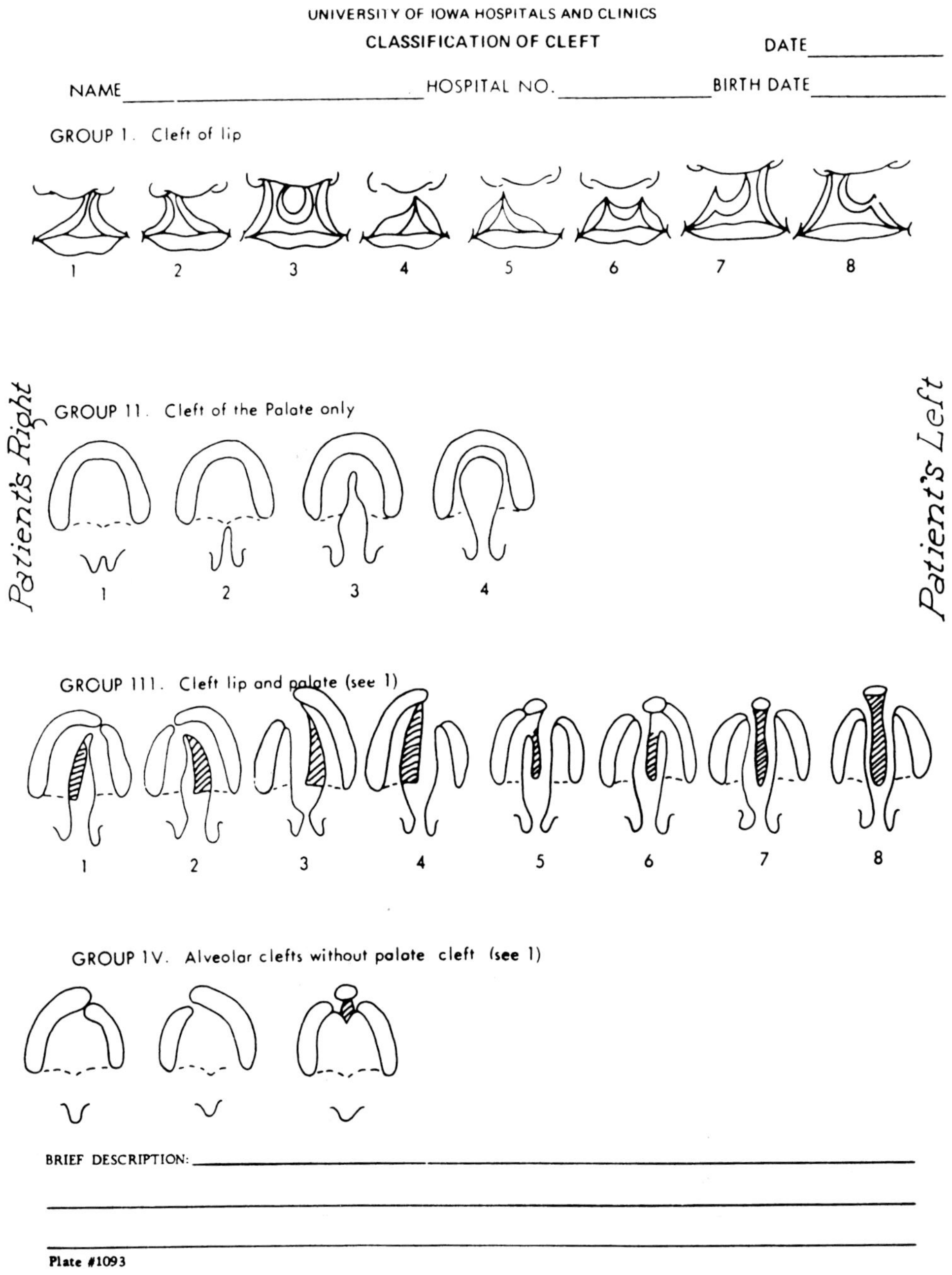

Figure 2–1. The University of Iowa Cleft Classification System. (From *Otolaryngology/Head and Neck Surgery*, by C. Cummings, Ed., 1997, Vol. 2, Figure 66–1. Copyright 1997 Elsevier Science. Reprinted by permission.)

suckling, and manual compression of the bottles allows increased flow into the infant's mouth. There are also special feeding devices that cover or obturate the cleft, thus reducing nasal regurgitation. It is also helpful to keep the child in the erect or upright position while feeding (Paradise, 1990).

The child with a cleft palate is also subjected not only to feeding and nutritional problems but also has a propensity to develop otological and audiological difficulties. It is estimated that at least half of cleft palate patients are affected by hearing loss in infancy, and this increases to an estimated 75% in older children and adults (Aschan, 1966; Pannbacker, 1969; Skolnick, 1958; Walton, 1973). The cause of the hearing loss is mostly middle ear in origin, such as perforations, cholesteatomas, scarring, and other sequelae of chronic effusions and otitis media. Stool and Randall described nearly 100% of children with unrepaired cleft palate had middle ear effusions and this finding has been confirmed in a vast number of studies (Frable, Brandon, & Theogara, 1925; Koch, Neveling, & Hartung, 1970; Stool & Randall, 1967). After surgical repair of the cleft palate, the incidence of middle ear effusion decreases but still presents problems into adulthood (Paradise & Bluestone, 1974). Although the exact cause of middle ear effusion in cleft palate patients is unknown, it is highly suspected that the eustachian tube does not function properly, leading to ventilation abnormalities of the middle ear, thereby leading to middle ear effusion and otitis media. Another proposed mechanism is, that due to velopharyngeal irregularities associated with cleft palate, there may be reflux of secretions into the eustachian tube, thereby causing the development of effusions and infections (Hubbard et al., 1985; McWilliams et al., 1973; Paradise, 1990).

Due to the chronicity of ear disease in these children, speech and language disorders are not uncommon. There have been studies that both demonstrate and repudiate decreases in cognitive and language skills in children suffering from hearing loss secondary to cleft abnormalities.

Due to the high incidence of middle ear effusion in cleft children, they should be treated aggressively with respect to avoiding middle ear effusions and hearing loss. Early myringotomy with placement of a pressure-equalizing tube is highly recommended. Although we adhere to this philosophy, some authors believe in close observation and waiting for effusions to develop before tube placement. The myringotomy and tube insertion is usually performed at the time of the cleft lip repair (at approximately 10 weeks of age).

Treatment of cleft lip and palate is usually managed by a team approach. The team usually consists of an orthodontist, social worker, speech pathologist, otolaryngologist and a plastic and reconstructive surgeon. The defect itself determines the type of surgical repair. The patient with a unilateral cleft lip and palate has deficiency of soft tissue in the lip region as well as at the alveolar and palatal bones. The classic description of the abnormality includes maxillary arch deviation towards the noncleft side which is caused by the unopposed pull of the cheek muscles rotating the maxilla away from the cleft. This action also pulls the septum, columella, nasal tip, and alar base towards the noncleft side. Another anatomic factor in the unilateral cleft lip is that the orbicularis oris muscle, which usually forms a complete circle around the lips, is not present. Muscular fibers also circle the mouth, inserting on the opposite philtral ridge, thus adding stability and oral competence. In the unilateral cleft lip, the muscle follows the cleft towards the nose, inserting at the alar base and columella (Figure 2–2). In patients with bilateral cleft lip the orbicularis musculature encircles the mouth but travels upwards into the base of the ala.

The surgeon must consider the muscles of the palate when evaluating cleft lip and palate patients. The tensor veli palatini arises from the base of the medial pterygoid plate, the spine of the sphenoid, and the cartilaginous portion of the eustachian tube. The muscle angles at the hamulus and then inserts on the oral aponeurosis in the center of the palate. Studies have demonstrated the tensor veli palatini's morphology and anatomy is normal in cleft patients (Latham, Lang, & Latham, 1980). Studies have also shown that the tensor muscle has no palatal role and its primary function is to dilate the eustachian tube. The levator palatini arises from the inferior petrous portion of the temporal bone, the border of the carotid canal, and the cartilage of the eustachian tube, and subsequently joins the palatopharyngeus muscle. The levator palatini is involved in lateral pharyngeal wall motion and velar displacement during swallowing. The palatopharyngeus originates from the thyroid cartilage, posterior and lateral pharynx, and inserts on the hamulus, cartilage of the eustachian tube, and the palatal aponeurosis. The palatopharyngeus medializes and contracts the palatopharyngeal arches, narrowing the pharyngeal in-

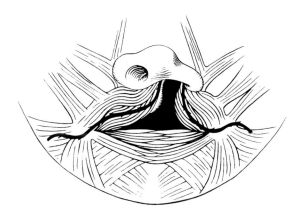

Figure 2–2. Muscular insertions in the unilateral cleft lip. The dark lines represent the arterial supply of the lip. (From *Otolaryngology/Head and Neck Surgery*, by C. Cummings, Ed., 1997, Vol. 2, Figure 66–7. Copyright 1997 Elsevier Science. Reprinted by permission.)

let. The anatomy and function of palatal muscle is greatly altered in cleft patients. The tensor and levator palatini muscles can not cross or attach in the midline and therefore the effectiveness and efficiency of their actions are reduced (Figure 2–3).

MANAGEMENT

Management of unilateral cleft lip and palate involves correction of the lip deformity and alignment of the alveolar arches, thereby creating a platform for the lip and nose as well as architecture for lip and nasal growth. Preoperative orthodontic devices assist in clo-

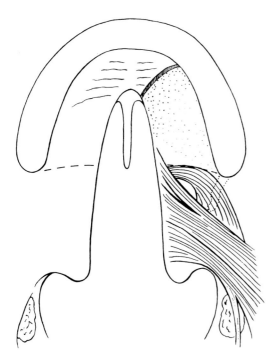

Figure 2–3. The musculature insertions in the cleft palate are demonstrated. Note the palatal musculature is positioned more posterior and is abnormally directed. (From *Otolaryngology/Head and Neck Surgery*, by C. Cummings, Ed., 1997, Vol. 2, Figure 66–9. Copyright 1997 Elsevier Science. Reprinted by permission.)

sure of the alveolar cleft and narrow the nasal floor. For wider clefts or bilateral clefts, some surgeons will use preoperative orthodontic devices. Finger pressure over the alveolar segment in the child by the parent can move maxillary segments into the proper position. Other techniques include taping the prolabium or using a hard helmet with an elastic premaxillary strap. A lip adhesion procedure may also be of benefit when a wide cleft is present (Figure 2–4).

There are many surgical treatments for cleft lip and palate. The surgical techniques are beyond the scope of this text but will be briefly described. Cleft closure described by Mirault (1844), Blair and Brown (1930), and Brown and McDowell (1945) was used in the past. LeMesurier described a modified version of the Hagedorn technique in 1949. This procedure created a neo-Cupid's bow by rotating a lateral quadrilateral flap produced by a medial releasing incision. Tennison describe and popularized the Blair/Brown modification by the addition of a Z-plasty. The maneuver placed the Cupid's bow in its normal position. Millard subsequently described the technique that is most commonly used in cleft lip repair today.

Traditional cleft lip repair occurs at 10 weeks and is part of the rule of 10s. The child must be 10 weeks old, weigh at least 10 pounds, and have a hemoglobin count greater than 10 gms. Recently, earlier repair at about 5 week in healthy children has demonstrated satisfactory results (Siebert & Bumsted, 1993). As stated earlier, the Millard rotation flap is frequently preferred at this time. The technique consists of a medially based flap that is rotated inferiorly and a laterally based flap that is advanced into the infranasal tissue defect (Millard, 1958) (Figure 2–5). This procedure recreates the philtral ridge at its "normal" location, medially repositions the alar base insertion, preserves tissue, and gives the surgeon the ability to intraoperatively modify the flap. The major disadvantage of the Millard flap is that excellent results require an experienced surgeon and there is difficulty in closing wide defects using this technique. Other minor disadvantages include nostril narrowing on the cleft side and the occasional need to sacrifice lip mucosa.

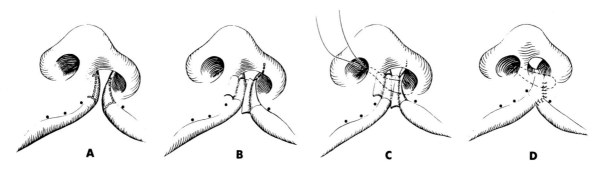

Figure 2–4. Lip adhesion. **A.** Diagram of flaps. **B.** Flap elevation. **C.** Permanent retention suture placement. **D.** Suture of skin flaps. (From *Otolaryngology/Head and Neck Surgery*, by C. Cummings, Ed., 1997, Vol. 2, Figure 66–14. Copyright 1997 Elsevier Science. Reprinted by permission.)

The Tennison-Randall flap is also commonly used for closure of cleft lip defects (Randall, 1959; Tennison, 1959) (Figure 2–6). This technique uses an inferolateral based triangular flap, which rotates medially across the defect. An advantage is that excellent results are obtained when used for wide tissue defects. This flap also preserves tissue and Cupid's bow. However, the incision does leave a Z-shaped scar at the philtral line and is relatively rigid in that the surgeon has little ability to modify or adjust the flap intra-operatively (Figure 2–7).

BILATERAL CLEFT LIP

The repair of the bilateral cleft lip is more complicated than the unilateral lip defect. The premaxilla is usually anteriorly displaced and is frequently rotated to one side or the other. It is not uncommon that the maxillary arches lateral to the premaxilla are collapsed medially, leaving little room for the premaxilla. Also, the prolabium is abnormal in that not only is it much smaller than usual, but muscular and vermilion tissue are usually deficient (Siebert & Bumsted, 1993).

Repair of bilateral cleft lip is accomplished in one or two stages. The one stage procedure repairs muscle continuity and mucosa, leading to a more symmetrical

lip, nose and cupid's bow. As described by Millard, a philtral flap is raised superiorly, as well as adjacent vermilion/mucosal and submucosal flaps. The ala are incised at their base and medialized, then fixed to the prolabium in the region of the nasal spine (Figures 2–8, 2–9, and 2–10). The medial edges of the lip, and both the mucosa/cutaneous portion and muscles, are approximated in the midline. The superiorly based prolabium flap is then reflected inferiorly and secured. This maneuver recreates the philtrum (Figures 2–11 and 2–12). The two-stage procedure is performed later at about 10–12 weeks, thus allowing time for tissue growth. The Millard or Tennison-Randall flaps may be used to correct the bilateral defect into a unilateral cleft. The second stage repair is usually undertaken at 2–3 months after the first stage.

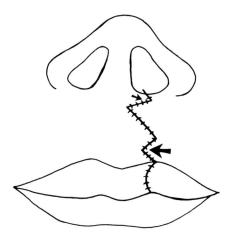

Figure 2–7. Modification of the Tennison-Randall flap. The flap consists of two interdigitated flaps. The superior flap (*small arrow*) is rotated laterally and the inferior flap (*large arrow*) is rotated medially. (From *Otolaryngology/Head and Neck Surgery*, by C. Cummings, Ed., 1997, Vol. 2, Figure 66–29. Copyright 1997 Elsevier Science. Reprinted by permission.)

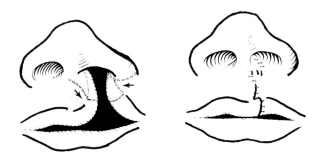

Figure 2–5. Millard rotation flap. Drawing of flaps for elevation. The flaps are rotated into the cleft and sutured. (From *Otolaryngology/Head and Neck Surgery*, by C. Cummings, Ed., 1997, Vol. 2, Figure 66–15. Copyright 1997 Elsevier Science. Reprinted by permission.)

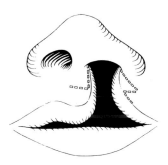

Figure 2–6. Tennison-Randall rotation flap. Incisions for the single laterally based flap. (From *Otolaryngology/Head and Neck Surgery*, by C. Cummings, Ed., 1997, Vol. 2, Figure 66–16. Copyright 1997 Elsevier Science. Reprinted by permission.)

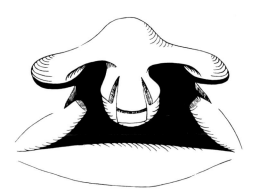

Figure 2–8. Repair of bilateral cleft lip. All flaps are incised and elevated. The prolabium provides the philtral flap. (From *Otolaryngology/Head and Neck Surgery*, by C. Cummings, Ed., 1997, Vol. 2, Figure 66–30. Copyright 1997 Elsevier Science. Reprinted by permission.)

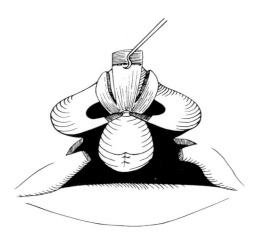

Figure 2–9. Tips of the nasal ala are deepithelialized and sutured medially to the base of the prolabium. Excess prolabial mucosa provides the medial lining of the labial sulcus. (From *Otolaryngology/Head and Neck Surgery*, by C. Cummings, Ed., 1997, Vol. 2, Figure 66–31. Copyright 1997 Elsevier Science. Reprinted by permission.)

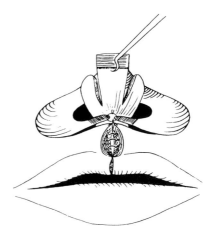

Figure 2–11. The orbicularis oris muscle and mucosa are approximated. (From *Otolaryngology/Head and Neck Surgery*, by C. Cummings, Ed., 1997, Vol. 2, Figure 66–33. Copyright 1997 Elsevier Science. Reprinted by permission.)

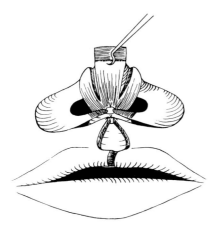

Figure 2–10. The tips of the flaps are sutured medially at the base of the prolabium. (From *Otolaryngology/Head and Neck Surgery*, by C. Cummings, Ed., 1997, Vol. 2, Figure 66–32. Copyright 1997 Elsevier Science. Reprinted by permission.)

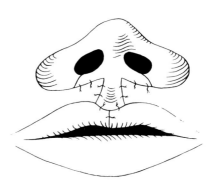

Figure 2–12. Placement of forked flaps in the nasal sil and final suturing. (From *Otolaryngology/Head and Neck Surgery*, by C. Cummings, Ed., 1997, Vol. 2, Figure 66–34. Copyright 1997 Elsevier Science. Reprinted by permission.)

CLEFT PALATE REPAIR

Cleft palate repair is usually performed at 6–8 months if there is only a soft palate defect and at 1–2 years for a hard palate cleft, although some surgeons propose earlier repair before the age of 12 months. The overall goal of palate repair is to separate the oral and nasal cavities, thus restoring function, including speech and feeding, and without compromising future facial skeletal growth. Once again the surgical technique of cleft palate repair is beyond the scope of this text but a brief description follow.

Primary veloplasty (Schweckendiek's technique) directly closes the soft palate mucosa and muscle (Siebert & Bumsted, 1993). This is usually followed by hard palate closure at 4–5 years old. The von Langenbeck palatoplasty involves the raising of bipedi-cled mucoperiosteal flaps and rotating each flap medially to close the central cleft. Although this method closes the defect, it fails to lengthen the palate (Siebert & Bumsted, 1993) (Figure 2–13). A V-Y pushback is based on the development of two posteriorly based flaps and an anteriorly based single palatal flap (Kilner, 1937; Wardill, 1937). The posteriorly based flaps are advanced medially and secured to each other, thus restoring the central and posterior levator sling; and the anteriorly based flap is advanced posteriorly to meet the other two flaps at the center of the Y (Figure 2–14). This technique lengthens the palate and produces less scar contracture. The two-flap palatoplasty is also used frequently. Two posteriorly based palatal flaps that extend to the alveolus are raised (Figures 2–15, 2–16, and 2–17). The muscle is approximated in the midline and the mucosal flaps are rotated medially and sutured.

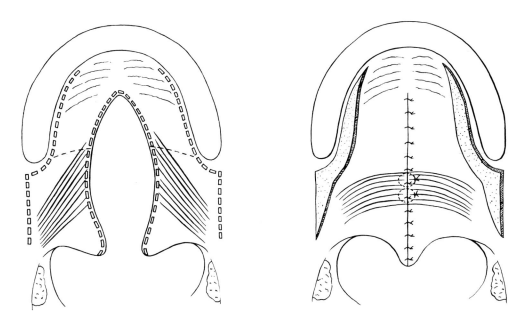

Figure 2–13. Von Langebeck's palatoplasty. Incisions are indicated by dashed lines. The levator sling is reconstructed by dissecting and repositioning the palatal musculature. Closure is obtained by the use of bipedicle mucoperiosteal palatal flaps. (From *Otolaryngology/Head and Neck Surgery*, by C. Cummings, Ed., 1997, Vol. 2, Figure 66–38. Copyright 1997 Elsevier Science. Reprinted by permission.)

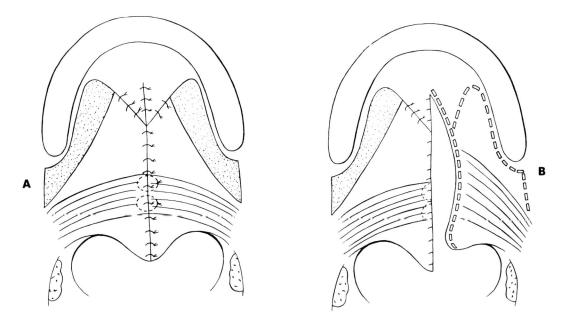

Figure 2–14. A. V-Y pushback palatoplasty as it would appear after completion of the procedure. The levator muscular sling is reconstructed and the palate is lengthened by the V-Y pushback. **B.** Theoretical amount of palatal lengthening. (From *Otolaryngology/Head and Neck Surgery*, by C. Cummings, Ed., 1997, Vol. 2, Figure 66–39. Copyright 1997 Elsevier Science. Reprinted by permission.)

SUMMARY

Cleft lip and palate disorders are not uncommon. These are complex medical, social, and surgical problems. Parents of children with these disorders frequently are distraught over the appearance of the child. They must be reassured early that both excellent cosmetic and functional results are the rule following appropriate management. This reassurance is necessary so that healthy parental-child bonding occurs normally.

The management of cleft lip and palate disorders requires a team approach and includes a reconstructive

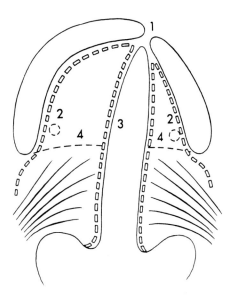

Figure 2–15. Two-flap palatoplasty. Landmarks and incisions: **1.** alveolar cleft; **2.** neurovascular bundle; **3.** vomer; **4.** posterior edge of hard palate. (From *Otolaryngology/Head and Neck Surgery*, by C. Cummings, Ed., 1997, Vol. 2, Figure 66–41. Copyright 1997 Elsevier Science. Reprinted by permission.)

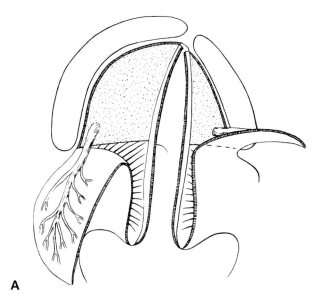

A

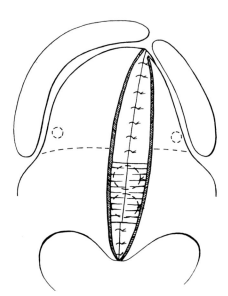

B

Figure 2–16. Two-flap palatoplasty. Nasal mucosa and mucoperiosteal closure **(A)** and levator reconstruction **(B)**. (From *Otolaryngology/Head and Neck Surgery*, by C. Cummings, Ed., 1997, Figures 66–42 and 66–43. Copyright 1997 Elsevier Science. Reprinted by permission.)

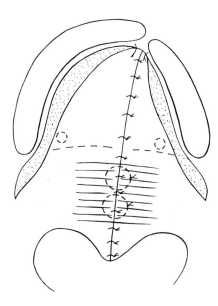

Figure 2–17. Two-flap palatoplasty. Oral layer closure. (From *Otolaryngology/Head and Neck Surgery*, by C. Cummings, Ed., 1997, Vol. 2, Figure 66–44. Copyright 1997 Elsevier Science. Reprinted by permission.)

surgeon, prosthodontist, otolaryngologist, speech pathologist, social worker, and other support members. With increased communication and an experienced team, reconstruction results in improved feeding, speech, and cosmesis. Children should be followed long-term due to the frequency of otologic problems that plague these patients throughout life, as well as for the need for "touch-up" procedures.

References

Aschan, G. (1966). Hearing and nasal function correlated to post-operative speech in cleft palate patients with velopharyngoplasty. *Acta Otolaryngology, 61,* 371.

Blair, V. P., & Brown, J. B. (1930). Mirault operation for single hairlip. *Surgey, Gynecology, and Obstetrics, 51,* 81.

Brown, J. B., & McDowell, F. (1945). Simplified design for repair of single cleft lips. *Surgery, Gynecology, and Obstetrics, 80,* 12.

Davis, J. S., & Ritchie, H. P. (1922). Classification of congenital clefts of the lip and palate. *Journal of the American Medical Association, 79,* 1323.

Drillen, C. M., Ingram, T. T. S., & Wilkerson, E. M. (1966). *The causes and natural history of cleft lip and palate.* Edinburgh, Scotland: L. & S. Livingston.

Frable, M. A., Brandon, G. T., & Theogaraj, S. D. (1985).Velar closure and ear tubing as a primary procedure in the repair of cleft palates. *Laryngoscope, 95,* 1044.

Fraser, F. C. (1970). The genetics of cleft lip and palate. *American Journal of Human Genetics, 22,* 336.

Hubbard, T. W., Paradise, J. L., McWilliams, B. J. et al. (1985). Consequences of unremitting middle-ear disease in early life: Otologic, audiologic and developmental findings in children with cleft lip and palate. *New England Journal of Medicine, 312,* 1529.

Johnston, M. C., Bronsky, P. T., & Millicovsky, G. (1990). Embryogenesis of cleft lip and palate. In J. G. McCarthy (Ed.), *Plastic surgery.* Philadelphia: W. B. Saunders.

Kilner, T. P. (1937). Cleft lip and palate repair technique. *St. Thomas Hospital Report. 2,* 12.

Koch, H. F., Neveling, R., & Hartung, W. (1970). Studies concerning the problems of ear disease in cleft palate children. *Cleft Palate Journal, 7,* 187.

Latham, R. A., Long, R. E., & Latham, E. A. (1980). Cleft palate velopharyngeal musculature in a five month old infant: A 3 dimensional histological reconstruction. *Cleft Palate Journal, 17,* 1.

LeMesurier, A. B. (1949). Method of cutting and suturing lip in complete unilateral cleft lip. *Plastic and Reconstructive Surgery, 4,* 1.

McCarthy, J. G., Cutting, C. B., & Hogan, V. M. (1990). Introduction to facial clefts in plastic surgery. In J. G. McCarthy (Ed.), *Plastic surgery.* Philadelphia: W. B. Saunders.

McWilliams, B. J., Morris, H. L., Shelton, R. L. et al. (1973). Speech, language, and psychological aspects of cleft lip and palate: The state of the art. *Asha, 9,* 1.

Millard, D. R. (1958). A radical rotation in single hairlip. *American Journal of Surgery, 95,* 318.

Mirault, G. (1844). Deux lettres sur l'operation du bec-de-lieure. *Malgaigne Journal de Chirurgie (Paris),* 2, 257.

Pannbacker, J. (1969). Hearing loss and cleft palate. *Cleft Palate Journal, 6,* 50.

Paradise, J. L. (1990). Primary care of infants and children with cleft palate. In C. D. Bluestone & S. E. Stool (Eds.), *Pediatric otolaryngology* (2nd ed.). Philadelphia: W. B. Saunders.

Paradise, J. L., & Bluestone, C. D. (1974). Early treatment of the universal otitis media of infants with cleft palate. *Pediatrics, 53,* 48.

Randall, P. (1959). A triangular flap operation for the primary repair of unilateral clefts of the lip. *Plastic and Reconstructive Surgery, 23,* 331.

Ross, R. B., & Johnston, M. C. (1972). *Cleft lip and palate.* Baltimore: Williams and Wilkins.

Siebert, R. W., & Bumsted, R. M. (1993). Cleft lip and palate. In C. W. Cummings, J. M. Fredrickson, L. A. Harker, C. J. Krause, & D. E. Schuller (Eds.), *Otolaryngology—head and neck surgery.* St. Louis, MO: Mosby-Year Book.

Skolnik, E. M. (1958). Otologic evaluation in cleft palate patients. *Laryngoscope, 68,* 1908.

Stool, S. E., & Randall. (1967). Unexpected ear disease in infants with cleft palate. *Cleft Palate Journal, 4,* 99.

Tennison, C. W. (1959). The repair of the unilateral lip by the stencil method. *Plastic and Reconstructive Surgery, 23,* 331.

Walton, W. K. (1973). Audiometrically normal conductive hearing loss among the cleft palate. *Cleft Palate Journal, 10,* 99.

Wardill, W. E. M. (1937). The technique of operation for cleft palate. *British Journal of Surgery, 25,* 117.

Zickenfoose, M. (1957). Feeding problems of children with cleft palate. *Children, 4,* 225.

3

Foreign Bodies of the Aerodigestive Tract in Children

Chris de Souza, M.S., D.O.R.L., D.N.B., F.A.C.S., and S. P. Wagh, M.S., D.O.R.L.

Technologic advances in the endoscopic removal of foreign bodies, safer pediatric anesthesia, better antibiotics, improved radiological imaging, and better public awareness have resulted in a 40% decrease in fatality rates (Baker & Fisher, 1980) in children presenting with foreign bodies in the aerodigestive tract. Choking, however, still remains the cause of 40% of accidental deaths of children under 1 year of age in the United States of America (Baker, O'Neill, & Ginsburg, 1992). The peak incidence of all foreign body ingestion and aspirations for children is between the ages of 9 months and 24 months and the risk continues to be present until the age of 6 years (Bannerjee, Rao, Khanna, Rao, & Deo, 1988). A second group of older children (average age: 10 years) has also been shown to be at risk and boys are more often at risk than girls.

Deaths from choking accidents occur in the home environment in more than 95% of children and the mean age at which a fatal outcome occurs is approximately 14 months (Reilly, Cook, Stool, & Rider 1996). Numerous studies confirm that coins and food form 80% of foreign bodies in children. Coins are generally lodged in the upper esophagus while food is likely to be aspirated. Toddlers are particularly at risk for choking on food. Incomplete deciduous dentition makes chewing of certain foods difficult. Ingestion or aspiration of foreign bodies follows a simple formula. Risk is the result of the hazard of the product multiplied by exposure (Reilly, et al., 1996).

DIAGNOSTIC EVALUATION

Pediatricians are usually the first medical personnel called on to evaluate a choking event. Sometimes the parents are unable to give a definite history of a foreign body ingestion. On occasion such children are brought in for a medical consultation long after such an incident may have occurred. This usually applies to aspirated foreign bodies. The child usually presents with a cough, fever, and pneumonia. Under these circumstances the pediatrician is usually not given a definite history of foreign body ingestion. To avoid being improperly blamed for a late diagnosis in these circumstances, treating pediatricians should explore the possibility of a foreign body as the cause of the child's symptoms.

Children who are witnessed to have choked on a foreign body usually present a straightforward diagnosis.

Foreign Bodies of the Digestive Tract

The child usually presents with drooling, painful swallowing, and dysphagia. In a child, a foreign body in the esophagus is usually easier to diagnose than a foreign body in the airway. An x-ray including the chest and abdomen in the posteroanterior and lateral planes should be taken (Figure 3–1). If the foreign body is not radiopaque a barium swallow is likely to be needed to demonstrate the presence and outline of the foreign body, as well as the level at which it is lodged.

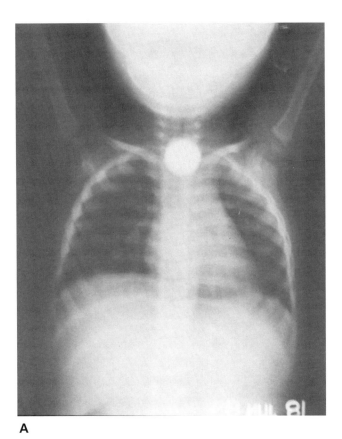

A

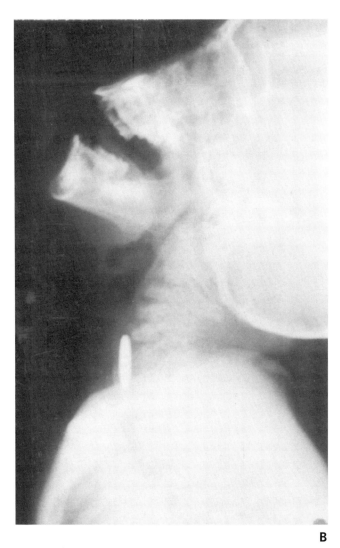

B

Figure 3–1. A. A radio-opaque foreign body in the upper esophagus. **B.** X-ray of the lateral aspect of the neck demonstrates a foreign body in the cricopharynx.

Foreign Bodies of the Respiratory Tract

Pointed questions related to persistent coughing, and sudden onset of wheezing should be asked in the case of a child without a history of asthma. These questions would help increase the index of suspicion regarding the presence of a foreign body in the respiratory tract. An ominous sign is stridor and cyanosis. The chest should be auscultated for the quality of breath sounds.

When a foreign body is suspected to be lodged in the respiratory tract, fluoroscopy of the airway is indicated. Airway fluoroscopy can emphasize subtle differences in aeration of the main bronchi and show atelectasis with mediastinal shifting. Plain x-rays of the chest are mandatory (Figure 3–2). X-ray examination of the child should be done in an upright position if possible and should include all structures from the nasopharynx to the tuberosities of the ischia in order to prevent overlooking a foreign body (Jackson & Jackson, 1936). Although Chevalier Jackson recommended this in 1936, the procedure still holds true today. X-rays of the chest should be taken during inspiration as well as expiration (Figure 3–3). This is sometimes difficult in young uncooperative children. An x-ray of the lateral aspect of the chest completes the examination. X-rays including anteroposterior and lateral views of the neck in a posi-

tion of extension should be taken to observe the upper airway.

CT scans are helpful (Berger, Kuhn, & Kuhns, 1980) when there is a suggestion of a localized obstructive object. CT scans are usually needed when x-rays of the chest are equivocal and the treating physician still strongly suspects the presence of a foreign body. Good quality x-rays of the chest usually help detect the presence of a foreign body in the bronchus.

Obstructive Emphysema

Obstructive emphysema is produced by a valvular obstruction to the expiratory phase of respiration. The obstruction is caused by a foreign body in the lumen of the bronchiolar passage. The air passages dilate on inspiration and contract on expiration. Air is trapped distal to the site of obstruction, and with each phase of respiration, more air is trapped and accumulates distal to the site of obstruction. There is a shift of the mediastinum to the unobstructed side of the chest. In atelectasis the opposite occurs, that is, the mediastinum shifts to the obstructed side.

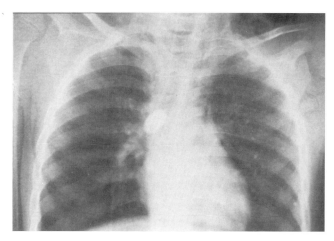

Figure 3–2. A radio-opaque foreign body (stone) lodged in the right main bronchus in a 12-year old child. Note a small pneumomediastinum on the left. The child also had surgical emphysema.

The exact role of MRI for locating and defining foreign bodies remains open. There is a possibility that ferromagnetic objects can get dislodged. Such objects would be visualized anyway on a good quality x-ray of the chest. Future reports in the literature will define the role of MRI for foreign bodies of the respiratory tract.

MANAGEMENT

When a foreign body is suspected to be present in the aerodigestive tract, endoscopy of these passages serves dual purposes. Endoscopy has both diagnostic and therapeutic value. Endoscopic inspection of the aerodigestive tract is the best way to confirm the presence of a foreign body and the best way to ensure its removal.

Sophisticated and accurate imaging modalities, refined anesthesia, and vastly improved endoscopes (Figure 3–4) have all contributed to improvement in the management of foreign bodies located in the aerodigestive tract. These tools cannot replace timely diagnosis, competence in management, and skillful techniques that must be employed to remove these foreign bodies.

All children suspected of having a foreign body lodged in the aerodigestive passages should be hospitalized. This is done with the intention of subjecting the child to endoscopic inspection of the passage in which a foreign body is thought to be present.

Foreign Bodies of the Esophagus

The rigid endoscope is the preferred instrument of choice. Anesthetists should use a slightly smaller tube when intubating the child to avoid compressing the foreign body. However, for foreign bodies in the hypopharynx, intubation may not be necessary. Such foreign bodies can be removed with an anesthetist's

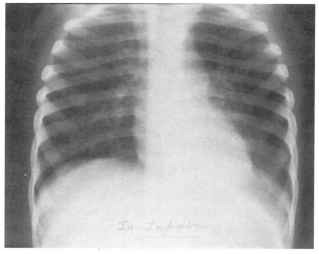

A

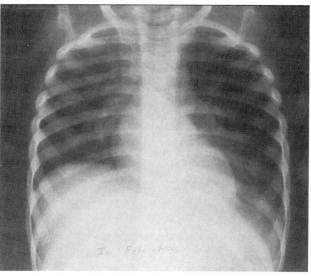

B

Figure 3–3. A. Plain x-ray of a 7-year-old child taken in *inspiration*. There is collapse of the left lower lobe, peripheral air trapping in the left middle zone and base, and hyperinflation of the rest of the left lung, which is typical of obstructive emphysema associated with a foreign body in the left bronchus. **B.** Plain x-ray of the same child taken in *expiration* demonstrating a shift of the mediastinum to the right.

laryngoscope. Muscle relaxants should be used only when the child is given a head low position. This avoids the foreign body slipping into the stomach, especially when the foreign body is located at the distal end of the esophagus. Foreign bodies that slip into the stomach have the potential to cause intestinal obstruction, which is a more serious complication.

TECHNIQUE

In our setup, the anesthetist administers ketamine (0.5 mg per kg body weight intravenously) followed by

2% halothane/98% oxygen through the mask. The child is then intubated and ventilated. The child's vital parameters are continuously monitored throughout the procedure.

The endotracheal tube is taped to the left side of the mouth. Ophthalmic ointment is introduced into the child's eyes and they are taped shut to avoid inadvertent injury. The teeth in the lower jaw are protected with a small piece of gauze. The endoscope is then introduced into the oral cavity from the right. The hypopharynx will usually need to be suctioned at this stage. The endotracheal tube can be seen entering the larynx. The child's neck is gently extended and the endoscope should be delicately insinuated between the arytenoids and the posterior pharyngeal wall. The cricopharynx can then be visualized and the endoscope is gently slid in. The beak of the endoscope should be directed upward and forward. The foreign body is usually seen at this stage and is delicately removed with the appropriate instrument. The forceps to be used for the extraction should be appropriate for the foreign body present. Foreign bodies larger than the lumen of the endoscope are grasped and brought to the tip of the endoscope, and the endoscope and foreign body are removed together. Sharp instruments like open safety pins are particularly dangerous foreign bodies. This is particularly so when the tip points away from the stomach (cephalad). The dictum of "advancing points perforate but trailing points do not" is true (Jackson & Jackson, 1936) and should be the philosophy when attempting to remove a sharp instrument from the aerodigestive tract.

Care should be taken against inadvertently dislodging loose teeth. Teeth that have been dislodged should be carefully retrieved.

Foreign bodies that have been lodged in the esophagus for more than 24 hours likely cause edema of the esophagus. This makes the mucosa of the esophagus friable, thus making endoscopy hazardous. Perforation of the esophagus is more likely under such circumstances. Antibiotics and steroids may be given to reduce edema prior to endoscopy. During endoscopy the area of the esophagus distal to the foreign body should be inspected for the presence of pathology.

Postprocedure the child is kept starving for 4 hours. The child is observed for symptoms indicative of perforation of the esophagus. The neck is palpated for surgical edema and the chest is auscultated for breath sounds. An x-ray of the chest is taken to determine the status of the chest and its contents. The presence of air in the mediastinum is indicative of perforation of the esophagus.

Management of Foreign Bodies of the Respiratory Tract

The instrument of choice is the rigid ventilating bronchoscope. Foreign bodies blocking the laryngeal inlet and those in the trachea present as dire emergen-

cies. The child presents with severe respiratory distress and may be cyanosed. Usually tracheotomy helps secure the airway and can be a life-saving procedure. On occasion it is possible to remove the foreign body with the aid of an anesthetist's laryngoscope. Large foreign bodies may have to be delivered through the tracheotomy (Svensson, Rah, Kim, Brooks, & Slazberg, 1985).

Postbronchoscopy steroids may be necessary as repeated passage of the endoscope may cause edema of the vocal cords (de Souza & Joshi, 1995). If a tracheotomy is present, steroids may still be necessary to reduce the edema of the bronchus and for the reduction of bronchospasm. Antibiotics may be necessary.

Instruments

Complete sets of ventilating bronchoscopes of various sizes with an optical forceps employing the Hopkins rod lens system are invaluable for bronchoscopy. These provide superior optics and illumination. The bronchoscopes are equipped with two side channels, one for ventilation and the other for instrumentation and suction. The disadvantage is that the side channel will permit the introduction of a very small forceps. The optical forceps come with different degrees of visualization so that all the bronchi may be satisfactorily inspected.

ANESTHESIA

Spontaneous anesthesia is frequently used. The patient is masked and halothane is given. When the patient is sufficiently anesthetized the larynx is sprayed with a solution of 4% xylocaine to prevent undue irritation of the larynx.

TECHNIQUE

All the vital parameters of the child are monitored. The child is then well oxygenated. The bronchoscope is held in the right hand and steadied with the left. The child's neck is gently extended. The teeth are protected and the larynx is identified. The beak of the laryngoscope is gently inserted parallel to the vocal cords and slid into the laryngeal inlet. The laryngeal inlet is carefully inspected for pathology. As the bronchoscope is being inserted into the larynx, the larynx and trachea are carefully inspected and evaluated by the endoscopist. When the right main bronchus is being inspected, the head should be tilted to the left so that the scope enters the right main bronchus from the left and vice versa for the left main bronchus. Before inspecting the bronchi the lungs are ventilated. The bronchi are carefully inspected. Both bronchi should be inspected to avoid missing a foreign body that may be lodged in both bronchi. From time to time the anesthetist carefully oxygenates the child and alerts the bronchoscopist if any of the parameters worsen. The optical forceps can be inserted when the foreign body is sighted to ensure safe complete removal.

Organic foreign bodies may prove difficult to remove, as they will likely have disintegrated. Patience and meticulous attention to detail aid complete removal of such foreign bodies. A check endoscopy a few days later is needed to confirm that the foreign body has been completely removed. This is particularly useful when the child does not do well following bronchoscopy or if the foreign body was not completely removed.

FUTURE GOALS

Prevention of aspiration or ingestion of foreign bodies is the goal of the future.

In the U.S.A. federal regulations over the last 25 years have forced manufacturers to restrict products intended for children below 3 years of age to a minimum size that exceeds the dimensions of the Small Parts Test Fixture (SPTF) (31.7 mm in diameter by 57.1 mm in depth) (*Federal Register*, 1973; Reilly, 1990). Although these regulations are useful and have served to eliminate dangerous objects that have the potential of becoming foreign bodies, they have still not eliminated certain objects that have the potential to cause fatal injuries (Reilly et al., 1995). Spherelike objects are the leading cause of mortality as they fit snugly into the hypopharynx and oropharynx (Rimell et al., 1995). To prevent being ingested, the minimum diameter for spherical objects should exceed 44.4 mm and for nonspherical objects the diameter should equal or exceed 36.8 mm (Reilly et al., 1996).

Finally, parents and those who look after children of various age groups should be instructed about the dangers of organic and inorganic foreign bodies. Appropriate foods should be given to children, especially infants. Appropriate measures should be taken, especially in the event of foreign body ingestion/aspiration.

References

Baker, S. P. & Fisher, R. S. (1980). Childhood asphyxiation by choking and suffocation. *Journal of the American Medical Association, 224*, 1343–1344.

Baker, S. P., O'Neill, B., & Ginsburg, M. J. (1992). LiG asphyxiation by aspiration and suffocation. In *Injury Fact Book* (2nd ed., p. 186). New York: Oxford University Press.

Bannerjee, A., Rao, K. S., Khanna, S. K. Rao, M. G., & Deo, S. K. (1988). Laryngotracheobronchial foreign bodies in children. *Journal of Laryngology and Otology, 102*, 1029–1032.

Berger, P. E., Kuhn, J. P., & Kuhns, L. R. (1980). Computed tomography and occult foreign body. *Radiology, 134*, 133–135.

de Souza C. E., & Joshi S. S. (1995). Foreign bodies and methods of inspection of the aerodigestive tract. In C. E. de Souza, M. V. Goycoolea, & C. B. Ruah (Eds.), *Textbook of the ear, nose and throat* (pp. 201–208). India: Orient Longman.

Federal Register. (1973, January 22). Banning of toys and other children's articles presenting choking, aspiration and/or ingestion hazards due to small parts. 38:14. 21 CFR Pt. 191 p. 2179.

Jackson, C., & Jackson C. L. (1936). *Diseases of the air and food passages of foreign body origin.* Philadelphia: W. B. Saunders.

Reilly, J.S. (1990). Prevention of aspiration in infants and young children. Federal regulations. *Annals of Otology, Rhinology and Laryngology, 99*,273–276.

Reilly, J. S., Cook, S. P., Stool, D., & Rider, G. (1996). Prevention and management of aerodigestive foreign body injuries in childhood. *Pediatric Clinics of North America, 43*, 1403–1411.

Reilly, J. S. (1990). Prevention of aspiration in infants and young children. Federal regulations. *Annals of Otology, Rhinology, and Laryngology, 99*, 273–276.

Reilly, J. S., Walter, M. A., Beste, R., & Johnson, M. K. (1995) Size/shape analysis of aerodigestive foreign bodies in children: A multi-institutional study. *American Journal of Otolaryngology, 16*, 190–194.

Rimell, F. L., Thome, A., Jr., Stool S., Reilly, J. S., Rider, G., Stool, D., & Wilson, C. L. (1995). Characteristics of objects that cause choking in children. *Journal of the American Medical Association, 274*, 1763–1765.

Svensson, E. E., Rah, K. H., Kim, M. C., Brooks, K., & Slazberg, A. M. (1985). Extraction of large tracheal foreign bodies through a tracheostome under bronchoscopic control. *Annals of Thoracic Surgery, 39*, 251–253.

4

Diseases of the Esophagus in Children

Philip Abraham, M.D., D.N.B.(GE), F.I.C.P.,
Shobna J. Bhatia, M.D., D.N.B.(GE), and
Prashant V. Bhandarkar, M.D., D.N.B.(Med), D.M., D.N.B.(GE)

GASTROESOPHAGEAL REFLUX DISEASE

The term gastroesophageal reflux disease (GERD) refers to any symptoms or esophageal mucosal damage that result from reflux of gastric contents into the esophagus. That backward flow of gastric contents into the esophagus can produce a clinical disorder was first recognized by Asher Winkelstein in 1935. The disease affects all ages and symptoms vary considerably with regard to both degree and profile.

Gastroesophageal reflux (GER) can be classified as physiologic, in which the infant is free of clinical sequelae, or as pathologic (GERD), in which gastrointestinal, pulmonary, or neuropsychiatric complications are present. In the pediatric age group, GER may also be classified according to the natural history. Thus, infantile GER, which results from a delay in maturation of upper gastrointestinal motility, usually resolves by 1 year of age. Childhood GER begins during infancy and has a chronic course similar to that in adults (Glassman, George, & Grill, 1995).

Pathophysiology

The antireflux barrier at the gastroesophageal junction is an anatomically complex zone whose functional integrity is maintained by one or more of its different components. These include the intrinsic lower esophageal sphincter (LES) pressure, extrinsic compression of the LES by the crural diaphragm, the intra-abdominal location of the LES, integrity of the phrenoesophageal ligament, and maintenance of the acute angle of His (angle between the lower end of the esophagus and the fundus).

Antireflux Barrier

The LES is the most important element protecting the esophagus against gastric contents (Holloway & Dent, 1990). It is a segment of circular smooth muscle capable of exerting sustained elevated pressure. In infants, the pressure generated by the LES increases with postnatal age and correlates with its length. However, some studies found that the LES is usually fully functional in the full-term infant. In the premature infant also, the LES may be competent (Omari et al., 1995). Maturation of LES function coincides with the clinical improvement seen in children with GER between ages 6 and 12 months (Vanderhoof, Zach, & Adriane, 1994). Infants with GER also have a shorter LES as compared to infants without GER.

The LES has intrinsic myogenic tone, which is modulated by neural and hormonal mechanisms. Alpha-adrenergic neurotransmitters or beta-blockers stimulate the sphincter, and alpha-blockers and beta-stimulants reduce its pressure. Vasoactive intestinal polypeptide and nitric oxide have been implicated as the mediators involved in LES relaxation.

Increases in gastric and abdominal pressures are associated with increases in LES pressure. The crural diaphragm contributes a phasic component to the tonic high pressure zone of the esophageal-gastric junction and plays a role in preventing reflux in conditions associated with increased intraabdominal pressure, particularly during coughing and Valsalva maneuver.

The phrenoesophageal ligament defines the limits of the intra-abdominal portion of the esophagus. Its integrity and site of insertion into the distal esophagus change the length of the intra-abdominal segment and the angle of His and influence the probability of reflux.

LES Incompetence and Transient LES Relaxations

Reflux of gastric contents can occur only through a relaxed or hypotonic sphincter. The traditional view was that reflux occurs as a consequence of LES hypotonia. It is now recognized that a majority of reflux episodes in children and infants occur during brief intermittent LES relaxation (transient lower esophageal sphincter relaxations [TLESRs]) rather than because of persistently defective LES tone (hypotonia) (Kawahara, Dent, & Davidson, 1997; Omari et al., 1997). Although the basal LES pressure is normal in infants, it falls significantly after feeding.

TLESRs are inappropriate relaxations of an otherwise normal LES that occur independent of swallowing. Decrease in the tone of the crural diaphragm during TLESR further compromises the reflux barrier. TLESRs are significantly longer in duration than swallow-induced LES relaxations. Their frequency is increased by distension of the stomach and by upright posture; they probably result from gastric distension or attenuated swallows that fail to initiate peristalsis. TLESRs are suppressed during sleep.

In normal subjects, about 40 to 50% of TLESRs are accompanied by acid reflux, compared with 60 to 70% in patients with reflux disease. Whether reflux occurs or not during TLESRs is influenced by abdominal straining, which increases the likelihood of reflux; the presence of hiatus hernia; and the degree of esophageal shortening.

Marked basal LES hypotension can also expose the esophagus to gastric acid. LES basal pressure of less than 6 mmHg is associated with severe and refractory GERD. However, a continuous reduction in LES pressure is observed in only 14% of children with GER.

Hiatus Hernia

Hiatus hernia is associated with anatomic disruption of the diaphragmatic sphincter. This increases the likelihood of reflux episodes during stress maneuvers. The hiatus hernia predisposes to reflux, impairs esophageal emptying by trapping the refluxate, and thus contributes to the development of esophagitis. The presence of hiatus hernia does not correlate with GER in adults, but children with this disorder are often refractory to medical therapy.

Gastric Emptying

Delayed gastric emptying, by virtue of increase in intragastric pressure and thus gastroesophageal pressure gradient and increase in number of TLESRs, can increase reflux. About 30% of children with GER have delayed gastric emptying. This occurs in children with GER and pulmonary symptoms, Down syndrome, and in older children with GER who are otherwise normal. Increase in intragastric pressure due to delayed gastric emptying is the cause of approximately 66% of reflux episodes in children (Fonkalsrud & Ament, 1996). It has also been implicated in the pathogenesis of infantile vomiting.

The Refluxate

The gastroesophageal refluxate is a heterogeneous mixture of hydrogen ions, pepsin, bile acid, trypsin, and food. Damage to the esophageal mucosa occurs at pH < 4. In infants, the rate of acid secretion is low, and there is hypergastrinemia and increased LES pressure; in addition, the buffering capacity of the feeds may temporarily neutralize gastric acid. After 2 months of age, acid secretion increases and LES pressure falls. Children with esophagitis may have hypersecretion of acid. The severity of esophagitis is related to the duration of acid exposure; however, the frequency and duration of exposure are not always predictive of the degree of esophageal injury, suggesting a role for other factors.

Patients with achlorhydria may also develop esophagitis, probably due to duodenal contents (bile). Patients with columnar-lined (Barrett's) esophagus are known to have greater concentration of bile acids in their gastric and esophageal contents than patients with simple reflux esophagitis.

At the cellular level, esophagitis results from hydrogen ion diffusion into the mucosa, leading to cellular acidification and necrosis.

Esophageal Defense

When an episode of reflux has occurred, it is important that the refluxed material be evacuated from the esophagus as early as possible. This clearance function is a two-stage phenomenon requiring first a reduction in volume by peristalsis (volume clearance) and then chemical neutralization by saliva (pH clearance).

Esophageal peristalsis is mainly responsible for the clearance of acid in both the upright and supine positions. Esophageal stimulation from gastric reflux and associated drop in pH can trigger secondary peristalsis, which can contribute to volume clearance. Ninety percent of the refluxed material is cleared after two peristaltic waves. Patients with reflux disease exhibit a defect in triggering secondary peristalsis. In preterm infants, the incidence of dysmotility and failed peristalsis is high (Omari et al., 1995). There is a high incidence of GER in children with esophageal motor dysfunction such as repaired esophageal atresia, connective tissue disorders, and static encephalopathy. Failed peristalsis and inadequate peristaltic amplitude in the distal esophagus result in inadequate volume clearance.

Whether peristaltic abnormalities are the cause or the consequence of esophagitis is not clear. Most studies indicate that the motor abnormalities remain unchanged after healing of esophagitis. Hiatus hernia impairs volume clearance by causing re-reflux because acid gets trapped in the hiatus.

In the upright posture, gravity helps in elimination of the refluxed material. Reflux in the supine posture therefore leads to more damage. Peristaltic dysfunction may further this damage.

Although most of the refluxate volume is cleared by peristalsis, the juxtamucosal pH remains low unless it is neutralized by alkali from swallowed saliva or esophageal secretion. There is no evidence of impaired salivary function in GERD. Salivary secretion is decreased during sleep, and this may contribute to esophageal damage from reflux.

Mechanisms of esophageal mucosal resistance are less well investigated. The layer of mucus carpeting the mucosa and mucosal bicarbonate constitute an important line of defense against acid injury. Blood supply also adapts in response to acid injury by bringing bicarbonate ions to eliminate some H^+ ions. If acid injury and cell necrosis occur, the rate of regeneration may play a role in determining the severity of lesions.

Associated Clinical Disorders

Children with neurologic disease appear to be at particular risk for GER. Approximately 10 to 15% of neurologically impaired children have vomiting, and associated GER is present in 65 to 75% of these children. The pathogenic factors implicated for GER in these patients include LES hypotonia, chronic supine posture, abdominal muscle spasticity, medications, and chronic nasogastric intubation.

Environmental tobacco smoke exposure, especially from smoking mothers, seems to be a significant factor in gastroesophageal reflux in children (Alaswad, Toubas, & Grunow, 1997).

Pathology

The normal esophageal mucosa is a 25- to 30-cell thick layer of nonkeratinized squamous epithelium functionally divided into a proliferating basal cell layer, a mid-zone layer of metabolically active squamous cells, and a 5- to 10-cell thick layer of dead cells. The epithelium also contains a few submucosal glands. The basal cell layer does not exceed 10% of the total thickness of the epithelium. Papillae extend upwards from the basal layer, less than two thirds of the distance to the surface of the mucosa. The criteria for chronic low-grade reflux esophagitis on esophageal biopsy are as follows: (1) the basal zone constitutes more than 15% of the total thickness of the epithelium and (2) papillae extend more than two thirds of the distance to the surface.

These changes are not found in infants because pathologic reflux has not caused sufficient injury.

High-grade changes are characterized by severe epithelial injury or destruction, commonly accompanied by mucosal infiltration by neutrophils, eosinophils, or both. Changes are usually confined to the epithelium, lamina propria, and muscularis mucosae. In children with predominant eosinophilic infiltration, a diagnosis of food intolerance should be considered especially if there is no response to GER treatment (Kelly et al., 1995). Pseudomembranes, inflammatory polyps, and reactive changes mimicking dysplasia sometimes occur.

Barrett's esophagus (columnar-lined esophagus [CLE]) is the most severe histologic consequence of chronic GER. The normal squamous lining undergoes metaplasia and resembles gastric fundal, gastric cardiac, or intestinal mucosa. It is now known that only small intestinal metaplasia is associated with adenocarcinoma of the esophagus. The abnormality should be above the LES and not confused with mucosa in a hiatal hernial sac.

As in adults, Barrett's esophagus in children is related to severe GERD. Approximately 3.3% of children with GER develop Barrett's esophagus (Eizaguirre, Tovar, Gorostiaga, Echeverry, & Torrado, 1993). Most of these children have severe neurologic impairment or have undergone previous surgery for esophageal atresia (Othersen, Ocampo, Parker, Smith, & Tagge, 1993). The mean age of development of Barrett's esophagus is 14 years. Associated gastroduodenal reflux is often present. Fortunately, adenocarcinoma, though reported in children, is rare (Cheu et al., 1992). Barrett's esophagus persists even after surgical treatment for GERD (Cheu et al., 1992).

Symptoms

In infants and young children, symptoms of GER are different from those in adults. It must be realized that GER physiologically occurs in all infants and is not as severe as pathologic reflux. The predominant symptom in young children is excessive regurgitation and spitting of the feeds, which may be associated with respiratory symptoms like apnea or aspiration pneumonia. Regurgitation of at least 1 episode a day is reported in half of 0- to 3-month-olds. This symptom decreases to 5% at 1 year; peak reported regurgitation of 67% is at 4 months and then decreases between 6 and 7 months of age (Nelson, Chen, Syniar, & Christoffel, 1997).

In adults, *heartburn* is the most frequent symptom and is almost synonymous with GER (Klinkenberg-Knol & Castell, 1992); this is not so in children. Heartburn is best defined as retrosternal burning pain that travels cephalad and is exacerbated by eating, bending, or lying down.

Regurgitation is described as effortless appearance of acid or a bitter taste in the mouth, or awakening from sleep because of coughing and strangulating sensation and noting secretions on the pillow. Effortless postprandial regurgitation is the typical symptom in infancy. A small number of these episodes result in vomiting. On scintigraphy, less than 20% of the refluxed material is regurgitated in infants with GER.

Chest pain as a manifestation of GER mainly occurs in older children. GER is the cause for idiopathic chest pain in 40 to 60% of cases. In children with mitral valve prolapse and asthma, GER is found in 75% of those who complain of chest pain. Reflux-induced motor abnormalities contribute to the onset and/or exacerbation of chest pain in pediatric patients with GER and esophagitis (Ganatra et al., 1995).

Major *pulmonary manifestations* are asthma and chronic cough. GER has been implicated in the pathogenesis of reactive airway disease, chronic bronchopulmonary disease, cough, and stridor. Nonseasonal asthma can be caused by either microaspiration of gastric contents into the lung or activation of the vagal reflex arc from the esophagus to the lung, causing bronchoconstriction.

Acid instillation in the esophagus has been shown to cause reduction in heart rate and forced respiratory vital capacity, and obstructive ventilatory defect in asthmatics. Similar changes occur after intraesophageal balloon distension. The character as well as the size of the refluxed material may thus influence respiratory function. About 75% of children with uncontrolled asthma without esophageal symptoms have evidence of GER.

Nocturnal wheezing, lack of family history of atopy, poor response to bronchodilators, and early onset of bronchopulmonary disease suggest that GER may be the causative factor. Healing of esophagitis in these children is usually associated with relief of pulmonary symptoms. In children with recurrent pulmonary infection, approximately 40% have silent GER; the rest have some suggestive symptoms. Clinical improvement occurs in 80% of children after antireflux therapy. Other respiratory manifestations which possibly occur due to GER are bronchopulmonary dysplasia, apnea, and stridor.

Drugs used in treatment of bronchial disorders like theophylline and oral β-agonists can decrease LES pressure and aggravate GER.

Other symptoms in infants, like atypical colic, irritability, and sleep disturbances, have been attributed to reflux. Esophageal inflammation may result in feeding disturbances and refusal to feed.

A wide range of extraesophageal manifestations are thought to result from abnormal GER. Otolaryngological manifestations include excessive salivation, hoarseness, postnasal drip, persistent coughing, sore throat, choking spells, laryngospasm, and posterior laryngitis. Reflux-related laryngitis (posterior laryngi-

tis) correlates with reflux extending into the proximal esophagus, especially nocturnal reflux. Reflux-related upper airway disease may also be due to proximal esophageal reflux (Conley, Werlin, & Beste, 1995)

There can be failure to thrive, iron-deficiency anemia, and dysphagia. Infants may present with bradycardia. Approximately 50% of infants presenting with apparent life-threatening events have associated reflux (McMurray & Holinger, 1997). Sandifer's syndrome is a movement disorder characterized by a peculiar head tilt with neck extension and rotation; it appears to be reflux-related.

Complications of GER result from severe disease and include peptic stricture and Barrett's esophagus.

Differential Diagnosis

Any disorder in children that delays gastric emptying or causes proximal small bowel obstruction can mimic GER. These include annular pancreas, pyloric stenosis, and milk protein enterocolitis.

Before performing any diagnostic test in children with GER, it is important to remember that almost all infants have physiologic reflux. This usually responds by the first birthday or at the latest by the age of 18 months (Fonkalsrud & Ament, 1996). Investigations should therefore be considered only in children with severe or atypical symptoms, symptoms of complications, or in those in whom other disorders of gastric emptying need to be ruled out. The age of the patient should also be considered. In children less than 2 months of age, vomiting is always considered significant.

Various diagnostic studies are available for the diagnosis of GER (Table 4–1). However, some of these are not specific, as they do not differentiate primary from secondary causes of GER; for example, a child with pyloric stenosis would also test positive for GER.

Barium Studies

A barium upper gastrointestinal series is more useful than a barium swallow, since it can also diagnose associated gastric and small bowel disorders like pyloric stenosis, annular pancreas, and intestinal webs, stenosis, and atresia, which may present with GER-like symptoms. The ability to accurately assess GER on barium studies requires an experienced pediatric radiologist; attention should be paid to the presence of hiatal hernia and esophageal stricture.

Esophagoscopy

Endoscopy is the most widely used method to diagnose esophagitis, although it is not required in most children with GER. It is indicated in the following situations: in the differentiation of GERD from other forms of esophagitis, in diagnosis and follow-up of severe

Table 4–1. Diagnostic tests for GER.

1. Is abnormal reflux present?
Barium upper gastrointestinal series
Gastroesophageal scintiscan
Standard acid reflux test
Ambulatory pH monitoring

2. What is the cause for reflux?
Barium upper gastrointestinal series
Endoscopy
Esophageal motility evaluation
Gastric emptying study

3. Is there reflux-related injury?
Air-contrast barium esophagogram
Endoscopy
Mucosal biopsy
Chest radiography (for pulmonary complications)
Extended intraesophageal pH and respiratory monitoring

4. Are symptoms due to reflux? (i.e., symptom correlation)
Bernstein test
pH monitoring

5. Can prognostic or preoperative information be obtained?
Esophageal motility evaluation
pH monitoring
Types of defect

GERD and its complications, and in assessment of reflux disease refractory to standard medical therapy.

Endoscopy has high sensitivity and specificity for the detection of mucosal injury. However, infants do not have esophagitis, and the primary role of endoscopy with them is to diagnose associated gastroduodenal disorders. The endoscopic features of esophagitis are erythema, linear erosions that may be confluent, ulcers, and, rarely, stricture and Barrett's esophagus. These changes are usually localized to the distal esophagus, but in severe disease the proximal part may also be affected. Various endoscopic grading systems for reflux esophagitis based on the presence and severity of lesions have been used. Strictures develop in around 15 percent of patients with reflux esophagitis. About 40% of patients may have histologic changes alone and can be diagnosed only with endoscopic biopsy.

Ambulatory Esophageal pH Monitoring

Ambulatory esophageal pH monitoring has emerged as the gold standard for the diagnosis of GER. Development of lightweight portable recorders and computerization have increased the popularity of this technique. A number of electrodes have been developed. Glass and antimony electrodes are the most frequently used.

The electrode is best placed 5 cm, 3 cm, and 2 cm above the manometrically defined LES in adults, children, and infants, respectively. In children, formulae to

determine the position of the LES with reference to the subject's height have been found to be useful (Staiano & Clouse, 1991); for children less than 2 years of age, the equation $L = 0.22(H) + 4.92$, where L is the location in centimeters from the nares and H is the height in centimeters correctly predicts LES location in 90% of patients; this equation is less useful in older children. Recording is carried out for 24 hours. The parent is advised to keep a diary documenting within minutes the start and finish of meals, the occurrence and nature of symptoms, and supine or upright posture. The child must be appropriately fed during the procedure to ensure gastric distension and simulate the physiologic state. Proton-pump inhibitors and H2-receptor antagonists should be stopped before the study. Double-probe pH monitoring (simultaneous esophageal and pharyngeal) is useful for patients with laryngeal abnormalities, pulmonary abnormalities, and emesis as manifestations of reflux; many of these children may have normal esophageal acid exposure times (Little et al, 1997).

In infants, acid secretion is inconsistent, and ambulatory pH monitoring may thus underdiagnose the intensity of GER. Simultaneous measurement of gastric pH helps to overcome this fallacy. Postprandial reflux is not accurately assessed by pH probe because of the pH buffering effect of the feeds.

Analysis of Data

The threshold of pH 4 is most widely used for the definition of episodes of GER. Simple calculation of the total 24-hour acid exposure (pH < 4) is the best single determinant to discriminate normal from abnormal reflux (Fonkalsrud & Ament, 1996; Varty, Evans, & Kapilas, 1993). Other measurements include total number of reflux episodes, duration of long episodes (> 5 minutes), total number of long episodes, and total reflux time in supine and in upright positions. A symptom index can also be calculated in older children. Ambulatory pH monitoring has a sensitivity and specificity in the detection of GERD of up to 96%.

Patients with symptoms typical of GERD and with documented esophagitis do not benefit from an initial pH study. Patients with atypical symptoms and children with respiratory symptoms may have clarification of their syndrome with pH testing. An additional use of pH testing is in the evaluation of patients whose symptoms continue while they receive therapy. In patients with suspected reflux-related laryngitis, the probe may be positioned in the proximal esophagus to assess proximal acid reflux.

Esophageal Manometry

Esophageal manometry measures intraluminal pressure and coordination of pressure activity in the muscles of the esophagus. It is necessary before pH monitoring to determine the level of the LES, especially in older children. Esophageal manometry may also be helpful to document the presence of effective peristalsis when antireflux surgery is being considered.

In GERD, LES function is an important determinant of acid reflux, and effective peristalsis is a critical determinant of acid clearance. It should be kept in mind, however, that peristaltic function is not mature in infants, especially in the premature ones (Omari et al., 1995). In contrast, the LES mechanisms seem well developed (Omari et al., 1995). Children with previous surgery for atresia also have severe dysmotility and poor acid clearing capacity.

Finding of a high percentage of abnormal contractions, the presence of hypotensive LES, or both not only suggests a more severe form of GERD, but also implies greater difficulty with long-term therapy. Other manometric abnormalities are short length of LES and excessive transient relaxation. However, none of these aberrations predicts the occurrence of clinically significant GERD.

In children, transient upper esophageal sphincter relaxations may occur during episodes of esophageal distension caused by GER; these have been implicated in esophagopharyngeal reflux (Willing, Furukawa, Davidson, & Dent, 1994). Esophageal motility studies thus provide useful diagnostic and prognostic information. Manometry is not indicated for making or confirming a suspected diagnosis of GERD; it is also not useful for predicting postoperative surgical outcome (Cullu et al., 1994).

Scintiscan

A ^{99}Tc scintiscan is a noninvasive technique to document GER, especially in children. After ingestion of a radionuclide feed, the child is placed under a gamma counter and counts over the esophagus are obtained in various views. Scintiscan is more easily available than ambulatory pH monitoring. It is, however, not as reliable as pH monitoring, but provides additional information regarding gastric emptying, and so is useful in postprandial reflux. It is also useful to detect pulmonary aspiration (Hillemeier, 1996). However, the evaluation is for short periods of time, and the specificity and reproducibility of the test are not good.

Medical Therapy of Gastroesophageal Reflux Disease

Treatment of GER in children depends on severity of symptoms. If the child is thriving well, and the main complaint is regurgitation and spitting, no therapy except postural and dietary advice needs to be given.

Drug therapy is required in patients with severe symptoms, complicated GER, and respiratory symptoms. A stepwise approach is useful, and consists of symptomatic therapy, reduction of acid exposure, pro-

kinetic drugs, and surgery. Surgery is required only in refractory cases and in patients with strictures.

Symptomatic Therapy

This includes elevation of the head-end of the bed, prone positioning, thickening of feeds, and diet/behavior modification.

The child should be placed head-high at an angle of 30° during and after feeds. In children with severe disease, this position may be necessary for longer durations. Prone positioning is also useful. In these positions, gravity helps in volume clearance of the esophagus, and decreases the acid-induced damage. The total number of reflux episodes, and their duration, decrease in the prone position. Recently, however, the prone position has been implicated in increased risk of sudden infant death syndrome.

Thickening of formula feeds with starch (rice, cereal) or inert noncaloric substances (carob) decreases regurgitation in patients with GER. It is not clear, however, whether the reflux actually decreases. It is observed, however, that the episodes of emesis, time spent crying, and time spent awake are reduced (Hillemeier, 1996).

Certain foods like chocolates, carminatives, and foods rich in fat, garlic, onion, and peppermint have been shown to relax the LES, and may increase reflux. Certain drinks with low pH or high osmolarity such as orange juice, tomato juice, and aerated drinks increase symptoms in patients with GER. Foods that increase GER should be avoided in children.

Alteration of the feeding schedule, that is, smaller and more frequent feeds, decreases gastric distention and hence GER.

Other measures like decreasing the gastroesophageal pressure gradient by weight loss and avoidance of tight-fitting clothes also lead to a decrease in reflux.

Reduction of Esophageal Acid Exposure

Drugs are to be used as an adjunct to symptomatic therapy in patients who do not respond to the same.

Topical Therapy

Antacids are safe and provide rapid and effective, but short-lasting relief of symptoms, and have to be given in frequent doses. Liquid formulations are better than tablets. In infants, they are given in the dose of 0.5 mL/kg between feeds. Magnesium-containing antacids lead to diarrhea, while those containing aluminum lead to constipation and aluminum absorption.

Alginic acid forms a viscous layer over gastric residue, protecting the esophagus from acid exposure. Thus the refluxate has a neutral pH, and does not cause esophageal damage. A combination of alginic acid and antacids is superior to antacids alone and equivalent to sucralfate and H$_2$-receptor antagonists (H$_2$RA) when used along with prokinetic agents.

Sucralfate has been found to be equivalent to H$_2$RA in the therapy of GERD. The benefit of sucralfate is maximum in patients with severe disease. This is because esophageal retention of the drug is greater. However, the drug has to be given at frequent intervals and compliance is low.

Acid Suppression

These drugs are the mainstay of therapy in GERD. Because acid is the final mode of insult to the esophageal mucosa, acid-suppressive therapy aids in healing of esophagitis even if the associated motor abnormalities are not corrected. However, therapy of GERD differs from that of peptic ulcer disease in that greater acid suppression is required for a longer time to produce healing of esophagitis. Also, acid suppression in GERD is required round-the-clock, necessitating long-acting drugs or more frequent dosing.

H$_2$-receptor Antagonists

Acid suppressive therapy with H$_2$-receptor blockers provides good healing and symptom relief; however, H$_2$RAs have to be administered at least two to three times daily since their duration of action is about 6–9 hours. H$_2$RAs in standard doses provide symptom relief in only 50 to 75% of patients, while endoscopic healing is seen in only 60% of patients after 12 weeks of therapy at high doses. High doses of ranitidine (20 mg/kg/day) may be required for children with refractory esophagitis (Cucchiara et al., 1993). The healing rates depend on the severity of esophagitis. H$_2$RAs are relatively free of side effects. Cimetidine has been shown to have antiandrogenic effects, neurological adverse events, and drug interactions. Side effects with ranitidine, famotidine, roxatidine, and nizatidine are rare.

Proton-Pump Inhibitors (PPI)

The discovery of profound suppressors of acid secretion has radically changed the management of patients with GERD. These drugs confer prolonged acid suppression (approximately 24 hours), making them ideal for GER treatment. PPI are irreversible inhibitors of H+K+ ATPase that is locally activated, thus providing targeted therapy. They are superior to all the other drugs used in the treatment of reflux disease.

Three PPI are currently available. Omeprazole (40 mg/day/1.73 m^2 surface area) produces 80% healing of endoscopic esophagitis at 8 weeks with superior symptom relief (Cucchiara et al., 1993). However, since the underlying motor abnormality remains uncorrected there is a high rate of recurrence, with more than 80% of patients developing endoscopic esophagitis within 6 months of discontinuing treatment. Lansoprazole and pantoprazole are recently added drugs to the armamentarium for GERD. Because they provide more acid suppression than omeprazole, they are ideal for patients with severe GERD and those not responding to omeprazole.

Prokinetic Agents

These drugs are physiologically most suited for the treatment of GER as they tend to correct some of the factors leading to reflux. They increase the LES pressure and esophageal contractility. They also increase gastric emptying, thus decreasing LES relaxation triggered by gastric fundal distention. The commonly used prokinetic agents include metoclopramide, domperidone, and cisapride.

Metoclopramide has both central and peripheral actions. It decreases transmission of dopamine, which is an inhibitory neurotransmitter in the gastrointestinal tract. It improves LES pressure and gastric emptying, but has no effect on peristalsis. The recommended dose is 0.1 mg/kg with a maximum of 0.5 mg/kg. The incidence of side effects (11–34%) such as anxiety, fatigue, and restlessness is high, especially in chidren less than 6 months of age, and is dose-dependent. Dystonic reactions also occur. Gynecomastia due to metoclopramide use has been reported in children (Madani & Tolia, 1997). Domperidone has only peripheral dopamine-antagonist action and has less neurological side effects. Its actions in the gastrointestinal tract are similar to those of metoclopramide, and is given in the dose of 0.3 to 0.6 mg/kg.

Cisapride increases the release of acetylcholine from the myenteric plexus and is relatively free of side effects. It increases LES pressure and accelerates gastric emptying; the effect on esophageal peristalsis is debatable. Cisapride is also known to stimulate salivary volume and increase the salivary protein output and salivary bicarbonate (Goldin et al., 1997). Cisapride (0.2 mg/kg q.i.d.) alone for 3 months relieves reflux and also respiratory symptoms in 80 percent of patients (Tucci et al., 1993). It is especially useful for nocturnal reflux, where it is administered at bedtime. There have been reports of prolongation of QT interval in infants after cisapride use (Lewin, Bryant, Fenrich, & Grifka, 1996). This cardiotoxicity increases when the drug is combined with ranitidine (Valdes et al., 1997).

All the prokinetic agents give good symptom relief, but poor endoscopic healing rates when used alone. They are useful in patients with symptoms suggestive of delayed gastric emptying or as an adjunct to acid suppressive therapy in those with severe GERD. A single dose of prokinetic agent may be used before bedtime in patients with persistent nocturnal symptoms.

Maintenance Therapy

Most children symptomatically improve as they reach 2 years of age. In children who develop late-onset symptoms, or do not improve by 2 years of age, GERD is a chronic disease, as in adults; acute short-term therapy is not expected to give lasting relief. Long-term maintenance with high-dose H₂RA or PPI may be required. Long-term acid suppression may increase the side effects due to hypochlorhydria (diarrhea, bacterial overgrowth). There is a potential for enterochromaffin cell hyperplasia to occur in patients on long-term PPI therapy. Patients not controlled in spite of maintenance therapy are candidates for surgical intervention.

Children who develop peptic strictures following GERD require esophageal dilatation. Results are usually good, but repeated dilatations combined with aggressive acid suppression are required in resistant cases. Some of these patients require surgery for GERD.

Surgery for Gastroesophageal Reflux Disease

The goal of surgery is to improve the mechanical barrier of the gastroesophageal junction and prevent reflux. Surgery is indicated in children with severe, refractory GER, especially when there is failure to thrive or respiratory impairment. Surgery is also indicated for peptic strictures that do not respond to dilatation.

The most commom surgery is fundoplication (Fonkalsrud & Ament, 1996) and its modification, an anterior wrap (Kazerooni, Van Camp, Hirschl, Drongowski, & Coran, 1994). Results are good in experienced hands, but the failure rate is about 40% at 5 years. After surgery, more than 80% of children experience relief of symptoms, even when they are operated at less than 2 years of age (Kazerooni et al., 1994). The uncut Collis modification of Nissen's fundoplication has also found to be a useful and effective surgery in children (Cameron, Cochran, & McGill, 1997). Recently, laparoscopic surgery has been done with good results. About 50% of small children undergoing fundoplication have underlying neurologic disease. In children who require esophageal replacement for congenital disorders, colonic replacement along with the ileocecal valve helps to prevent GER (Touloukian & Tellides, 1994).

ACHALASIA CARDIA

The term achalasia denotes failure to relax. The earliest clinical description of achalasia cardia was published by Thomas Willis in 1674, who recounted a patient with a dilated esophagus and was successfully treated by dilation with a whale bone.

Pathogenesis

Achalasia cardia is characterized by absence of propulsive peristalsis in the distal esophageal body and failure of the LES to completely relax on deglutition and esophageal hypersensitivity to a cholinergic drug. Resting LES pressures may also be elevated.

There is degeneration and reduction in the number of ganglion cells in Auerbach's plexus, with patchy fibrosis and scarring in the esophageal musculature. These changes tend to be more commonly identified in the body of the esophagus than in the LES, and are more marked in patients with longstanding disease. On electron microscopy, muscle changes suggestive of denervation atrophy have been observed. Occasional intracytoplasmic inclusions (Lewy bodies) in the dorsal motor nucleus of the vagus and myenteric plexus have also been found. In postmortem specimens, esophagi of patients having symptoms for longer than 10 years have fewer ganglion cells than those with symptoms of lesser duration. The earliest pathological changes consist of myenteric inflammation with injury to and subsequent loss of ganglion cells and injury to and fibrosis of myenteric nerves (Goldblum, Rice, & Richter, 1996).

Vagal nerve abnormalities have been found on electron microscopy. There is reduction in the number of nerve cells in the dorsal motor nucleus of the vagus and in the caudal portion of the nucleus ambiguus. Following stimulation or after sham feeding there is delayed response in gastric acid secretion, suggesting vagal dysfunction.

Other neurologically mediated reflexes such as transient LES relaxation are altered. There is significantly less LES relaxation in achalasia patients versus normals following gastric distention. There is also an abnormal belch reflex of the upper esophageal sphincter.

The inhibitory mechanisms of the circular LES muscle are impaired. There is LES hypersensitivity to exogenous gastrin in achalasia. Relaxation of the LES is mediated through nonadrenergic noncholinergic (NANC) inhibitory neurons. Currently, nitric oxide seems to be the most important mediator of LES relaxation (Anand & Paterson, 1994). Loss of NO-synthase containing neural elements has been observed in achalasia (Gaumnitz et al., 1995).

No etiologic agent has been identified as yet, and the cause of the disease is still unknown. A similar disturbance of esophageal motility resulting from damage to the myenteric nerve plexus has been seen in patients infected with *Trypanosoma cruzi* in some South American countries (especially Brazil). In contrast to achalasia, other viscera are also often involved.

Histologically, epithelial thickening with basal cell hyperplasia, papillary elongation, widening of the stratified zone, and pathologic cornification have been reported, and in longstanding achalasia, small ulcers may extend into the submucosa or muscularis.

Incidence

It has been estimated that each year approximately 0.5–1.0 per 100,000 population are affected with the disease. Only 2 to 5% of the patients are under 14 years of age; apart from these, 3 to 5% of the adults are able to trace their symptoms back to childhood. In our center, 3% of achalasia patients presented in childhood. The disease is uncommon under 12 months of age.

Three general etiologic categories of achalasia exist: (1) idiopathic achalasia, which represents approximately 98% of all cases; (2) familial achalasia; and (3) achalasia associated with degenerative neurologic diseases.

Familial achalasia represents less than 1% of the achalasia population (Wong & Maydonovitch, 1992). Over 75 cases have been reported in the literature. In all these cases symptoms first appeared during adult life. Most of these cases are horizontally transmitted, occurring in the pediatric age group in siblings and even in monozygotic twins. Many of these result from consanguinous unions. In familial achalasia males are more commonly affected, in contrast to sporadic achalasia where both sexes are equally affected. Although these familial cases suggest that in some instance the disorder may have an inherited basis, no precise mode of inheritance is evident.

Achalasia cardia may occur in association with other disorders like Sjögren's syndrome; a neurological syndrome characterized by mental deficiency, cerebellar ataxia, and bilateral optic atrophy; a syndrome characterized by congenital deafness, short stature, vitiligo and muscle wasting; and glucocorticoid deficiency and impaired tear production. Achalasia has also been described in association with Down syndrome (Preiksaitis, Miller, Pearson, & Diamant, 1994).

Clinical Features

Difficulty with swallowing and regurgitation of retained esophageal contents during or after a meal are the main complaints. Dysphagia is usually most evident with solid food though some children find equal difficulty in swallowing liquids. In older children, dysphagia is described as a fullness in the chest during a meal, with a filling and even overflow sensation as the meal progresses. Older children may also complain of a choking sensation or of food sticking in the region of the lower sternum or, less often, at the level of the cricoid. A child may endeavor to promote emptying of the esophagus by drinking or by employing a variety of maneuvers such as deep breathing, straining, exerting pressure with a finger over the suprasternal notch, and crouching forward while swallowing. Alternatively, he or she may regurgitate the offending food. The presence in the "vomit" of undigested food eaten many hours previously is characteristic. Unlike gastric outlet obstruction, where the vomitus is sour due to gastric acid, the vomit in achalasia is bland.

The onset is insidious and symptoms fluctuate in severity, especially during the early stages of the dis-

ease. The best historical estimates of dysphagia are indicated by changes in the length of time it took to eat a meal and drink liquids during a meal, before and after symptom onset.

The second most commonly described symptom (66%) is regurgitation. Regurgitated food is undigested, nonbilious (nongreen), and nonacidic. However, fermented intraesophageal contents may taste acidic.

Aspiration of regurgitated esophageal contents may give rise to recurrent pulmonary infections and suppuration. These respiratory symptoms may in fact constitute the principal clinical complaint, particularly in young children. Nocturnal regurgitation can cause spasms of coughing and result in undigested food and mucus being found on the child's pillow in the morning.

Pain is not a common complaint; when it occurs it is seen in the early phases of the disease due to the increased sensitivity of the nondilated esophagus. Some patients with achalasia also have abnormalities in the upper esophageal sphincter which may result in difficulty in belching (Ali, Hunt, Jorgensen, deCarle, & Cook, 1995). Failure to thrive is common; in longstanding cases loss of weight and malnutrition may occur.

Diagnosis

Chest x-ray is useful only in severe cases where a paracardiac shadow (mediastinal widening) with a fluid level in the posterior mediastinum on lateral radiograph may be seen. In patients with respiratory complications, pulmonary changes due to aspiration pneumonia may be seen. The fundic gas bubble is absent in 40% of cases.

During a *barium swallow*, the classic appearance of a dilated, aperistaltic esophagus with distal narrowing and "bird-beak" appearance is seen in 80% of cases. In severe cases, the esophagus may be dilated and tortuous, giving the "sigmoid" appearance. Rarely, regurgitation into the trachea may be seen in severe cases. In early cases, the disease may be missed because of lack of dilatation; fluoroscopy may help in these cases to detect lack of peristalsis and the intermittent obstruction at the LES.

Esophageal manometry is the gold standard for the diagnosis of achalasia. Manometric features are esophageal aperistalsis following swallows, high or normal basal LES pressure, incomplete LES relaxation on swallowing, and baseline esophageal pressure higher than gastric pressure. Occasionally, high-amplitude nonperistaltic waves are seen. It is important to remember that sedation cannot be given during the procedure, since the patients need to be given swallows of water. The test is therefore difficult to perform in very small or uncooperative children.

Endoscopy does not contribute to the diagnosis; in achalasia cardia it is done more to rule out mechanical obstruction due to peptic stricture or a carcinoma. In longstanding achalasia and dilated esophagus with retained food, mucosal ulceration may be seen.

Differential Diagnosis

Achalasia cardia needs to be differentiated from causes of mechanical obstruction like peptic stricture, and esophageal or gastric fundus malignancy, both of which are rare in childhood.

Treatment

The treatment of achalasia is directed towards relief of dysphagia, such as decreasing the resistance of the LES to passage of food.

Medical Therapy

Drugs like calcium-channel blockers and nitroglycerine transiently decrease LES pressure and can be administered before a meal to decrease dysphagia. These are useful only as short-term measures and need to be administered prior to every meal. Their long-term use has not been evaluated in children.

Botulinum toxin injection into the LES is a recent addition to the therapy of achalasia. The toxin acts through a paralytic action on the LES by binding to the presynaptic cholinergic nerve terminals. Initial results have been promising, but more than one-third of patients relapse with dysphagia at 6 months.

Balloon Dilatation

The principle of balloon dilatation is to stretch and rupture only enough circular LES muscle as to decrease dysphagia without the complication of GER or perforation. Unfortunately it is very difficult to accurately adhere to this principle.

Various types of balloons are available, and the advent of over-the-wire Rigiflex dilators has made the procedure safe. The dilatation may be done at one sitting or in a graded manner while increasing the pressure and the outer diameter of the balloon. Various trials have evaluated the optimum pressure required, the balloon diameter, and the duration of dilatation; no consensus is available however. Most of these studies have evaluated adult patients.

Factors that affect the success of dilatation are: diameter of the balloon, pressure applied, and duration of dilatation. Unfortunately, these are also the factors that influence the complication rate. Approximately 5% of patients develop significant GER following dilatation. The incidence of perforation is less than 5% in experienced hands. Most perforations are limited to the mucosa or the muscle layer and can be conserva-

tively managed. Transmural perforations need surgical management.

Most individuals experience relief of dysphagia after dilatation. Repeat dilatation is required for those who do not respond. Over the long term, relief persists in 60% and 25% of patients after 1 and 5 years, respectively.

Surgery

Patients who do not respond to two or three successive dilatation sessions and fail to thrive require surgical intervention. Heller's myotomy with or without an antireflux procedure is the accepted surgery for achalasia cardia. Results are better than balloon dilatation in the long-term. The incidence of GER is 20%.

CORROSIVE STRICTURES OF THE ESOPHAGUS

Caustic injury of the esophagus occurs accidentally most often following ingestion of strong alkali or acid (Clausen, Nielsen, & Fogh, 1994). Most affected children are between 1 and 4 years of age. Tragic accidents are attributable to storage of caustic fluids in containers carelessly left within the reach of young children.

Corrosive substances are ubiquitous and vary in strength and composition. Most corrosives are available as over-the-counter drain cleaners. The corrosive substance is most commonly some form of alkali, such as sodium hydroxide.

Alkaline Injury

Sodium hydroxide is the most frequent cause of injury. In experimental animals, 3.8% NaOH can cause necrosis of the muscular layer even after a 10-second contact time; most corrosives available have a higher concentration. Other alkaline corrosives include hypochlorite and ammonia. In contrast to granule form, the liquid form tends to coat the mucosa more uniformly and results in more extensive injury.

Small button-type alkaline batteries contain potassium or sodium hydroxide within a plastic seal that joins the cathode and anode. Damage results from an electrolyte reaction, is localized at a point where the battery gets lodged, and may be severe enough to cause perforation.

Alkali provokes full-thickness liquefaction or saponification necrosis of the esophageal wall. In the initial stage, there is an acute inflammatory response with mucosal necrosis, followed by sloughing of necrotic tissue and ulceration over 4 to 15 days. After 3 to 4 weeks, cicatrization begins. Significant esophageal strictures develop only when there is circumferential damage.

Acid Injury

Hydrochloric and sulfuric acids are the common acids available in the form of drain bowl cleaners. The effect of acid is similar to that of alkalis, but penetration into the deeper layers is limited by rapid transit through the esophagus with superficial coagulation necrosis and eschar formation. Isolated esophageal injury is less common than after alkali ingestion; associated gastric injury is more common.

The amount, nature, and concentration of the swallowed corrosive and the duration of tissue contact determine the extent of injury.

Clinical Features

Symptoms of caustic ingestion depend on the type and concentration of the ingested agent (Browne & Thompson, 1992). Crystals or solid forms of lye, or substances with foul odor or taste tend to be taken in small quantities, and the child may spit out the offending agent, limiting the injury to the mouth, pharynx, and larynx. A tasteless liquid would be swallowed and would result in severe injury.

Symptoms include burning pain in the mouth and throat, odynophagia, excessive salivation, stridor, hoarseness, dysphagia, and chest pain. Gastric involvement leads to abdominal pain and vomiting, and occasionally symptoms and signs of perforation. About 20 to 60% of patients with oropharyngeal injuries do not have esophageal damage; on the other hand, 20% of patients with esophageal injuries do not have oropharyngeal damage.

There is often edema and ulceration of the lips, tongue, and pharynx. Airway obstruction from severe epiglottic and laryngeal edema may result. Patients with this feature tend to have severe esophageal damage as well. Airway obstruction is more frequent in children because of the small size of the larynx.

The postcricoid region of the pharynx and the lower third of the esophagus (the esophageal sphincters) are the sites most commonly affected. In severe cases there may be perforation into the mediastinum or pleural cavity, development of a tracheoesophageal fistula, or gastric involvement with necrosis.

As the acute inflammatory reaction subsides, odynophagia and dysphagia decrease; with the development of esophageal stricture, dysphagia gradually returns, usually within 1 to 3 months after the accident. The more penetrating the esophageal damage the more likely a fibrous stricture will develop. Difficulty in swallowing is confined at first to solid food, but later even fluids may be regurgitated.

Investigations

The initial investigations focus on verification of the ingested agent and assessing the severity of damage and complications. Standard pH test paper may be used to test the remains of the substance.

A chest x-ray may help to define a pulmonary complication or mediastinitis. Laryngoscopy (preferably flexible) should be done to assess the pharynx and larynx in terms of mucosal injury and edema.

There is a controversy on the role of early esophagoscopy in the management of caustic injury. It is a safe procedure if undertaken within the first 24 hours and if no attempt is made to advance the esophagoscope beyond an area of circumferential injury. Endoscopy should not be done in patients with compromised vital parameters and in those with symptoms/signs of visceral perforation. Three degrees of damage have been described and graded:

Grade 0: normal appearance of esophageal mucosa.

Grade I: mucosal edema and hyperemia.

Grade IIa: friability, hemorrhage, erosion, blistering, whitish membranes, exudates, superficial ulceration.

Grade IIb: features of IIa plus deep, discrete, or circumferential ulceration.

Grade III: multiple ulcers and necrosis evidenced by brownish-black or gray areas of discoloration.

Patients with Grade 0-IIa injury have no complications. Over the long term, strictures develop in patients with Grade IIb or III injury. Death occurs mainly with Grade III injury (Zargar et al., 1991).

Examination by barium swallow and fluoroscopy during the acute stage is usually not indicated, as the degree of injury may be misinterpreted due to severe edema and sloughing. Additionally, there is a risk of aspiration. Barium swallow after 2 to 3 months helps to define the stricture length and diameter, especially in cases where the endoscope cannot negotiate the stricture.

Treatment

Acute Phase

The aim of therapy is to maintain an adequate airway, resuscitation, and supportive care. Tracheostomy is necessary when there is severe respiratory distress due to laryngeal edema; intravenous fluids, gastrostomy feedings, or total parenteral nutrition may sometimes be required. Gastric lavage increases the risk of aspiration and, like induced emesis, reexposes the esophagus to the caustic substance. Neutralization of the caustic agent by buffering substances is not effective, because the agent is usually not active by the time the patient is seen by a physician. In cases of acid ingestion, neutralization may increase gastric injury because of the chemical reaction which is generated (Spiegelman & Rogers, 1996).

Steroids, although advised at one time, are not recommended at present. Antibiotic therapy is required only if secondary infection sets in. Prophylactic antibiotics have not been found to be useful.

Some authors recommend placement of a nasogastric tube in the acute phase itself. This helps to maintain enteral nutrition as well as acting as a guide to future dilatation. Early dilatation has been associated with a high risk of perforation, and is therefore no longer recommended. Antacids, sucralfate, and omeprazole may be helpful to control the inflammation; no proof of their efficacy has yet been established.

Surgery may be required in patients who develop perforation of the esophagus. In patients with severe injury, where transmural esophageal or gastric injury develops, early laparotomy with esophagogastroectomy has been recommended by some authors.

Patients with mild injury should undergo endoscopy after 3 to 6 weeks to assess if any severe esophageal damage was missed in the initial endoscopy.

Chronic Phase

Stricture of the esophagus is the major long-term complication. Caustic strictures are often extensive and multiple, involving most of the lower esophagus. In general, corrosive strictures respond to antegrade dilatation, but not as well as peptic strictures (Broor et al., 1996). In severe cases, retrograde dilatation may be done. Repeated dilatation is necessary, though the frequency of dilatation may decrease over some time. Self-bougienage may be practiced by a well trained patient. Esophageal resection with a colon or gastric tube replacement may be necessary in cases where the lumen is too small for dilatation, or in cases of extensive damage. A single narrow stricture may respond to balloon dilatation.

Esophageal squamous cell carcinoma is a potential long-term complication of corrosive injury. The risk of developing carcinoma is 1,000 times that of the general population. The latency period from the time of injury to carcinoma is approximately 40 years. Carcinoma develops at the site of previous stricture. Because many of these patients present at a younger age, and spread of carcinoma is limited by the surrounding fibrous tissue, their response to therapy is good. Surveillance by endoscopy is recommended by some authors.

HIATUS HERNIA

That the stomach and other abdominal viscera could herniate through an enlarged esophageal hiatus in the diaphragm was recognized by postmortem examinations in the 18th and 19th centuries. A clinical diagnosis was not possible until the advent of contrast radiography, but there was a poor correlation between symptoms and demonstration of a hiatus hernia. It was believed that an upwardly displaced stomach must be due to a congenitally short esophagus or trauma (Haubrich, 1996).

Pathophysiology

Herniation through the esophageal hiatus occurs in two forms: (1) an axial or sliding type in which both the distal esophagus and a varying portion of the stomach (i.e., the entire esophagogastric junction) are situated above the diaphragm and (2) a paraesophageal or rolling type in which the lowermost esophagus and the esophagogastric junction retain their position below the diaphragm, while a portion of the proximal stomach protrudes into the thorax alongside the esophagus. It is now recognized that the problem of hiatus hernia lies not in its anatomic displacement, but in the functional consequence of gastroesophageal reflux.

Normally, decussation of the crura results in a slit-like hiatus that tends to compress the terminal esophagus in an elliptic fashion, with the axis extending anteriorly from the right and posteriorly to the left. Fibroelastic elements from these lamellae extend at the hiatus to form the phrenoesophageal membrane that penetrates the wall of the esophagus along a varying extent adjacent to the hiatus. This tends to fix the lower esophagus (about 3 cm) within the abdomen.

Two basic types of hiatus hernia are recognized. In the common type 1 (axial or sliding) hiatus hernia, there is expansion of the muscular tunnel and laxity of the phrenoesophageal membrane circumferentially. This allows the cardiac portion of the stomach to herniate upward through the hiatus. The lax phrenoesophageal membrane remains intact, and its level of insertion marks the distal esophagus. The typical sliding hiatus hernia is small and consists of only the terminal esophagus and a portion of the gastric cardia. It is unusual for more than 3 cm to 5 cm of the gastric pouch to herniate through the esophageal hiatus. The size of the hernia alone does not predict the presence or severity of symptoms; larger, more longstanding hernias are more likely to be associated with symptomatic GER. Some authors prefer to refer to hiatus hernia in children as "partial thoracic stomach" to differentiate it from the one occurring in adults.

The less common paraesophageal or rolling hernia is marked by the normal position of the esophagogastric junction and protrusion of the gastric fundus through an expanded hiatus. This allows the less than atmospheric intrathoracic pressure to be directly transmitted through the pleura to the peritoneal sac. With positive intra-abdominal pressure exerting an upward push, this hernia tends to progressively enlarge. Indeed, the entire stomach, and rarely, the transverse colon, segments of the small bowel, or the spleen may enter the hernial sac. Eventually the phrenoesophageal membrane becomes so lax that the previously fixed esophagogastric junction migrates above the level of the diaphragm. This accounts for what appears to be a combined sliding and paraesophageal hernia. Paraesophageal hernia is rarely seen in children.

The typical paraesophageal hernia is rarely associated with GER; however, because of incarceration and strangulation, the herniated gastric pouch can bleed.

Almost all newborn infants are notably liable to regurgitation, and in a few cases, a sliding hiatus hernia can be demonstrated.

Associated Congenital Disorders

In congenital hiatus hernia, there is an overall 1 in 12 chance that a young sibling will be similarly affected. About 10% of these infants have other major congenital malformations and an additional 5% have minor associated anomalies. The majority of these defects involve the central nervous system and skeletal structures. The association with mental handicap is particularly noteworthy. The incidence of hypertrophic pyloric stenosis is approximately 15 times the expected frequency. Low birth weight (< 2,500 g) among babies with a partial thoracic stomach is about twice the expected frequency.

A similar association of pyloric muscular hypertrophy with hiatus hernia has been noted in adults. The frequency of congenital hiatus hernia of sliding type is approximately 10 per 10,000 live births.

Clinical Features

The clinical features are considered in terms of the age of the child. Some authors have classified patients with sliding hiatus hernia as Group I (early infancy) and Group II (early childhood).

Persistent vomiting is the principal complaint in early infancy. In 75% of patients, vomiting starts within the 1st week and in another 10% between the 1st and 6th weeks of life. It is usually copious during or shortly after feeding. Occasional brown staining of the vomit due to bleeding is a characteristic feature. Large hematemesis is extremely rare. Bile staining may suggest the possibility of intestinal obstruction. Due to persistent vomiting, the majority of these infants are underweight, dehydrated, and hungry and take feeds greedily. Infants with a large hiatus hernia are susceptible to recurrent episodes of aspiration pneumonia. In the majority of patients, vomiting tends to spontaneously subside during the early months of life.

In late infancy and childhood, the two principal complaints are vomiting and difficulty with swallowing solid food. Vomiting typically occurs at night; usually little food is contained in it. Dysphagia occurs in patients who develop a peptic stricture. Difficulty in swallowing solid food is also experienced by patients with minimal or no esophageal narrowing; the reason for this is not fully understood. A number of mechanisms like intramural inflammation and edema with neuromuscular dysfunction may be responsible. An occasional child may have bizarre contortions and posturing of the head and neck; these probably constitute maneuvers aimed at relieving discomfort.

If an esophageal stricture does not develop, there is a gradual spontaneous lessening of both complaints with advancing age.

Children whose vomiting improves either before or coincidentally with the introduction of a semisolid diet follow a benign clinical course and are free of symptoms by 1 to 2 years of age. These patients represent about two thirds of all affected infants and have been classified as Group IIa. In the remainder (Group IIb), symptoms either show no improvement or are aggravated at the time of introducing mixed feeds. Most of these latter children tend to have troublesome symptoms for up to 4 years and longer. About one in seven of this group (i.e., 5% of all patients) develop a stricture.

On follow-up after 20 years, all Group I and 80% of Group IIa patients (i.e., those without a stricture) are symptom-free, but a partial hiatus hernia can still be radiologically demonstrable in about 50%. In a long-term prospective evaluation of children with this condition, Carré found that most became asymptomatic at 6 to 9 months of age; when reexamined later as young adults, a surprising finding was that a majority had a normal esophagogastric junction (Carré, 1987).

Investigations

In uncomplicated cases, a barium swallow is the only investigation required. The intrathoracic stomach is seen well on barium swallow examination. However, it may be seen transiently, and would be recognized only on fluoroscopy. A contracted LES offers resistance to the flow of barium, and allows demarcation of the cardioesophageal junction. In infants with severe reflux and a lax LES, the hiatus hernia may not be recognized, due to difficulty in locating the LES. Paraesophageal hernia can also be diagnosed by barium meal study. In patients with complications, endoscopy is required to assess a stricture.

Treatment

A majority of infants become symptom-free by the 1st year, and require no specific treatment. Treatment is directed toward control of the GER and consists mainly of posture therapy and small frequent feeds. Response to therapy can be assessed by monitoring the frequency of vomiting, weight gain, and pulmonary symptoms.

Surgical therapy is required only in children who develop a stricture or those who persist to have troublesome symptoms even after 18 months of age. It is estimated that 50% of children who do not respond to therapy by 18 months require surgery.

ESOPHAGEAL ATRESIA AND TRACHEOESOPHAGEAL FISTULA

Esophageal atresia (EA), usually with an associated tracheoesophageal fistula (TEF), is the most common congenital anomaly of the esophagus; it is also the most serious (Holder, 1986). The anomaly was first described by Thomas Gibson in 1697; TEF without EA was first simultaneously described by Lamb and Pinard in 1873 (Carré, 1987).

Survival was not reported with this disorder till 1939, when Ladd and Levin independently described the first two survivors who had been treated with a combination of operations: feeding gastrostomy and cervical esophagostomy, followed by esophagus reconstruction (Ladd, 1944; Levin, 1941). Haight and Towsley (1943) described the first successful primary repair with division and suture of the TEF and direct esophageal anastomosis.

The etiology of EA and TEF is not known; a genetic contribution is likely (Chen, Goei, & Hertzler, 1979). The incidence of EA and/or TEF is about 1 in 3000–4500 births (Myers, 1974). Males and females are equally affected

Various classification systems have been proposed for these disorders; Table 4–2 shows a commonly used classification system described by Gross (1953). Type C (EA with distal TEF) is the most common anomaly, accounting for 85–90% of all cases. Here the upper esophagus terminates in a blind pouch while the lower esophageal segment has a fistulous connection with the trachea. This anomaly is further divided into two types: (1) with a long atretic segment of the esophagus and (2) where the upper and lower portions of the esophagus either overlap or are separated only by a narrow gap (Roberts, Carré, & Inglis, 1955). A long gap between the two ends of the esophagus makes esophageal reconstruction technically difficult.

TEF without esophageal atresia (type E), or "H" type TEF, most often occurs at or above the level of the second thoracic vertebra. There may be multiple fistulas, but they are rare.

These anomalies have recently been classified as a part of communicating bronchopulmonary foregut malformations (Srikanth, Ford, Stanley, & Mahour, 1992).

Pathogenesis

The esophagus and trachea have a common origin from the embryonic foregut (Gray & Skandalakis,

1972). The trachea and lungs normally develop from a linear groove on the ventral aspect of the foregut, the laryngotracheal groove, which appears on day 21-23. A single foregut tube is divided into two tubes by the inward growth and eventual fusion of lateral septa; the separation progresses in a caudocranial direction. Misdirection of the lateral ridges can obliterate a portion of the developing esophagus (atresia); incomplete separation of the trachea and esophagus can result in a TEF (Smith, 1957).

Associated Abnormalities

Maternal polyhydramnios is a commonly associated condition. This is expected because the normal swallowing of amniotic fluid by the fetus and its subsequent absorption from the fetal gastrointestinal tract, and transfer to the maternal circulation via the placenta, are interrupted (Gray, Nesten, & Plentl 1956; Swenson, Lipman, Fisher, & Deluca, 1962).

Associated anomalies are present in nearly half of the infants (Table 4–3). Serious among them are congenital heart disease and intestinal or anal atresia (Spitz, 1993). Patent ductus arteriosus and septal defects (atrial and ventricular) are the most common cardiac anomalies (Ein, Shandling, Wesson, & Filler, 1989). A right aortic arch (seen in approximately 5% of cases with EA) can present technical problems at the time of repair. Heart disease is a major cause of mortality.

Duodenal atresia is the most commonly associated intestinal atresia. Anorectal malformations are also very common (Andrassy & Mahour, 1979; Briard, Frezel, Kaplan, Nihaul-Fekete, & Valyer, 1977). Jejunal or ileal atresia, Meckel's diverticulum, intestinal malrotation and, uncommonly, hypertrophic pyloric stenosis (Czernik & Raine, 1982) and congenital esophageal stenosis (Mortensson, 1975) have been described. Cleft lip, cleft palate, and hypospadias have also been reported.

Table 4–2. Classification of EA and/or TEF: relative frequency.

Type	Anatomic Management	Frequency (%)
A	EA without TEF	8
B	EA with proximal TEF	1
C (i and ii)	EA with distal TEF	86
D	EA with proximal and distal TEF	1
E	TEF without EA	4

Table 4–3. Incidence of associated anomalies.

Anomaly	Incidence (%)
Congenital heart disease	10
Gastrointestinal	23
Musculoskeletal	15
Pulmonary	1.5
CNS	3
Genito-urinary	10
Chromosomal	2.5
Other	4

Source: Data from "Esophogeal Atresia and Tracheoesophageal Fistula: A Survey of Pediatrics," by T. M. Holder, D. T. Cloud, J. E. Lewis, Jr., and G. E. Pilling IV, 1964. *Pediatrics, 34,* 542-549.

One pattern of associated anomalies, the VATER association (Kirkpatrick, Wagner, & Pilling, 1965; Quan & Smith, 1973), includes vertebral defects, anal atresia, TEF with EA, and radial and renal dysplasia. Not all the defects may be present in a given patient.

Clinical Features

Babies with EA have a higher incidence of intrauterine growth retardation (Cozzi & Wilkinson, 1969); about one third of them weigh less than 2500 g. They are symptomatic since birth, presenting with constant drooling of saliva (sometimes blood- or bile-stained) because of inability to swallow. Attacks of regurgitation, choking, coughing, dyspnea, and cyanosis are common, especially on attempting oral feeds. Recurrent pulmonary infections and atelectasis are serious complications. Pulmonary complications are more common in patients with distal fistula (Waterston, Bonham-Carter, & Aberdeen, 1963).

In patients with TEF, the abdomen can become grossly distended, with excessive burping and flatus, due to air being forced through the fistula into the stomach when the baby cries. In patients with narrow TEF without EA, symptoms may be slight or absent in early childhood and the diagnosis may be delayed till late childhood or even adulthood, the main symptom being recurrent chest infections.

Diagnosis

The presence of maternal polyhydramnios should always raise the suspicion of EA in the fetus. If the diagnosis is suspected in a newborn, a relatively stiff radioopaque 10 Fr plastic catheter should be passed through the nose (or mouth) and its position checked by a chest radiograph. Ability to put the catheter into the stomach rules out EA; in patients with EA the catheter will get stuck 10–12 cm from the nares in the blind proximal esophageal pouch.

A radiograph of the chest and abdomen will also reveal the state of the lungs, heart, intestinal gas pattern, and the presence of vertebral anomalies. In types A and B anomalies, there will be no gas in the abdomen.

Additional radiological investigations are usually not needed, but studies using nonionic, water-soluble contrast through an esophageal catheter or via a gastrostomy tube, or both, may be done if required.

TEF without EA (type E) may be difficult to diagnose. The fistula may be demonstrated on esophageal contrast studies under cinefluoroscopy, or by bronchoscopy with or without instillation of methylene blue into the esophagus. Alternatively, an esophagoscopy can be done.

A clever method of demonstrating an H-type fistula has been proposed. The patient is ventilated with 100% oxygen and intragastric and intraesophageal oxygen concentration is measured. An elevation in oxygen concentration will be found as the sampling electrode is withdrawn from the stomach into the esophagus (Powers, 1979).

Treatment

Preoperative Management

As soon as a diagnosis of EA is established (or suspected), all feeding should be stopped and the proximal pouch should be decompressed with a sump tube attached to continuous low suction (Replogle, 1963). Infants with distal TEF should be nursed with head and shoulders elevated. Hypothermia and hypoglycemia should be prevented. Antibiotic treatment and/or respiratory assistance may be needed.

Healthy babies weighing over 1300 g who have no pneumonia or major associated anomaly should undergo prompt repair. Pulmonary complications, low birthweight (< 1,300 g) in a premature baby, and associated cardiac anomalies, imperforate anus, or intestinal atresia may all delay definitive surgery. Decompression of the proximal pouch along with a gastrostomy are necessary in such cases before primary repair can be undertaken.

Surgical Correction

The aim of surgical treatment is to achieve closure of the fistula and establish esophageal continuity as far as possible. Extrapleural approach by thoracotomy is preferred to a transpleural approach as any esophageal anastomotic leak is well confined. Additional cervical incision may be necessary.

Type C (ii)

After dividing the TEF, primary end-to-end anastomosis without undue tension is usually easy as the two ends of the esophagus are close to each other.

Types A, B, and C (i)

Primary anastomosis between the upper and lower ends of esophagus is difficult as they are separated by a wide gap. The gap can be bridged in some cases by performing circular myotomy on the upper esophageal pouch and lengthening the esophagus (Janik, Simpson, & Filler, 1981; Rescorla, West, Scherer, & Grosfeld, 1994; Ricketts, Luck, & Raffensperger, 1981). In other cases, only the TEF is divided and gastrostomy is performed in the first stage. Primary esophageal anastomosis is undertaken after 2 to 3 months during which time the esophageal pouches naturally lengthen (Puri, Blake, O'Donnell, & Guiney, 1981) or by daily manual bougienage of the upper pouch (Mahour, Woolley, &

Gwinn, 1974). Rarely, it may be necessary to use colonic, gastric, or jejunal interposition to establish esophageal continuity; this is associated with considerable morbidity (Cohen, Middleton, & Fletcher, 1974; Ein & Friedberg, 1981; Raffensperger, Luck, Reynolds, & Schwartz, 1996; Spitz, 1992).

Type D

A separate cervical approach is recommended for closure of the proximal fistula (Rehbein, 1964).

Type E

Accurate localization of the fistula determines the surgical approach. Most patients require a transcervical approach (Andrassy et al., 1980; Bedard, Girvan, & Schandling, 1974).

Postoperative Care

Particular attention should be paid to respiratory complications. Transanastomotic nasogastric catheter, gastrostomy, jejunal tube feeding, or total parenteral nutrition are the options available to maintain nutrition. After an uncomplicated surgery, oral fluids can be commenced on the fifth postoperative day.

Complications

Anastomotic leak is the most frequent serious early postoperative complication, responsible for about a fifth of all postoperative deaths (Buker, Box, Pauling, & Sietter, 1972). Leaks developing after an extrapleural approach fare far better than those after a transpleural approach. Traditionally, leaks are managed by doing a cervical esophagostomy with gastrostomy. Leaks can also be managed by reoperation with primary repair, use of intercostal muscle flap with or without pleural patch, and/or drainage allowing the native esophagus to be preserved, with a good outcome (Chavin, Field, Chandler, Tagge, & Othersen, 1996).

Recurrent fistula can develop in about 10% of cases, and needs surgical correction. Anastomotic stricture is a common late complication and generally responds well to esophageal dilatation.

Esophageal motor abnormalities, detectable by esophageal manometry studies, are by far the main cause of dysphagia and recurrent aspiration pneumonitis (Duranceau et al., 1977; Orringer, Kirsh, & Sloan, 1977; Tovar et al., 1995; Werlin, Dodds, Hogan, Glicklich, & Arndorfer, 1981). Symptoms gradually improve with age although manometric abnormalities may persist. The motor abnormalities are thought to be inherent with the disease rather than due to surgical trauma.

GERD is another significant complication, at times aggravating an anastomotic stricture. Reflux disease can be conservatively managed in the majority (Carré 1987; Pieretti, Shandling, & Stephens, 1974; Tovar et al., 1995).

Prognosis

Factors adversely affecting survival include low birthweight, pulmonary complications, and associated congenital abnormalities. Congenital heart disease is a leading cause of mortality. Early diagnosis and improved management have resulted in overall survival rates between 75% and 85% (Holder & Ashcraft, 1981; Spitz, Kiely, & Brereton, 1987) in the absence of major associated congenital abnormalities (Louhimo & Lindahl, 1983; Touloukian, 1992).

DEVELOPMENTAL ANATOMY AND CONGENITAL MALFORMATIONS OF THE ESOPHAGUS

Developmental Anatomy

The esophagus, trachea, lungs, and stomach develop from the primitive foregut (Amoury, 1986). The foregut differentiates into the esophagus and a ventrally placed respiratory diverticulum (lung bud) at 22–23 days of development. With further elongation of the esophagus and respiratory diverticulum, the laryngotracheal groove is formed on the ventral aspect of the esophagus. By the 5th week, the pharynx, esophagus, stomach, and the two lung buds can be identified. The lateral ridges that form along the posterior rim of the trachea begin to proliferate, grow inward and fuse in the midline, forming two tubes (trachea and esophagus) from a single foregut tube. The esophagus continues to elongate with the linear growth of the embryo (Scherer & Grosfeld, 1986).

The esophageal mucous membrane is derived from the foregut endoderm. During the 7th and the 8th weeks of development, a rapid proliferation of the epithelial cells nearly fills the esophageal lumen, except for areas of vacuoles. The vacuoles coalesce by the end of the 10th week to form a hollow tube (Bremer, 1944).

Congenital Malformations

Congenital malformations of the esophagus, with the exception of esophageal atresia and tracheoesophageal fistulae, are relatively rare disorders. As a group, they present a significant challenge with respect to both diagnosis and treatment (Esophageal atresia and tracheoesophageal fistula are discussed in another section in this chapter.)

Congenital Esophageal Stenosis

Congenital stenosis of the esophagus is uncommon, the reported incidence being 1 in 25,000 to 1 in 50,000 live births (Murphy, Yazbeck, & Russo, 1995). Esophageal atresia is seen in one third of cases. Acquired stricture due to reflux esophagitis is the most common cause of esophageal stenosis in infancy (Scherer & Grosfeld, 1986).

Congenital stenosis usually affects the lower esophagus (Carré, 1987). Three main types have been described: (1) segmental stenosis, (2) membranous web or diaphragm with a central or eccentric aperture, and (3) intramural rests of tracheobronchial tissue (Marmuse et al., 1993). Histologically, segmental hypertrophy and membranous web contain only mucosal and submucosal components. Esophageal stenosis can occasionally be associated with a tracheoesophageal fistula or esophageal atresia and other extraesophageal congenital anomalies.

Clinical Presentation

A complete web presents like esophageal atresia, with symptoms of excessive salivation, choking spells, and respiratory distress in the neonatal period. Esophageal stenosis presents with symptoms of incomplete obstruction including dysphagia, regurgitation, recurrent respiratory infections, vomiting during meals, and failure to thrive. Symptoms may be delayed to introduction of semisolid food in late infancy. Sudden-onset dysphagia due to food impaction is not an uncommon presentation.

Diagnosis

Barium esophagogram and esophagoscopy are useful in the diagnosis. An endoscopic biopsy beyond the stenotic area may be helpful in excluding stricture due to reflux esophagitis as inflammatory changes are minimal or absent in congenital stenosis and the epithelium is squamous in type. GER may need to be excluded by pH testing or radioisotope studies.

Treatment

Esophageal dilatation is the first line of therapy (Allmendinger et al., 1996). For an impassable stricture, initial gastrostomy is needed. A string is then passed antegrade through the gastrostomy site and serves as a guide for subsequent dilatation of the stenotic segment. Rarely, if dilatation fails, either resection of the stenotic area with end-to-end anastomosis or some form of esophagoplasty is required (Vidne & Levy, 1970). Esophageal dilatation is, however, usually not successful and can actually be dangerous in patients with esophageal stenosis due to tracheobronchial remnants.

The chances of perforation are high (Deiraniya, 1974) and surgical resection of the stenotic segment with primary esophageal anastomosis is the treatment of choice.

An esophageal web has been endoscopically incised using electrocautery followed by esophageal dilatation (Huchzermeyer, Burdelski, & Hruby, 1979). Rupture of a membranous web, combined with dilatation, is also an effective form of treatment (Petit, Borde, Gubler, & Tourane, 1970).

Foregut Duplication

Intrathoracic foregut anomalies can be classified into three categories: bronchogenic cysts, intramural esophageal cysts, and enteric cysts (neurenteric cysts) (Gray & Skandalakis, 1972). The term neurenteric cyst appropriately describes the origin of this anomaly. (Bronchogenic cysts are not considered in the present discussion.)

Intramural esophageal cysts or duplication share a common wall and may or may not communicate with the lumen of the normal esophagus. The cyst wall consists of one or more layers of muscularis and includes a myenteric plexus. The epithelial lining may be ciliated columnar, squamous, or gastric. The lesion is thought to arise from a defect in the vacuolization process during the 7th to 10th week of gestation. A rapid proliferation of the esophageal epithelial cells takes place during the 6th week of gestation, and may occlude the esophageal lumen. Normally, the lumen is reestablished by the formation and coalescence of vacuoles. Chains of vacuoles may fuse separate from the main lumen, resulting in esophageal duplications (Scherer & Grosfeld, 1986).

Neurenteric cysts occur in the posterior mediastinum, adjacent or adherent to the esophagus and vertebral column. The notochord forms from specialized cells of the ectoderm, in the 3rd week of gestation, and migrates dorsally. An adhesion may form between the notochord and the entoderm before the dorsal migration, giving rise to two possible anomalies: (1) failure of vertebral column to close ventrally in the region of that somite and (2) an entodermal tract or diverticulum associated with the notochord and foregut, resulting in the formation of a neurenteric cyst. The cyst wall of the neurenteric cyst is composed of the same histologic elements as an intramural cyst, but the embryologic origin is different.

A neurenteric cyst may have an intra-abdominal component, often attached to the duodenum or jejunum and sometimes communicating with their lumen. It may also communicate with the spinal canal as a mass or a patent canal of Kovalevski.

Associated Anomalies

Common anomalies associated with neurenteric cyst include spina bifida, hemivertebrae, fused vertebrae, or intraspinal mass in the region of the lower cervical or upper thoracic regions. A majority of neurenteric cysts show only fibrous attachment to the vertebral column, but may communicate within the dura (Rahaney & Barclay, 1959; Superina, Ein, & Humphreys, 1984). Vertebral anomalies are present in 80% of cases with neurenteric cysts and intraspinal anomalies in 25%. The second most common anomaly is an additional duplication of the small intestine (Bower, Cieber, & Kiesewetter, 1978).

Clinical Presentation

Patients with esophageal duplication and neurenteric cysts present in infancy and childhood. Respiratory and gastroesophageal symptoms are common, though older infants and children with middle and lower mediastinal lesions may be asymptomatic, detected only as mediastinal widening on a plain X ray of the chest.

Respiratory symptoms, seen in 50 to 90% of reported cases, include stridor, pneumonia, hemoptysis, chest pain, cough, and occasionally severe respiratory distress in the newborn. Gastroesophageal symptoms (seen in 10 to 15%) include epigastric pain, vomiting, hematemesis, and dysphagia (Scherer & Grosfeld, 1986). Hemorrhage can occur as a result of ulceration of ectopic gastric mucosa lining the cyst wall, and can rarely prove fatal (Ahmed, Jolleys, & Dark, 1972; Grosfeld, O'Neill, & Clatworthy, 1970). A majority of the esophageal duplication cysts and all neurenteric cysts do not communicate with the esophageal lumen, but they may cause compression by attaining a large size as a result of fluid secreted by the lining epithelium. A typical triad of neurenteric cyst, consisting of respiratory symptoms, a mediastinal mass, and a vertebral anomaly, is seen in 70% of patients.

Diagnosis

A plain roentgenogram can demonstrate a mediastinal mass with or without air-fluid level, and associated vertebral anomaly. A barium esophagogram (Youngblood & Blumenthal, 1983), ultrasonography to detect the solid or cystic nature of the mass (Teele, Henschke, & Tapper, 1980), and computerized tomography scan to delineate anatomic details and extensions (Weiss, Fagelman, & Warhit, 1983) are other useful diagnostic modalities. Myelography may be abnormal in 25% of cases with neurenteric cysts (Superina et al., 1984).

Ectopic gastric mucosa can be picked up on radioisotope technetium scan. Magnetic resonance imaging can be useful in the differential diagnosis of mediastinal masses. Differential diagnosis includes a variety of benign and malignant tumors (Filler, Simpson, & Ein, 1979). The risk of malignancy in a mediastinal mass in childhood is 40%.

Treatment

Complete surgical removal of the cyst, if possible, preserving all vital structures, is the treatment of choice. If this is not possible, stripping of the mucosa from the muscularis in order to get rid of the mucus-producing tissues and ectopic gastric mucosa should be performed. Transdiaphragmatic and intraspinal extensions should be taken care of (Tarnay, et al., 1970). Transesophageal needling of the cyst and rarely spontaneous rupture and disappearance of the cyst have been reported (Kuhlman, Fishman, Wang, & Siegelman, 1985; Nakahara et al., 1990).

Diverticulum of the Esophagus

Congenital true diverticulum of the esophagus, that is, containing all the walls of the esophagus, is rare. Esophageal diverticula usually present in late infancy and early childhood with features of recurrent respiratory infection and progressive dysphagia (Scherer & Grosfeld, 1986). Lesions higher in the pharyngoesophageal region can mimic esophageal atresia with symptoms like excessive salivation, regurgitation, cough while feeding, and, rarely, cyanosis. Very rarely, a tracheoesophageal fistula may be present.

A barium esophagogram is the method of choice for the diagnosis; endoscopy may also be helpful. Single-stage surgical excision is the treatment of choice.

References

Ahmed, S., Jolleys, A., & Dark, J. F. (1972). Thoracic enteric cysts and diverticulae. *British Journal of Surgery, 59,* 963.

Alaswad, B., Toubas, P. L., & Grunow, J. E. (1996). Environmental tobacco smoke exposure and gastroesophageal reflux in infants with apparent life-threatening events. *Journal of the Oklahoma State Medical Association, 89,* 233–237.

Ali, G. N., Hunt, D. R., Jorgensen, J. O., deCarle, D. J., & Cook, I. J. (1995). Esophageal achalasia and coexistent upper esophageal sphincter relaxation disorder presenting with airway obstruction. *Gastroenterology, 109,* 1328–1332.

Allmendinger, N., Hallisey, M. J., Markowitz, S. K., Hight, D., Weiss, R., & McGowan, G. (1996). Balloon dilation of esophageal strictures in children. *Journal of Pediatric Surgery, 31,* 334–346.

Amoury, R. A. (1986). Structure and function of the esophagus in infancy and early childhood. In K. W. Asharaft, T. M. Holder (Eds.), *Pediatric esophageal surgery* (pp. 1–28). Orlando, FL: Grune & Stratton.

Anand, N., & Paterson, W. G. (1994). Role of nitric oxide in esophageal peristalsis. *American Journal of Physiology, 266,* G123–G131.

Andrassy, R. J., Ko, P., Hanson, B. A., Kubota, E., Hays, D. M., & Mahour, G. H. (1980). Congenital tracheoesophageal fistula without esophageal atresia. *American Journal of Surgery, 140,* 731–733.

Andrassy, R. J., & Mahour, G. H. (1979). Gastrointestinal anomalies associated with esophageal atresia or tracheoesophageal fistula. *Archives of Surgery, 114,* 1125–1128.

Bedard, P., Girvan, D. P., & Shandling, B. (1974). Congenital H-type tracheoesophageal fistula. *Journal of Pediatric Surgery, 9,* 663–668.

Bower, R. J., Cieber, W. K., & Kiesewetter, W. B. (1978). Alimentary tract duplications in children. *Annals of Surgery, 188,* 669.

Bremer, J. L. (1944). Diverticula and duplications of the intestinal tract. *Archives of Pathology, 38,* 132.

Briard, M. L., Frezel, J., Kaplan, J., Nihaul-Fekete, C., & Valyer, J. (1977). Les malformations ano-rectales et l'atresie de l'oesophage. *Archives of Franco Pediatrics, 34,* 172–183.

Broor, S. L., Lahoti, D., Bose, P., Ramesh, G. N., Raju, G. S., & Kumar, A. (1996). Benign esophageal strictures in children and adolescents: Etiology, clinical profile, and results of endoscopic dilatation. *Gastrointestinal Endoscopy, 43,* 474–477.

Browne, J. D., & Thompson, J. N. (1992). Caustic injuries of the esophagus. In D.O. Castell, (Ed.). *The esophagus* (pp. 669–685). Boston: Little, Brown.

Buker, R. H., Box, W. A., Pauling, F. W., & Sietter, G. (1972). Complications of congenital tracheoesophageal fistula. *American Journal of Surgery, 124,* 705–710.

Cameron, B. H., Cochran, W. J., & McGill, C. W. (1997). The uncut Collis-Nissen fundoplication: Results for 79 consecutively treated high-risk children. *Journal of Pediatric Surgery, 32,* 887–891.

Carré, I. J. (1987). Disorders of the oropharynx and oesophagus. In C. M. Anderson, V. Burke, & M. Gracey, (Eds.), *Pediatric gastroenterology.* (2nd ed, pp. 32–77). Melbourne: Blackwell Scientific.

Chavin K., Field G., Chandler J., Tagge E., & Othersen H. B. (1996). Save the child's esophagus: management of major disruption after repair of esophageal atresia. *Journal of Pediatric Surgery, 31:*48–51.

Chen, H., Goei, G. S., & Hertzler, J. H. (1979). Family studies on congenital esophageal atresia with or without tracheoesophageal fistula. *Birth defects: Original Article Series, 15,* 117–244.

Cheu, H. W., Grosfeld, J. L., Heifetz, S. A., Fitzgerald, J., Rescorla, F., & West, K. (1992). Persistence of Barrett's esophagus in children after antireflux surgery: Influence on follow-up care. *Journal of Pediatric Surgery, 27,* 260–264.

Clausen, J. O., Nielsen, T. L., & Fogh, A. (1994). Admission to Danish hospitals after suspected ingestion of corrosives. A nationwide survey (1984–1988) comprising children aged 0–14 years. *Danish Medical Bulletin (Denmark), 41,* 234–237.

Cohen, D. H., Middleton, A. W., & Fletcher, J. (1974). Gastric tube esophagoplasty. *Journal of Pediatric Surgery, 9,* 451–460.

Conley, S. F., Werlin, S. L., & Beste, D. J. (1995). Proximal pH-metry for diagnosis of upper airway complications of gastroesophageal reflux. *Journal of Otolaryngology, 24,* 295–298.

Cozzi, F., & Wilkinson, A. W. (1969). Intrauterine growth rate in relation to anorectal and oesophageal anomalies. *Archives of Disabled Children, 44,* 59–62.

Cucchiara, S., Minella, R., Iervolino, C., Franco, M. T., Campanozzi, A., Franceschi, M., D'Armiento, F., & Auricchio, S. (1993). Omeprazole and high dose ranitidine in the treatment of refractory reflux esophagitis. *Archives of Disabled Children, 69,* 655–659.

Cullu, F., Gottrand, F., Lamblin, M. D., Turck, D., Bonnevalle, M., & Farriaux, J. P. (1994). Prognostic value of esophageal manometry in antireflux surgery in childhood. *Journal of Pediatric Gastroenterology and Nutrition, 18,* 311–315.

Czernik, J., & Raine, P. A. M. (1982). Oesophageal atresia and pyloric stenosis—an association. *Zeitschrift für Kinderchirurgie, 35,* 18–20.

Dieraniya, A. K. (1974). Congenital oesophageal stenosis due to tracheobronchial remnants. *Thorax, 29,* 720.

Duranceau, A., Fisher, S. R., Flye, M. W., Janes, R. S., Postlethwait, R. W., & Sealy, W. C. (1977). Motor function of the esophagus after repair of esophageal atresia and tracheoesophageal fistula. *Surgery, 82,* 116–123.

Ein, S. H., & Friedberg, J. (1981). Esophageal atresia and tracheoesophageal fistula: Review and update. *Otolaryngology Clinics of North America, 14,* 219–249.

Ein, S. H., Shandling, B., Wesson, D., & Filler, R. M. (1989). Esophageal atresia with distal tracheoesophageal fistula: associated anomalies and prognosis in the 1980s. *Journal of Pediatric Surgery, 24,* 1055.

Eizaguirre, I., Tovar, J. A., Gorostiaga, L., Echeverry, J., & Torrado, J. (1993). Barrett esophagus in children. Presentation of 12 cases. *Circle of Pediatrics, 6,* 66–68.

Filler, R. M., Simpson, J. S., & Ein, S. H. (1979). Mediastinal masses in infants and children. *Pediatric Clinics of North America, 26,* 677.

Foglia, R. P. (1994). Esophageal disease in the pediatric age group. *Chest Surgery Clinics of North America, 4,* 785–809.

Fonkalsrud, E. W., & Ament, M. E. (1996). Gastroesophageal reflux in childhood. *Current Problems in Surgery, 33,* 1–70.

Ganatra, J. V., Medow, M. S., Berezin, S., Newman, L. J., Glassman, M., Bostwick, H. E., Halata, M., & Schwarz, S. M. (1995). Esophageal dysmotility elicited by acid perfusion in children with esophagitis. *American Journal of Gastroenterology, 90,* 1080–1083.

Gaumnitz, E. A., Bass, P. P., Osinski, M. A., Sweet, M. A., & Singaram, C. (1995). Electrophysiological and pharmacological responses of chronically denervated lower esophageal sphincter of the opossum. *Gastroenterology, 109,* 789–799.

Glassman, M., George, D., & Grill, B. (1995). Gastroesophageal reflux in children. Clinical manifestations, diagnosis, and therapy. *Gastroenterology Clinics of North America, 24,* 71–98.

Goldblum, J. R., Rice, T. W., & Richter, J. E. (1996). Histopathologic features in esophagomyotomy specimens from patients with achalasia. *Gastroenterology, 111,* 648–654.

Goldin, G. F., Marcinkiewicz, M., Zbroch, T., Bityutskiy, L. P., McCallum, R. W., & Sarosiek, J. (1997). Esophagoprotective potential of cisapride. An additional benefit for gastroesophageal reflux disease. *Digestive Disorder Science, 42,* 1362–1369.

Gray, M. J., Neslen, E. D., & Plentl, A. A. (1956). Estimation of water transfer from amniotic fluid to fetus. *Processes of Social and Experimental Biological Medicine, 92,* 463–464.

Gray, S. W., & Skandalaki, J. E. (Eds.). (1972). *Embryology for surgeons* (pp. 69–79). Philadelphia: W. B. Saunders.

Grosfeld, J. L., O'Neill, J. A., & Clatworthy, H. W. (1970). Enteric duplications in infancy and childhood: An 18-year review. *Annals of Surgery, 172,* 83.

Gross, R. E. (1953). *The surgery of infancy and childhood* (pp. 103–113). Philadelphia: W. B. Saunders.

Haight, C., & Towsley, H. A. (1943). Congenital atresia of the esophagus with tracheoesophageal fistula and end to end anastomosis of esophageal segments. *Surgery in Gynecology and Obstetrics, 76,* 672–688.

Haubrich, W. (1996). Diaphragmatic hernias. In W. S. Haubrich, F. Schaffner, & J. E. Berk (Eds). *Bockus' gastroenterology* (pp. 437–444). Philadelphia: W. B. Saunders.

Hillemeier, A. C. (1996). Gastroesophageal reflux. Diagnostic and therapeutic approaches. *Pediatric Clinics of North America, 43,* 197–211.

Holder, T. M. (1986). Esophageal atresia (Ed). *Pediatric esophageal surgery* (pp. 29–52). Orlando: Grune & Stratton.

Holder, T. M., & Ashcraft, K. W. (1981). Developments in the care of patients with esophageal atresia and tracheoesophageal fistula. *Surgical Clinics of North America, 61,* 1051–1061.

Holder, T. M., Cloud, D. T., Lewis, J. E. Jr., & Pilling, G. P. I. V. (1964). Esophageal atresia and tracheoesophageal fistula. A survey of its members by the surgical section of the American Academy of Pediatrics. *Pediatrics, 34,* 542–549.

Holloway, R. H., & Dent, J. (1990). Pathophysiology of gastroesophageal reflux: Lower esophageal sphincter dysfunction in gastroesophageal reflux disease. *Gastroenterology Clinics of North America, 19,* 517.

Huchzermeyer, H., Burdelski, M., & Hruby, M. (1979). Endoscopic therapy of a congenital oesophageal stricture. *Endoscopy, 4,* 259.

Janik, J. S., Simpson, J. S., & Filler, R. M. (1981). Wide gap esophageal atresia with inaccessible upper pouch. *Journal of Thoracic and Cardiovascular Surgery, 82,* 198–202.

Kawahara, H., Dent, J., & Davidson, G. (1997). Mechanisms responsible for gastroesophageal reflux in children. *Gastroenterology, 113,* 399–408.

Kazerooni, N. L., VanCamp, J., Hirschl, R. B., Drongowski, R. A., & Coran, A. G. (1994). Fundoplication in 160 children under 2 years of age. *Journal of Pediatric Surgery, 29,* 677–681.

Kelly, K. J., Lazenby, A. J., Rowe, P. C., Yardley, J. H., Perman, J. A., & Sampson, H. A. (1995). Eosinophilic esophagitis attributed to gastroesophageal reflux: Improvement with an amino acid-based formula. *Gastroenterology, 109,* 1503–1512.

Kirkpatrick, J. A., Wagner, M. L., & Pilling, C. P. (1965). A complex of anomalies associated with tracheoesophageal fistula and esophageal atresia. *American Journal of Roentgenology Radium Therapy and Nuclear Medicine, 95,* 208–211.

Klinkenberg-Knol, E., & Castell, D. O. (1992). Clinical spectrum and diagnosis of gastroesophageal reflux disease., In D. O. Castell (Ed.), *The esophagus* (pp. 441–447). Boston; Little Brown.

Kuhlman, J. E., Fishman, E. K., Wang, K., & Siegelman, S. S. (1985). Esophageal duplication cyst: CT and transesophageal needle aspiration. *American Journal of Rhinology, 145,* 531.

Ladd, W. E. (1994). The surgical treatment of esophageal atresia and tracheoesophageal fistula. *New England Journal of Medicine, 230,* 625–637.

Levin, N. L. (1941). Congenital atresia of the esophagus with tracheoesophageal fistula: Report of successful extrapleural ligation of fistulous communication and cervical esophagostomy. *Journal of Thoracic Surgery, 10,* 648–657.

Lewin, M. B., Bryant, R. M., Fenrich, A. L., & Grifka, R. G. (1996). Cisapride-induced long QT interval. *Journal of Pediatrics, 128,* 279–281.

Little, J. P., Matthews, B. L., Glock, M. S., Koufman, J. A., Reboussin, D. M., Loughlin, C. J., & McGuirt, W. F. Jr. (1997). Extraesophageal pediatric reflux: 24-hour double-probe pH monitoring of 222 children. *Annals of Otology, Rhinology, and Laryngology, 169(Suppl.),* 1–16.

Louhimo, I., & Lindahl, H. (1983). Esophageal atresia: Primary results of 500 consecutively treated patients. *Journal of Pediatric Surgery, 18,* 217–229.

Mahour, G. H., Woolley, M. M., & Gwinn, J. L. (1974). Elongation of the upper pouch and delayed anatomic reconstruction in esophageal atresia. *Journal of Pediatric Surgery, 9,* 373–383.

Marmuse, J. P., Cavillon, A., Mrejen, G., Toublanc, M., Potet, F., & Benhamou, G. (1993). Congenital stenosis of the esophagus due to tracheobronchial heterotopia. Review of the literature. Apropos of a case. *Annals of Chiropractics, 47,* 190–195.

McMurray, J. S., & Holinger, L. D. (1997). Otolaryngic manifestations in children presenting with apparent life-threatening events. *Otolaryngology—Head & Neck Surgery, 116,* 575–579.

Mortensson, W. (1975). Congenital oesophageal stenosis distal to oesophageal atresia. *Pediatric Radiology, 3,* 149–151.

Murphy, S. G., Yazbeck, S., & Russo, P. (1995). Isolated congenital esophageal stenosis. *Journal of Pediatric Surgery, 30,* 1238–1241.

Myers, N. A. (1974). Oesophageal atresia: The epitome of modern surgery. *Annals of the Royal College Surgery in England, 54,* 277.

Nakahara, K., Fujii, Y., Miyoshi, S., Yoneda, A., Miyata, M., & Kawashima, Y. (1990). Acute symptoms due to huge duplication cyst ruptured into the esophagus. *Annals of Thoracic Surgery, 50,* 309.

Nelson, S. P., Chen, E. H., Syniar, G. M., & Christoffel, K. K. (1997). Prevalence of symptoms of gastroesophageal reflux during infancy. A pediatric practice-based survey. Pediatric Practice Research Group. *Archives of Pediatric Adolescent Medicine, 151,* 569–572.

Omari, T. I., Miki, K., Davidson, G., Fraser, R., Haslam, R., Goldsworthy, W., Bakewell, M., & Dent, J. (1997). Characterisation of relaxation of the lower oesophageal sphincter in healthy premature infants. *Gut, 40,* 370–375.

Omari, T. I., Miki, K., Fraser, R., Davidson, G., Haslam, R., Goldsworthy, W., Bakewell, M., Kawahara, H., & Dent, J. (1995). Esophageal body and lower esophageal sphincter function in healthy premature infants. *Gastroenterology, 109,* 1757–1764.

Orringer, M. B., Kirsh, M. M., & Sloan, H. (1977). Long-term esophageal function following repair of esophageal atresia. *Annals of Surgery, 186,* 436–443.

Othersen, H. B. Jr., Ocampo, R. J., Parker, E. F., Smith, C. D., & Tagge, E. P. (1993). Barrett's esophagus in children. Diagnosis and management. *Annals of Surgery, 217,* 676–680.

Petit, P., Borde, J., Gubler, J. P., & Touraine, P. (1970). Les retrecissements congenitaux de l'oesophage. Á propos de 21 observations. *Annals of Chiropractics for Infants, 11,* 153–170.

Pieretti, R., Shandling, G., & Stephens, C. A. (1974). Resistant esophageal stenosis associated with reflux after repair of esophageal atresia: a therapeutic approach. *Journal of Pediatric Surgery, 9,* 355–357.

Powers, W. F. (1979). Further experience with intragastric oxygen measurement to diagnose H-type tracheoesophageal fistula. *Pediatrics, 63,* 668.

Preiksaitis, H. G., Miller, L., Pearson, F. G., & Diamant, N. E. (1994). Achalasia in Down's syndrome. *Journal of Clinical Gastroenterology, 19,* 105–107.

Puri, P., Blake, N., O'Donnell, B., & Guiney, E. J. (1981). Delayed primary anastomosis following spontaneous growth of esophageal segments in esophageal atresia. *Journal of Pediatric Surgery, 16,* 180–183.

Quan, L., & Smith, D. W. (1973). The VATER association. *Journal of Pediatric Surgery, 82,* 104–107.

Raffensperger, J. G., Luck, S. R., Reynolds, M., & Schwartz, D. (1996). Intestinal bypass of the esophagus. *Journal of Pediatric Surgery, 31,* 38–46.

Rahaney, K., & Barclay, G. P. T. (1959). Enterogenous cysts and congenital diverticula of the alimentary canal with abnormalities of the vertebral column and spinal cord. *Journal of Pathology and Bacteriology, 77,* 457.

Rehbein, F. (1964). Oesophageal atresia with double tracheoesophageal fistula. *Archives of Disabled Children, 39,* 138–142.

Replogle, R. I. (1963) Esophageal atresia: plastic sump catheter for drainage of the proximal pouch. *Surgery, 54,* 296–297.

Rescorla, F. J., West, K. W., Scherer, L. R., III., & Grosfeld, J. L. (1994). The complex nature of type A (long gap) esophageal atresia. *Surgery, 116,* 658–664.

Ricketts, R. R., Luck, S. R., & Raffensperger, J. G. (1981). Circular esophagomyotomy for primary repair of long-gap esophageal atresia. *Journal of Pediatric Surgery, 16,* 365–369.

Roberts, K. D., Carré, I. J., & Inglis, J. M. C. N. (1955). The management of congenital atresia and tracheo-oesophageal fistula. *Thorax, 10,* 45–52.

Scherer, L. R., & Grosfeld, J. L. (1986). Congenital esophageal stenosis, esophageal duplication, neurenteric cyst and esophageal diverticulum. In K. W. Ashcraft & T. M. Holder (Eds.), *Pediatric esophageal surgery* (pp. 53–71). Orlando, FL: Grune & Stratton.

Smith, E. I. (1957). The early development of the trachea and esophagus in relation to atresia of the esophagus and tracheoesophageal fistula. *Contr Embryology Carnegie. Inst Wash #245, 36,* 41.

Spiegelman, G. A., & Rogers, A. I. (1996). Chemical injury of the esophagus. In W. S. Haubrich, F. Schaffner, & J. E. Berk, (Eds.). *Bockus' gastroenterology* (pp. 483–491). Philadelphia: W. B. Saunders.

Spitz, L. (1992). Gastric transposition for esophageal substitution in children. *Journal of Pediatric Surgery, 27,* 252–257.

Spitz, L. (1993). Esophageal astresia and tracheoesophageal fistula in children. *Current Opinions in Pediatrics, 5,* 347–352.

Spitz, L., Kiely, E., & Brereton, R. J. (1987). Esophageal atresia: five years experience with 148 cases. *Journal of Pediatric Surgery, 22,* 103–108.

Srikanth, M. S., Ford, E. G., Stanley, P., & Mahour, G. H. (1992). Communicating bronchopulmonary foregut malformations: classification and embryogenesis. *Journal of Pediatric Surgery, 27,* 732–736.

Staiano, A., & Clouse, R. E. (1991). Value of subject height in predicting lower esophageal sphincter location. *American Journal of Disabled Children, 145,* 1424–1427

Superina, R. A., Ein, S. H., & Humphreys, R. P. (1984). Cystic duplications of the esophagus and neurenteric cysts. *Journal of Pediatric Surgery, 19,* 527.

Swenson, O., Lipman, R., Fisher, J. H., & Deluca, F. G. (1962). Repair and complications of esophageal atresia and tracheoesophageal fistula. *New England Journal of Medicine, 267,* 960–963.

Tarnay, T., Chang, C. H., Nugent, R. G., & Warden, H. E. (1970). Esophageal duplication (foregut cyst) with spinal malformation. *Journal of Thoracic and Cardiovascular Surgery, 59,* 293–298.

Teele, R. L., Henschke, C. I., & Tapper, D. (1980). The radiographic and ultrasonic evaluation of enteric duplication cysts. *Pediatric Radiology, 10,* 9.

Touloukian, R. J. (1992). Reassessment of the end-to-side operation for esophageal atresia with distal tracheoesophageal fistula: 22 year experience with 68 cases. *Journal of Pediatric Surgery, 27,* 562–567.

Touloukian, R. J., & Tellides, G. (1994). Retrosternal ileocolic esophageal replacement in children revisited. Antireflux role of the ileocecal valve. *Journal of Thoracic and Cardiovascular Surgery, 107,* 1067–1072.

Tovar, J. A., Diez-Pardo, J. A., Murcia, J., Prieto, G., Molina, M., & Polanco, I. (1995). Ambulatory 24-hour manometric and pH metric evidence of permanent impairment of clearance capacity in patient with esophageal atresia. *Journal of Pediatric Surgery, 30,* 1224–1231.

Tucci, F., Resti, M., Fontana, R., Novembre, E., Lami, C. A., & Vierucci, A. (1993). Gastroesophageal reflux and bronchial asthma: prevalence and effect of cisapride therapy. *Journal of Pediatric Gastroenterology and Nutrition, 17,* 265–270.

Valdes, L., Champel, V., Olivier, C., Jonville-Bera, A. P., & Autret, E. (1997). Syncope with long QT interval in a 39-day-old infant treated with cisapride (Malaise avec allongement de l'espace QT chez un nourrisson de 39 jours traité par cisapride) *Archives of Pediatrics (France), 4,* 535–537.

Vanderhoof, J. A., Zach, T. L., & Adriane, T. E. (1994). Gastrointestinal disease. In G. B. Avery, M. A. Fletcher, & M. G. Macdonald, (Eds.). *Neonatology. Pathophysiology and management of the newborn.* (44th ed, pp. 605–629). Philadelphia: J. B. Lippincott.

Varty, K., Evans, D., & Kapila, L. (1993). Paediatric gastro-esophageal reflux: Prognostic indicators from pH monitoring. *Gut, 34,* 1478–1481.

Vidne, B., & Levy, M. J. (1970). Use of pericardium for esophagoplasty in congenital esophageal stenosis. *Surgery, 68,* 389–392.

Waterston, D. J., Bonham-Carter, R. E., & Aberdeen, E. (1963). Congenital tracheo-oesophageal fistula in association with oesophageal atresia. *Lancet, ii,* 55–57.

Weiss, L. M., Fagelman, D., & Warhit, J. M. (1983). CT demonstration of an esophageal duplication cyst. *Journal of Computer Assistance in Tomography, 7,* 716.

Werlin, S. L., Dodds, W. J., Hogan, W. J., Glicklich, M., & Arndorfer, R. (1981). Esophageal function in esophageal atresia. *Digestive Disorder Sciences, 26,* 796–800.

Willing, J., Furukawa, Y., Davidson, G. P., & Dent, J. (1994). Strain induced augmentation of upper esophageal sphincter pressure in children. *Gut, 35,* 159–164.

Willis, T. (1674). *Pharmaceutice rationalis sive diatride de medicamentorum operationibus in human corpore.* London: A Leers.

Wong, R. K. H., & Maydonovitch, C. L. (1992). Achalasia. In D. O. Castell (Ed.), *The esophagus* (pp. 233–260). Boston; Little Brown.

Youngblood. D., & Blumenthal. B. I. (1983). Enteric duplication cyst. *Southern Medical Journal, 76,* 670.

Zargar, S. A., Kochhar, R., Mehta, S., & Mehta, S. K. (1991). The role of fibreoptic endoscopy in the management of corrosive ingestion and modified endoscopic classification of burns. *Gastrointestinal Endoscopy, 37,* 165–169.

5

Congenital and Developmental Anomalies of the Neck

Edward Wood, M.D.

Embryonic development of head and neck structures is an intricate process dependent on the occurrence of many complex interrelated events. Therefore, any errors in the orderly progression of these events may lead to a congenital or developmental malformation within the neck. Collectively, these malformations are not uncommon. Although they may become clinically apparent at any age, the majority present at birth or during early childhood. Most of these lesions are obvious to the well-trained clinician. Some, however, are quite enigmatic. Accurate diagnosis and proper management of these lesions is dependent on a thorough understanding of their embryology, anatomy, and clinical presentation.

EMBRYOLOGY OF THE NECK

The branchial or pharyngeal apparatus begins to develop around the 2nd week of fetal life and is usually complete by week 7. The branchial arch system consists of five transversely aligned mesodermal arches, which develop in the lateral foregut wall and are externally separated by ectodermally lined clefts and internally by pouches lined with endoderm (Figure 5–1). A branchial plate separates clefts from pouches which do not communicate at any time. The five arches are cranially to caudally numbered. The rudimentary 5th arch does not appear on the surface and by convention is called the 6th arch. Developing branchial arches contain a cartilaginous skeleton, primitive muscle, nerve, and artery.

First Branchial Arch

Cartilage of the first arch consists of a dorsal portion known as the maxillary process and a ventral portion, the mandibular process or Meckel's cartilage. Membranous ossification of maxillary process mesenchyme gives rise to the premaxilla, maxilla, zygomatic bone, and a portion of the temporal bone (Table 5–1). Similar ossification of Meckel's cartilage gives rise to the mandible. Two small portions of the dorsal ends of each persist and form the incus and malleus, respectively.

First arch musculature is destined to become the muscles of mastication (temporis, masseter, and pterygoids) as well as the anterior belly of the digastric, mylohyoid, tensor tympani, and tensor velij palatini. The nerve of the first arch supplies all its muscles and is the mandibular branch of the trigeminal nerve.

Second Branchial Arch

Second arch cartilage, or Reichart's, gives rise to the stapes, styloid process of the temporal bone, stylohyoid ligament, and lesser cornu and upper part of the hyoid bone. Second arch muscles include the stapedius, stylohyoid, posterior belly of the digastric, the auricular, and muscles of facial expression. All of these muscles are innervated by the nerve of the second arch, the seventh (facial) cranial nerve.

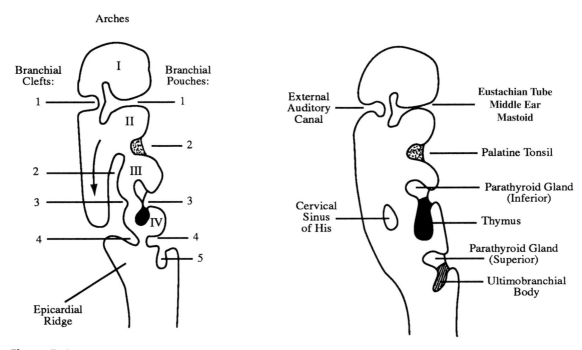

Figure 5–1. Schematic representation of the development of the pharyngeal clefts and pouches. The second arch overgrows the third and fourth arches; as a consequence the second, third, and fourth clefts coalesce, forming the cervical sinus of His. (Adapted from "Head and Neck," by J. Langman, 1981, p. 268. In: J. Langman, ed. *Medical embryology*, 4th ed. Baltimore: Williams & Wilkins.)

Table 5–1. Branchial arches.

Arch	Nerve	Artery	Skeletal Structure	Muscles
First (Mandibular)	Trigeminal (V)	Atrophies	Maxilla Mandible Malleus Incus	- Muscles of mastication - Mylohyoid - Anterior digastric - Tensor tympani - Tensor veli palatini
Second (Hyoid)	Facial (VII)	Stapedial (Atrophies)	Styloid Lesser cornu of hyoid Upper body hyoid Stapes	- Muscles of facial expression - Stylohyoid - Posterior digastric - Stapedius
Third	Glossopharyngeal (IX)	Internal carotid Common carotid	Greater cornu of hyoid Lower body hyoid	- Stylopharyngeus - Upper pharyngeal constrictors
Fourth	S. laryngeal N. (X)	Aortic arch Right subclavian	Epiglottis, thyroid and cuneiform cartilage	- Inferior pharyngeal constrictor - Cricothyroid
Sixth	R. laryngeal N. (X)	Ductus arteriosus Pulmonary artery	Corniculate, arytenoid, cricoid cartilages	- Intrinsic laryngeal muscles

Third Branchial Arch

Cartilage of this arch is destined to form the greater cornu and the lower part of the body of the hyoid.

Musculature is confined to the stylopharyngeus as well as the superior and middle pharyngeal constrictors. These muscles are innervated by the nerve of the third arch, the ninth (glossopharyngeal) cranial nerve.

Fourth Branchial Arch

Fourth arch muscles include the cricothyroid, levator palatini, and inferior pharyngeal constrictor. They are innervated by the fourth arch nerve, the tenth (vagus) cranial nerve, most notably its superior laryngeal branch. Cartilaginous components of this arch are laryngeal and include the epiglottis, thyroid, and cuneiform cartilages.

Sixth Branchial Arch

All intrinsic laryngeal muscles represent sixth arch musculature and are supplied by the recurrent laryngeal branch of the tenth cranial nerve. Cartilages are laryngeal and include the cricoid, arytenoids, and corniculates.

BRANCHIAL POUCHES

The human embryo has five paired branchial pouches, the last of which is often considered as part of the fourth. Pouches are lined with endoderm and give rise to several important organs with important endocrine and immunologic function (Table 5–2).

First Pharyngeal Pouch

The first pouch forms an elongated diverticulum (tubotympanic recess), which becomes incorporated into the temporal bone. The most lateral aspect of this pouch contacts the epithelial lining of the first branchial cleft, which will become the future external auditory canal.

The first branchial pouch is destined to become the middle ear and mastoid cavity, as well as the eustachian tube. The lining of the tympanic cavity contributes to the formation of the tympanic membrane.

Second Branchial Pouch

The endodermal layer of this pouch forms the epithelial lining of the palatine tonsil. Mesenchymal elements contribute to the formation of tonsillar tissue. Part of the pouch remains and is found in the adult as the tonsillar fossa.

Third Branchial Pouch

The third branchial pouch is subdivided into dorsal and ventral wings. Epithelium of the dorsal wing differentiates into cells that eventually become the inferior parathyroid gland. Ventral wing epithelium forms thymic tissue. Thymic tissue then migrates caudally and medially in the neck to assume its final position in the mediastinum, where it fuses with its counterpart from the contralateral side forming the thymus gland. Parathyroid tissue destined to become the inferior parathyroid gland accompanies the thymus in its migration and normally comes to rest on the dorsal surface of the thyroid gland.

Fourth Branchial Pouch

The fourth pouch is also divided into dorsal and ventral wings. Although the ultimate fate of the ventral aspect of the pouch remains in question, it is generally

Table 5–2. Branchial clefts and pouches.

	Cleft (Ectoderm)	*Pouch (Endoderm)*
First	External auditory canal Tympanic membrane	Eustachian tube Tympanic cavity Mastoid cavity Tympanic membrane
Second	Cervical sinus of His	Palatine tonsil Tonsillar fossa
Third	Cervical sinus of His	Inferior parathyroid Thymus Pyriform fossa
Fourth	Cervical sinus of His	Superior parathyroid ? Thymus
Fifth		Ultimobranchial body (usually considered part of fourth pouch)

felt to give rise to a small portion of thymic tissue. Epithelium of the dorsal wing forms parathyroid tissue destined to become the superior parathyroid gland.

Fifth Branchial Pouch

This pouch is generally considered part of the fourth pouch and gives rise to the ultimobranchial body. Cells of the ultimobranchial body give rise to parafollicular cells of the adult thyroid, which secrete calcitonin, a hormone involved in calcium regulation.

BRANCHIAL CLEFTS

At the 5th week of fetal development, there are four pharyngeal clefts. Only the first cleft contributes to any definitive structure. This cleft penetrates underlying mesoderm, ultimately giving rise to the external auditory canal. Epithelium medially also contributes to the formation of the tympanic membrane.

Proliferation of second arch mesoderm causes it to overlap the third and fourth arches. In so doing it fuses with the epicardial ridge, thereby causing the second, third, and fourth clefts to lose their outside contact. These clefts coalesce, temporarily forming an ectodermally lined cavity, the cervical sinus of His, which normally disappears completely with further development. The epicardial ridge represents mesodermal rudiments of the sternocleidomastoid, trapezius, infrahyoid, and lingual musculature.

BRANCHIAL CYSTS, SINUSES, AND FISTULAE

Branchial anomalies exist in one of three forms: sinuses, fistulae, or cysts. A sinus tract has an external opening (skin) or internal opening (foregut), but not both. Sinuses terminate within deep tissues of the neck. An external opening is theorized to represent a vestigial cleft, an internal opening a vestigial pouch. Persistence of both cleft and pouch with dissolution of the branchial plate represents a fistula which connects skin to foregut.

Should the second branchial arch not completely overgrow the third and fourth arches, remnants of the second, third, and fourth clefts may communicate externally by means of a sinus. Should their respective pouch persist with dissolution of the branchial plate, a fistula would form. Cysts might arise secondary to obstruction of a sinus or fistula, as well as persistence of the cervical sinus of His.

EMBRYOLOGY OF THE THYROID GLAND

The embryonic thyroid gland develops as an epithelial proliferation in the floor of the pharynx between the first and second pouches at a point later to become the tuberculum impar. The bilobed thyroid diverticulum then descends into the neck anterior to the pharyngeal gut. During its descent the gland remains connected to the tongue by a thin connection termed the thyroglossal duct (Figure 5-2). The thyroid reaches the level of the trachea by the 7th week. The thyroglossal duct normally obliterates. Should the thyroglossal duct persist, the eventual formation of a thyroglossal duct cyst may occur. Such cysts may be found anywhere along the migratory path of the thyroid. Similarly, aberrant thyroid tissue may be found anywhere along this migratory path. When the primordial thyroid fails to descend, it may persist in the tongue base as a lingual thyroid.

EMBRYOLOGIC DEVELOPMENT OF NECK MUSCULATURE

Much of the neck musculature is formed by branchial arch mesenchyme, as previously discussed. The precise development of the sternocleidomastoid and trapezius muscles is uncertain. Most feel these muscles are formed primarily from branchiomeric tissue within the epicardial ridge. However, there may be contribution in part from primordial muscle cells which migrate

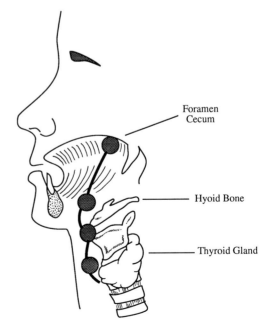

Foramen
Cecum

Hyoid Bone

Thyroid Gland

Figure 5–2. Migratory path of the thyroid gland with common sites of thyroglossal cyst occurrence.

from occipital somites. These muscles are innervated by the spinal accessory nerve. Infrahyoid muscles are somatic in origin and are innervated by the hypoglossal nerve with contribution of fibers from the first and second cervical nerves by way of the ansa cervicalis.

EMBRYOLOGIC DEVELOPMENT ARTERIES

The aortic arch and its major branches are formed from the primitive branchial arches. Five symmetrically paired branchial arch arteries arise from mesoderm and are formed sequentially in a cranial to caudal direction. The paired arteries arise from the ventral aorta in the roof of the pericardium and pass dorsally through each arch to unite with the dorsal aorta on its respective side. At a caudal level, the dorsal aortas fuse to form a single midline dorsal aorta. The initial arrangement of arch arteries is subsequently remodeled by fusion and atrophy of various vessels.

First and second branchial arch vessels degenerate at about the time third and fourth vessels commence to mature. The dorsal segment of the second arch artery does temporarily persist during fetal life as the stapedial artery, which passes through the crura of the stapes. This artery rarely persists into adulthood.

The proximal portion of the internal carotid artery is derived from the third arch artery with the remaining portion of the internal carotid artery developing from the dorsal aorta. The external and common carotid arteries are also derived from the third arch artery. The fourth arch artery becomes the proximal aorta on the left and the proximal subclavian on the right. The sixth arch artery on the left persists as the ductus arteriosus and the pulmonary artery on the right (Langman, 1981).

BRANCHIAL ANOMALIES OF THE NECK

First Branchial Anomalies

Anomalies of the first branchial cleft account for about 5% of all branchial anomalies. Work (1972) has described the most recognized classification of first branchial cleft anomalies and categorized these lesions into two types. Type I anomalies contain only ectodermal elements. They present as duplication anomalies of the external auditory canal. Type II anomalies, which are also known as cervicoauricular fistulae, are more common. They contain ectodermal and mesodermal elements and as such are thought to represent a duplication anomaly of the external auditory canal and pinna. Either anomaly may present as a cyst, sinus, or fistulous tract connecting skin and the external auditory canal. Rare communication with the middle ear has been reported.

Type I lesions (Figure 5–3) typically appear in the periauricular region, usually anterior or posterior to the pinna, and course parallel to the external auditory canal. In contrast, type II (Figure 5–4) anomalies usually are located posterior or inferior to the mandibular angle but superior to the hyoid bone. The tract of either type, but most notably type II, may have an unpredictable relationship to the facial nerve, lying deep, superficial, or passing between its branches. Type I anomalies most often are lateral to the facial nerve.

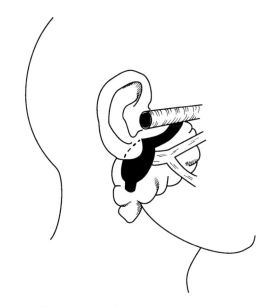

Figure 5–3. Type I first branchial anomaly.

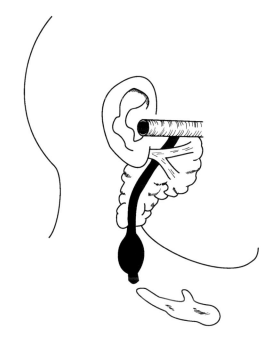

Figure 5–4. Type II first branchial anomaly (cervicoauricular fistula).

Definitive excision of first branchial cleft anomalies, particularly type II, requires identification and preservation of the facial nerve. This is best accomplished by utilizing a parotidectomy incision, which allows wide exposure with facial nerve identification (Finn, Buchalter, Sarti, & Romo, 1987). A first branchial cleft cyst without apparent tract or fistula might masquerade as a parotid tumor and should also be addressed in this fashion.

Second Branchial Anomalies

Second branch cleft anomalies account for the vast majority (90%) of all branchial lesions (Figures 5–5 and 5–6). A cyst or external opening is characteristically

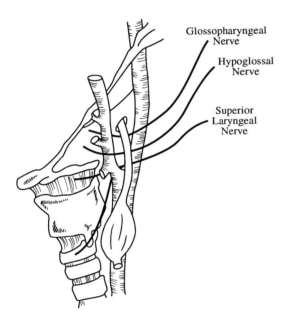

Figure 5–5. Classic course of second branchial cyst/fistula. The tract courses between the external and internal carotid arteries superior to the glossopharyngeal and hypoglossal nerves, penetrating the middle constrictor muscle terminating in the tonsillar fossa.

found along the anterior border of the sternocleidomastoid muscle at or below the level of the hyoid bone. An epithelial-lined fistula or sinus tract courses superiorly, lateral to the carotid artery and hypoglossal and glossopharyngeal nerve, and then courses in the medial direction between the internal and external carotid arteries. Sinus tracts may terminate deep within the neck, most often in close proximity to the middle constrictor muscle. Fistula will open internally in the region of the tonsillar fossa. Cysts may occur anywhere along the course of sinuses or fistula but most commonly present in the anterior neck along the sternocleidomastoid muscle, as described.

Complete identification of the cyst, fistula, or sinus tract is of importance in avoiding recurrence. This necessitates dissection of neural and vascular structures and possibly opening the pharynx. Complete excision of tracts is greatly facilitated by catheterization with a small embolectomy catheter. As dissection is carried cephalad, a second "stepladder" (Figures 5–7 and 5–8) incision may be necessary. This avoids a large disfiguring cervical scar. Many feel that complete excision may require a unilateral tonsillectomy.

Although excision of asymptomatic branchial cysts, sinuses, and fistula is somewhat elective, surgery is nonetheless advocated. Cystic lesions can sometimes enlarge dramatically. Secondary infection is also common and at times difficult to manage. Infection-related fibrosis of surrounding tissue makes ultimate excision more challenging and increases the possibility of incomplete resection with subsequent recurrence. If infection is active, it is desirable, when possible, to allow total resolution prior to definitive surgery.

Third and Fourth Branchial Anomalies

Third and fourth branchial anomalies are unusual. Similarities include their common pyriform fossa origin and frequent clinical presentation as suppurative thy-

Labels on Figure 5–5: Glossopharyngeal Nerve, Hypoglossal Nerve, Superior Laryngeal Nerve

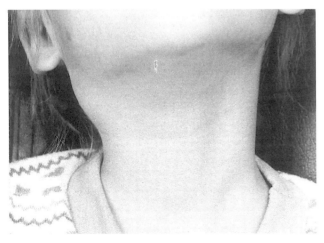

Figure 5–6. Nine-year-old with second branchial cyst.

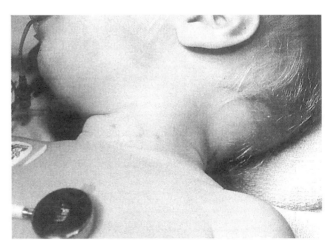

Figure 5–7. Infant with bilateral cervical pits.

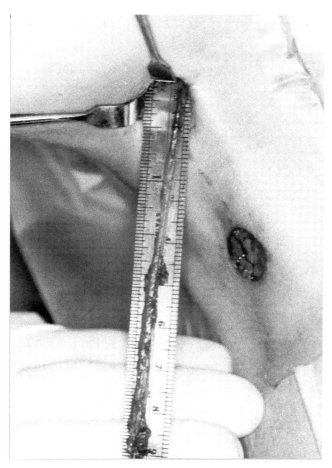

Figure 5–8. Stepladder technique used to excise a second branchial fistula.

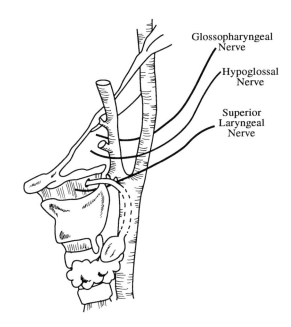

Figure 5–9. Anatomic relationships of a vestigial third branchial cyst/sinus. The tract emerges from the rostral pyriform and courses superior to the superior laryngeal nerve.

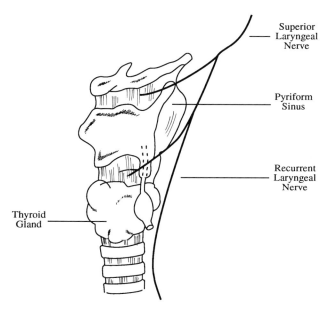

Figure 5–10. Anatomic relationships of a vestigial fourth branchial cyst/fistula. The tract courses from the caudal pyriform sinus beneath the superior laryngeal nerve and anterior to the cricothyroid joint. It then emerges along the border of the inferior constrictor muscle, terminating in the superior pole of the thyroid gland.

roiditis or neck abscess (Har-El, Sasaki, Prager, & Krespi, 1991).

A third branchial fistula (Figure 5–9) exists at the rostral aspect of the pyriform sinus, penetrates the thyrohyoid membrane rostral to the superior laryngeal nerve and inferior constrictor, then descends caudally between the common carotid and vagus nerve, terminating lateral to the thyroid gland.

Although a complete fistula of the fourth arch is a theoretical possibility, only the portion corresponding to the pharyngobranchial duct has been consistently described (Figure 5–10). After originating near the pyriform apex caudal to the superior laryngeal nerve, the tract descends translaryngeally under the thyroid ala emerging beneath the inferior constricture muscle to exit the larynx in proximity to the cricothyroid joint. The tract then descends lateral to the recurrent laryngeal nerve, terminating paratracheally or within the thyroid gland (Rosenfeld & Biller, 1991; Rosenfeld, Grundfast, & Milmoe, 1993).

The most effective treatment of both third and fourth branchial anomalies entails complete tract excision including their pyriform attachment. In doing so, recurrent laryngeal nerve identification is important. This is best achieved by utilizing a standard thyroidectomy in-

cision, thus exposing the thyroid gland, larynx, and lateral neck. Laryngoscopy should be performed at the time of excision, which can be greatly facilitated if the pyriform sinus ostium can be identified and cannulated with a small catheter. Complete resection may necessitate an ipsilateral thyroidectomy.

Cervical Thymic Anomalies

The thymus and parathyroid glands originate from the third and fourth pharyngeal pouches. As the thymic primordia caudally descends into the mediastinum, it maintains an epithelial-lined connection to the third pouch, which is called the thymopharyngeal duct. This duct normally involutes. It is theorized that remnants of this structure give rise to cervical thymic cysts. Ectopic cervical thymic tissue may occur as a consequence of normal thymic migration or arrest of descent. It would appear that this is not an uncommon event, as the reported incidence of asymptomatic thymic tissue in the neck of children at autopsy is 30%. Enlargement of this tissue may present as a cervical mass. Cervical thymic anomalies (Figures 5–11 and 5–12) have been well described and should be considered in the differential of all neck masses (Nguyen, de Tar, Wells, & Crockett, 1996). These lesions usually present in childhood as a slow growing painless mass anterior or deep to the sternocleidomastoid muscle. Distinguishing these lesions from a branchial cleft cyst or cystic hygroma may prove difficult. Thymic cysts may be unilocular or multilocular and may also coexist with solid thymic tissue. Pressure-related symptoms include hoarseness, dysphagia, and stridor. Respiratory distress has been described in neonates (Wagner, Vincour, Weintraub, & Golladay, 1988).

Complete surgical excision is the recommended treatment. Extension into the mediastinum has been described. Diagnosis can be made preoperatively by fine needle aspiration with identification of Hassall's corpuscles. This may be particularly helpful in the management of infants, as excision of this benign lesion should not be performed without radiographic docu-

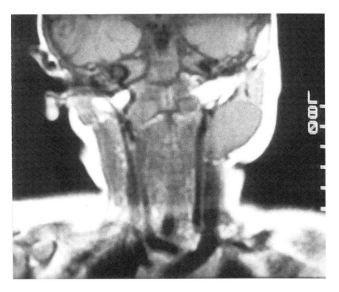

Figure 5–12. MRI of thymic lesion shown in Figure 5–11.

mentation of mediastinal thymus for fear of rendering such a patient athymic with disastrous immunologic sequelae.

Thyroglossal Duct Anomalies

Thyroglossal duct cysts are the result of an aberration in the normal embryologic development of the thyroid gland. The thyroid primordium descends from the foramen cecum of the tongue base along the anterior midline of the neck, attaining its final anatomical position anterior to the trachea. During its descent, the thyroid remains connected to the floor of the pharynx by

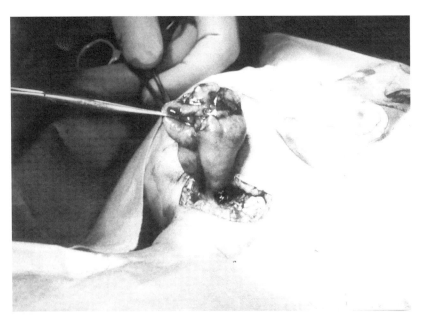

Figure 5–11. Excision of cervical thymus from a 15-month-old.

the thyroglossal duct, which eventually involutes. Persistence of this duct may lead to formation of a thyroglossal duct cyst. Further, arrest in the normal descent of the thyroid gland results in ectopic thyroid tissue (Batsakis, 1979b).

A thyroglossal duct cyst typically presents as an asymptomatic cystic midline neck mass (Figures 5–13 and 5–14). As the embryonic thyroglossal duct is intimately associated with the hyoid bone, these lesions are typically located in close proximity to this structure. These lesions may move vertically with swallowing and tongue protrusion. Childhood is the usual age of presentation with lesser prevalence in adulthood. Cystic size is variable. Enlargement is common and fluctuation of size is not unusual, particularly with upper respiratory tract infections. Secondary bacterial infection is not unusual and may at times prove chronic. Fistula formation may result from a surgical drainage procedure or spontaneous rupture of the cyst. Treatment of thyroglossal duct cysts is surgical. An unacceptable high rate of recurrence (50%) has been associated with local excision. The method advocated by Sistrunk in 1920 is widely accepted as the procedure of choice and entails excision of the cyst, central portion of the hyoid bone, and all duct remnants up to the tongue base. The rate of recurrence reportedly drops to 3% with this approach.

The preoperative evaluation of patients clinically suspected to have a thyroglossal duct cyst is debated. Conventional wisdom has been to ensure a clinically suspected thyroglossal duct cyst is not in actuality aberrant thyroid tissue, the removal of which may render a patient athymic. Traditionally this has been accomplished with thyroid scanning. The same goal may, however, be achieved noninvasively with ultrasound documentation of normal thyroid tissue (Sherman, Rosenburg, & Heyman, 1985).

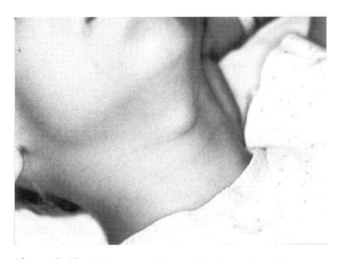

Figure 5–13. Eight-year-old boy with a thyroglossal duct cyst.

Dermoid Cyst

Dermoid cysts also present as midline neck masses. The clinical distinction between a thyroglossal duct and dermoid cyst may prove difficult. Unlike thyroglossal duct cysts, dermoid cysts typically do not elevate with swallowing or tongue protrusion. Dermoid cysts are most often attached to and move with skin. These lesions are lined by epidermis and contain epidermal appendages, such as hair follicles, sweat, and sebaceous glands with the cyst wall. This differentiates these lesions from simple epidermal or sebaceous cysts, which contain solely ectodermal elements. Cervical dermoids are theorized to arise along embryologic fusion lines (McAvoy & Zuckerman, 1976).

Most often, these lesions are easily delineated at surgery and, in contrast to thyroglossal duct cysts, require only local excision. However, should there be any confusion as to the exact nature of the lesion, a formal Sistrunk procedure should be considered and is advocated by many for the uniform treatment of all midline cystic masses deep to the strap muscles.

Cervical Teratomas

The most common location of childhood teratomas include the sacrococcygeal region, gonads, and mediastinum. Teratomas of the head and neck region, including the basicranial and cervical forms, are uncommon, accounting for 7 to 9% of reported cases. These tumors, derived from pleuripotential cells, are comprised of mature elements of ectoderm, mesoderm, endoderm, and immature embryonal tissue. These lesions have been associated with maternal polyhydramnios, stillbirth, prematurity, and fetal malposition.

Congenital cervical teratomas can present in a dramatic fashion. Most newborns with large cervical tumors present with acute respiratory distress secondary to tracheal compression. Prenatal ultrasound may allow

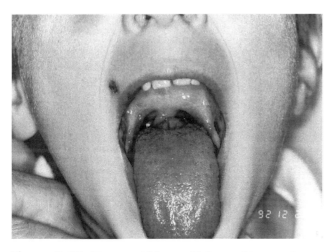

Figure 5–14. Six-year-old boy with base of tongue thyroglossal duct cyst.

assessment of these tumors *in utero*, thus assisting in strategy formation of airway management at birth. Treatment is complete surgical excision, if possible. Although most pediatric cervical teratomas are histologically benign, morbidity and mortality can be significant. Further, a malignant teratoma may develop after previous resection of a benign teratoma. Prolonged careful follow-up is, therefore, advised (Abemayor, Newman, & Dudley, 1984).

Lymphangioma (Cystic Hygroma)

Lymphangioma and cystic hygroma are theorized to arise from embryonic lymphatic channels or secondary to congenital obstruction of regional lymphatic drainage. Lymphangiomas are usually present at birth (50 to 60%) with 80 to 90% evident by the 2nd year of life. Less than 10% occur in adulthood. Lymphangiomas may present anywhere in the body, with most arising in the head and neck region.

These lesions may be classified on the basis of their lymphatic space size. "Simple lymphangiomas" or lymphangioma simplex are categorically composed of capillary-sized, thin wall lymphatics. "Cavernous lymphangiomas" are composed of dilated lymphatic channels whereas "cystic hygromas" have large multiloculated cysts. Mixed patterns may be encountered within a single lesion, promoting the concept of a collective lesion, referred to by many as a lymphatic malformation (Kennedy, 1989).

Lymphangiomas typically present as a painless, soft, compressible mass in neonates or infants. Size can be quite variable. Lesions may be isolated and confined to a particular anatomic location, for example, the posterior neck or extensive with involvement of contiguous regions (Figure 5–15). Such extensive cervicofacial cystic hygromas are typically suprahyoid and may involve the parotid and submandibular regions, parapharynx, floor of mouth, and tongue. Lesions may enlarge when secondarily infected or when traumatized secondary to hemorrhage within the mass. Clinical symptoms imparted by the lesion or its enlargement are most dependent on mass location. Airway obstruction and/or feeding difficulties are usually associated with suprahyoid lesions.

Conservative surgical management has been established as the treatment of choice since spontaneous involution, as occurs with hemangiomas, is not to be anticipated. Vital structures should not be sacrificed in an attempt at complete excision, which can prove formidable. A staged approach may be necessary for large lesions or those involving the floor of mouth, tongue, and larynx. Dependent on the lesion, airway securement with a tracheotomy and gastrostomy tube for nutritional support may be indicated (Ricciardelli & Richardson, 1991).

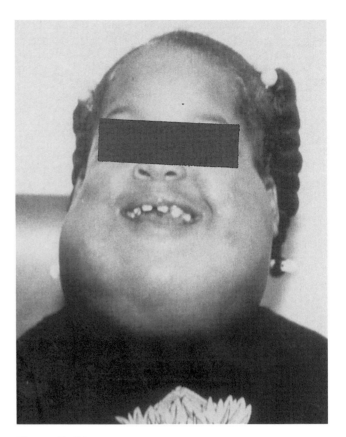

Figure 5–15. Ten-year-old girl with large cervicofacial cystic hygroma.

The incidence of recurrence and surgically related complications is higher in patients with suprahyoid lesions, particularly if they are bilateral. Lingual involvement may necessitate debulking or partial resection of the tongue. The carbon dioxide laser can prove helpful for the management of selected mucosal disease of the aerodigestive tract. Irradiation, cyst aspiration, diathermy, and sclerosing agents play no role in the contemporary management of these lesions.

Hemangiomas

Hemangiomas constitute the most common head and neck neoplasms in children. Most hemangiomas are not difficult to diagnose, presenting as a red or bluish, soft multilocular mass involving skin or mucosa (Figure 5–16). They may, however, occur deeply within subcutaneous tissues, facial layers, muscle, and parotid gland without associated dermal involvement. These lesions have been classified by histological appearance as capillary, cavernous, or juvenile (proliferative). Capillary hemangiomas may increase in size with straining or crying. MRI and CT scanning can be useful in establishing the diagnosis and demonstrating the extent of involvement. Fine needle aspiration with demonstration of blood and endothelial cells is helpful when the diagnosis is in question.

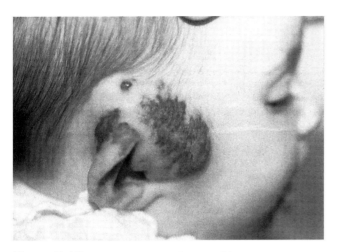

Figure 5–16. Two-year-old with parotid hemangioma.

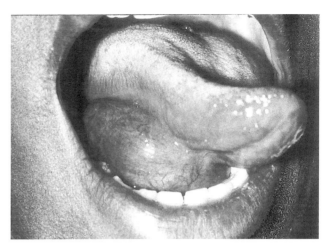

Figure 5–17. Intraoral floor of mouth ranula.

Characteristically, these lesions proliferate rapidly during the 1st year of life and subsequently undergo spontaneous slow involution. Complete resolution can be anticipated in 50% of children by 5 years of age and 70% by 7 years. Consequently, these lesions are treated conservatively unless there is associated functional impairment, bleeding, or consumptive coagulopathy. Surgery or laser therapy may also be indicated if disfiguring residual hemangioma persists (Stal, Hamilton, & Spira, 1986).

Steroid therapy, α-interferon, and/or chemotherapy may be indicated for patients with massive hemangioma that are life-threatening, especially when there is associated visceral involvement. Low-dose radiation therapy, once a popular modality, is no longer recommended except in extreme life-threatening situations. Sclerotherapy and cryotherapy are unpredictable and have been associated with considerable scarring (Hellman, Myer, & Pranger, 1992).

Plunging Ranulas

Ranulas are benign lesions of sublingual gland origin. An intraoral or simple ranula is a true retention cyst characterized by a bluish, translucent cystic swelling within the floor of mouth (Figure 5–17). A history of spontaneous rupture with liberation of viscid fluid is common. A cervical or plunging ranula (Figure 5–18) presents as a soft compressible neck mass most often suprahyoid and in the submental and/or submandibular regions. Cervical ranulas are pseudocysts and are thought to arise following mucous extravasation into soft tissue and fascial planes of the neck. These lesions may be isolated or associated with an intraoral component (Batsakis, 1979a). History or clinical evidence of an intraoral ranula would make the diagnosis obvious. When uncertainty exists, fine needle aspiration with demonstration of protein and amylase on fluid analysis would support the diagnosis.

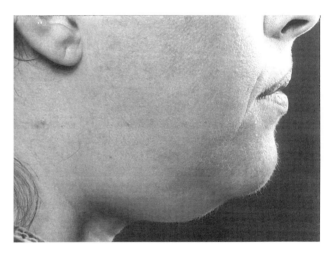

Figure 5–18. Cervical or plunging ranula.

Most physicians advocate transcervical excision of the sublingual gland as the treatment of cervical ranulas. This is greatly facilitated by submandibular gland excision. Some, however, recommend intraoral excision of the sublingual gland with oral drainage of the cervical component. The cervical approach, however, provides greater exposure and protection of the lingual nerve than can be achieved by an intraoral approach.

Laryngoceles

The laryngeal ventricle is the space found between the false and true vocal folds. The saccule is a small blind pouch opening into the anterior third of the ventricle and ascending vertically between the false cord and inner surface of the thyroid cartilage. The saccule is lined with serous and mucous glands and functions to provide lubrication for the true vocal fold.

Laryngoceles are abnormal, air-containing dilatations of the saccule. When a laryngocele becomes obstructed, mucous-filled, and no longer communicates with the larynx, it is called a saccular cyst. Laryngoceles are classified as "internal" if they are within the confines of the larynx, "external" if they extend through the thyrohyoid membrane into the neck, and "combined" if they extend internally and externally (Civantes & Hollinger, 1992).

External laryngoceles typically present in the neck in the region of the lateral thyrohyoid membrane. When internal or combined, an abnormal cry, hoarseness, and respiratory distress may occur. External laryngoceles are soft and compressible and when so examined may elicit a gurgling or hissing sound (Bryce's sign). Swelling within the neck may, however, be noted only during periods of increased intralaryngeal pressure. In contrast, external laryngopyoceles (infected laryngoceles) are firm and tender and may present as an acute inflammatory cervical process. Indirect laryngoscopy or fiberoptic nasolaryngoscopy will demonstrate the endolaryngeal component of combined lesions. A CT scan can prove helpful in confirming the diagnosis by demonstrating a paralaryngeal air-filled mass penetrating the thyrohyoid membrane into the neck.

Asymptomatic laryngoceles require no treatment. Symptomatic external laryngoceles and laryngopyoceles should be excised by a lateral neck approach with dissection of the distended saccule to the thyrohyoid membrane, which is then incised along the superior border of the thyroid ala. Blunt dissection exposes the internal component. Removing a portion of the thyroid ala may infrequently be necessary for exposure. A laryngofissure is not necessary and a tracheotomy can most often be avoided.

Congenital Muscular Torticollis

Congenital muscular torticollis is a fibrous contraction of the sternocleidomastoid muscle with resultant tilting of the head toward the side of the shortened muscle and contralateral rotation of the chin. The torticollis may be isolated or associated with an apparent neck mass, which classically presents as a hard fusiform olivelike mass within the distal sternocleidomastoid muscle. Infants are usually normal at birth, but at 2–4 weeks of age the sternocleidomastoid muscle "pseudotumor" initially appears. The etiology remains a mystery; however, association of this malady with intrauterine positioning disorders, such as hip dysplasia and club foot, suggests that intrauterine head tilting can selectively injure the sternocleidomastoid muscle, leading to the development of a compartment syndrome. The fibrotic muscle mass usually persists for several months and then gradually resolves. The nature of the mass can be easily determined by CT scan, MRI, or ultrasound. Satisfactory results can usually be achieved with exercises designed to passively stretch the muscle. Nonoperative management beyond 1 year of age is not usually suc-

cessful; and surgery, therefore, may be indicated. Although excision of the sternocleidomastoid muscle has been employed in the past, simple lysis of the distal muscle and associated platysmal banding is probably just as effective (Brandenkamp, Hoover, & Burke, 1990).

UNUSUAL HEAD AND NECK ABNORMALITIES

Bronchogenic Cyst

Bronchogenic cysts are congenital malformations which are ordinarily encountered in the thorax. The laryngotracheal diverticulum embryologically arises from the ventral foregut, divides, and branches into lung buds with subsequent evolution of the respiratory tract. Isolation of cells with formation of nonfunctional cysts is theorized to be the etiology of this lesion. Life-threatening respiratory distress is the typical clinical presentation in neonates and infants, although it is often asymptomatic in older children and adults.

Bronchogenic cysts rarely present outside the thorax as a neck mass. When encountered, they typically present in the lower neck as a cystic mass. In young children and infants, compressive symptoms of airway obstruction and dysphagia may occur. These cysts are easily remove, although possible injury to the recurrent laryngeal nerve is a concern as bronchogenic cysts tend to occupy the laryngotracheal and esophagotracheal grooves (Cohen, 1985; Dolgin, 1995).

Cervical Salivary Gland Heterotopia

Cervical salivary gland heterotopia (choristoma) is unusual. Patients have been described with discrete neck masses as well as with draining sinuses associated with these lesions. Heterotopic cervical salivary gland tissue usually presents below the hyoid bone along the anterior border of the sternocleidomastoid muscle. Fifty percent of these lesions are present at birth. There are no distinguishing clinical features. Surgical excision is usually curative and diagnosis is made following histological examination of excised tissue (Nash, Cho, & Cohen, 1988).

Internal Jugular Vein Phlebectasia

A markedly dilated jugular vein may present as an apparent cystic swelling anterior to the border of the sternocleidomastoid muscle. Size might increase with crying or Valsalva. Most patients present within the first decade of life. Jugular vein obstruction in the neck or mediastinum should be suspected, but most often there is no identifiable etiology. MRI or CT scan can confirm the diagnosis and exclude an obstructive cause.

Asymptomatic phlebectasia requires no treatment (Bowdler & Singh, 1989).

Branchial Arch Cartilage Anomalies

Isolated remnants of branchial arch cartilage rarely persist within the neck. Such patients typically present with a small mass of cartilage within the superficial soft tissue of the neck along the anterior border of the sternocleidomastoid muscle. These lesions are usually asymptomatic, pose no functional problems, and are easily excised.

References

Abemayor, E., Newman, A., & Dudley, J. (1984). Teratomas of the head and neck in childhood. *Laryngoscope, 94,* 1489–1492.

Batsakis, J. G. (1979a). Non-neoplastic disease of the salivary glands. In J. G. Batsakis (Ed.), *Tumors of the head and neck: Clinical and pathological considerations* (2nd ed., p. 100). Baltimore: Williams and Wilkins.

Batsakis, J. G. (1979b). Parenchymal cysts of the neck. In J. G. Batsakis (Ed.), *Tumors of the head and neck: Clinical and pathological considerations* (2nd ed., p. 233). Baltimore: Williams and Wilkins.

Bowdler, D. A., & Singh S. D. (1989). Internal jugular phlebectasia. *International Journal of Pediatric Otolaryngology, 12,* 165–171.

Brandenkamp, J. K., Hoover, L. A., & Burke, G. S. (1990). Congenital muscular torticollis. *Archives of Otolaryngology—Head and Neck Surgery, 116,* 212–216.

Civantes, F. J., & Hollinger, L. D. (1992). Laryngoceles and saccular cysts in infants and children. *Archives of Otolaryngology—Head and Neck Surgery, 118,* 296–300.

Cohen, S. R., Thompson, J. W., & Brennan, L. P. (1985). Foregut cysts presenting as neck masses. *Annals of Otology, Rhinology, and Laryngology, 94,* 433–436.

Dolgin, S. E., Groisman, G. M., & Shah, K. (1985). Subcutaneous bronchogenic cysts and sinuses. *Otolaryngology—Head and Neck Surgery, 112,* 763–766.

Finn, D. G., Buchalter, I. H., Sarti, E., & Romo, T. (1987). First branchial cysts: Clinical update. *Laryngoscope, 97,* 136–140.

Har-El, G., Sasaki, C. T., Prager, D., & Krespi, Y. P. (1991). Acute suppurative thyroiditis and the branchial apparatus. *American Journal of Otolaryngology, 12,* 6–11.

Hellman, J. R., Myer, C., & Prenger, P. C. (1992). Therapeutic alternatives in the treatment of life-threatening vasoformative tumors. *American Journal of Otolaryngology, 13,* 48–53.

Kennedy, T. L. (1989). Cystic hygroma/lymphangioma: A rare and still unclear entity. *Laryngoscope, 99*(Suppl. 49).

Langman, J. (1981). Head and neck. In J. Langman (Ed.), *Medical embryology* (4th ed., p. 268). Baltimore: Williams & Wilkins.

McAvoy, J. M., & Zuckerman, L. (1976). Dermoid cysts of the head and neck in children. *Archives of Otolaryngology 102,* 529–531.

Nash, M., Cho, H., & Cohen, J. (1988). Salivary choristomas of the neck. *Otolaryngology—Head and Neck Surgery, 99,* 590–593.

Nguyen, Q., de Tar, M., Wells, W., & Crockett, D. (1996). Cervical thymic cysts: Case reports and review of the literature. *Laryngoscope, 106,* 247–252.

Ricciardelli, E. J., & Richardson, M. A. (1991). Cervicofacial cystic hygroma patterns of recurrence and management of the difficult case. *Archives of Otolaryngology—Head and Neck Surgery, 117,* 546–553.

Rosenfeld, R. M., & Biller, H. F. (1991). Fourth branchial pouch sinus: Diagnosis and treatment. *Otolaryngology—Head and Neck Surgery, 105,* 44–50.

Rosenfeld, R. M., Grundfast, K. M., & Milmoe, G. J. (1993). Occult sinus of the pyriform fossa. *Otolaryngology—Head and Neck Surgery, 109,* 126–128.

Sherman, N. H., Rosenburg, H. K., & Heyman, S. (1985). Ultrasound evaluation of neck masses in children. *Journal of Ultrasound Medicine, 4,* 127.

Sistrunk, W. E. (1920). The surgical treatment of cysts of the thyroglossal tract. *American Journal of Surgery, 70,* 121–126.

Smith, J. H., Burke, D. K., Sato, Y., Poust, R. I., Kimura, K., & Bauman, N. M. (1996). Therapy for lymphangiomas. *Archives of Otolaryngology—Head and Neck Surgery, 122,* 1195–1199.

Stal, S., Hamilton, S., & Spira, M. (1986). Hemangiomas, lymphangiomas and vascular malformations of the head and neck. *Otolaryngologic Clinics of North America, 19,* 769.

Wagner, C. W., Vincour, C. D., Weintraub, W. H., & Golladay, E. S. (1988). Respiratory complications in cervical thymic cysts. *Journal of Pediatric Surgery, 23,* 657–660.

Work, W. (1972). Newer concepts of first branchial cleft defects. *Laryngoscope, 82,* 1581–1593.

6

Infectious and Inflammatory Illness of the Oral Cavity and Pharynx

David H. Darrow, M.D., D.D.S.

The oral cavity and pharynx are anatomic regions that are highly predisposed to infectious and inflammatory processes. These areas are commonly exposed to external influences during speech, mastication, deglutition, and oral respiration, and the thin oral mucosa offers little protection against penetrating trauma, multiplying organisms, or erupting bullae. Additionally, children use the oral cavity as an organ of exploration as well as a means of social contact, and the immaturity of their immune system may place them at even greater risk for local infection and inflammation.

The following chapter is by no means intended as a comprehensive discussion of all inflammatory disorders of the oral cavity and pharynx. Rather, it serves to review the classification, diagnosis, and management of a subset of these pathologic entities most commonly encountered by the otolaryngologist in children. The interested reader is referred to other sources for a complete discussion of normal oral and oropharyngeal physiology and immunology. Space infections of oral and oropharyngeal origin and neoplastic processes are covered elsewhere in this text.

CLASSIFICATION

Because the oral mucosa is so easily damaged, infectious and inflammatory processes may present in similar ways in their early stages, and distinguishing them from one another may be difficult. Table 6–1 provides a classification of some these disorders based on their appearance, duration, and recurrence rate. Table

6–2 categorizes these disorders as either stomatitis (originating primarily in the oral cavity) or pharyngitis, and subdivides them by etiology. The latter is the classification used in this chapter.

STOMATITIS

Bacterial Infections

Acute Necrotizing Ulcerative Gingivitis (ANUG) and Noma (Cancrum Oris)

ANUG is a necrotizing infection of the oral tissues believed to result from an overgrowth of bacteria commonly present in the oral cavity. In the past, the disease was known as "trench mouth," owing to its prevalence among troops in the trenches during World War I, and was felt to be contagious. Over the last several decades, however, ANUG has been recognized as a noncontagious disease of patients with hematologic disease or immune deficiency associated with fusiform bacilli and spirochetes. Progression of the disease to involve the soft and hard tissues of the face is known as noma or cancrum oris.

Epidemiology and Pathogenesis

Among children, ANUG is primarily a disease of adolescents with a prevalence of about 1–5%. Many affected patients have systemic disorders associated with leukocytic dysfunction, such as leukemia, aplastic ane-

Table 6–1. Classification of infectious and inflammatory disease of the oral cavity and pharynx in children by lesion.

Disorders with multiple acute oral lesions
  Herpes simplex
  Varicella zoster
  Herpangina
  Hand-foot-mouth disease
  Erythema multiforme
  Allergic stomatitis
  Ulceration secondary to chemotherapy
  Acute necrotizing ulcerative gingivitis
  Candidiasis
Disorders with recurring oral lesions
  Recurrent aphthous stomatitis
  Recurrent herpes simplex infection
  Zoster
  Cytomegalovirus
  Systemic lupus erythematosis
  Leukemia
Disorders with multiple chronic oral lesions
  Inflammatory bullous disease
  Geographic tongue
  Hairy leukoplakia
  Malnutrition
Disorders with single oral lesions
  Trauma
Disorders with generalized pharyngeal inflammation
  Viral pharyngitis
  Infectious mononucleosis
  Streptococcal pharyngitis
  Gonorrhea
  Diphtheria
  Kawasaki disease

Source: From "Ulcerative, Vesicular, and Bullous Lesions," by M. S. Greenberg, 1994, p. 11. In M. A. Lynch, V. J. Brightman, and M. S. Greenberg (Eds.), *Burket's Oral Medicine—Diagnosis and Treatment* (9th ed., pp. 11–50). Philadelphia: J. B. Lippincott. Reprinted with permission.

Table 6–2. Classification of infectious and inflammatory disease of the oral cavity and pharynx in children by site and etiology.

STOMATITIS
  Bacterial infections
    Acute necrotizing ulcerative gingivitis/Noma
  Viral infections
    Herpes simplex
    Varicella-zoster
    Cytomegalovirus
    Coxsackie virus
    Hairy leukoplakia
  Trauma/idiopathic diseases/other causes
    Trauma
    Recurrent aphthous stomatitis
    Erythema multiforme
    Candidiasis
    Inflammatory bullous diseases
    Geographic tongue
    Drug-induced and allergic stomatitis
    Leukemia
    Systemic lupus erythematosis
    Malnutrition
PHARYNGITIS
  Common bacterial and viral infections
    Adenovirus, influenza virus, parainfluenza virus, enterovirus
    Group A β-hemolytic streptococcus
    Infectious mononucleosis (Epstein-Barr virus)
  Other bacterial and viral infections
    Gonorrhea
    Diphtheria
    Kawasaki disease

mia, malnutrition, or human immunodeficiency virus (HIV). Risk factors in the absence of systemic disease include poor oral hygiene, smoking, and emotional stress.

The organisms felt to be responsible for ANUG are anaerobes, including *Treponema* sp., *Selenomas* sp., *Fusobacterium* sp., and *Bacteroides melaninogenicus* ssp *intermedius* (Loesche, Syed, Laughon, & Stoll, 1982). Destruction of the gingiva is thought to be the result of endotoxins elaborated by these bacteria, which act either directly on the tissue, or indirectly by initiating inflammatory or immunologic responses.

Clinical Features and Diagnosis

ANUG usually presents acutely with symptoms of gingival pain, tenderness, and bleeding, as well as increased salivation. Many patients report a metallic taste or loss of taste. Physical examination will commonly reveal gingival bleeding, and inflammatory changes in the interdental papillae, ranging from blunting to

punched-out ulcerations (Figure 6–1). Ulceration may also be noted elsewhere in the soft tissues of the oral cavity and oropharynx, and may extend to the alveolar processes resulting in sequestration of bone. The teeth may be stained, and severe halitosis is generally present. Cervical adenopathy is also common.

Patients with noma may present with rapid and severe facial disfigurement. The maxilla is most frequently involved (50%), followed by the maxilla and mandible combined (37%) and about two-thirds of cases are bilateral. The diagnosis must be distinguished from other necrotizing disorders including "lethal midline granuloma," Wegener's granulomatosis, carcinoma, and a variety of other infectious etiologies, including mucormycosis and invasive fungal disease.

Treatment

In patients with ANUG due to systemic illness, appropriate consultation should be obtained in order to treat the underlying disorder while local therapy is instituted. This usually includes hydration, improved nutrition, and elimination of risk factors. Local treatment typically includes aggressive debridement including periodontal curettage and irrigation. Antibiotics are not recommended for mild cases; however, chlorhexidine

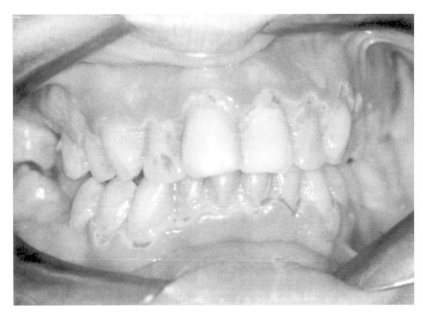

Figure 6–1. Gingival ulceration and blunting of the interdental papillae in a patient with ANUG. (Photo courtesy of Dr. John Svirsky)

rinses and systemic therapy with clindamycin or metronidazole may be useful adjuncts in more severely affected patients. Patients with noma generally require long-term intravenous antibiotic therapy for control of the disease. Bony destruction or facial involvement may require reconstructive surgery once the disease is locally and systemically controlled.

Viral Infections

Herpes Simplex Virus

Among the various herpes viruses associated with oral disease in children, herpes simplex (HSV) is by far the most common. This virus contains double-stranded DNA protected by three layers: a protein capsid, a tegument, and a lipid envelope derived from the nuclear membrane of host cells. Two subtypes, HSV-1 and HSV-2, may be distinguished by endonuclease restriction analysis, and each has a propensity to affect different anatomic areas. Most often, infection by the virus is manifest as vesicular and ulcerative lesions limited to the oral mucosa and skin; however, a variety of organ systems may be secondarily affected.

Epidemiology

Transmission of HSV requires intimate contact, since the enveloped virus is relatively unstable under normal atmospheric conditions. In most cases, the virus is acquired from other children via body fluids such as saliva, or by direct contact with infected skin or mucous membranes. However, transmission by infected adults

may also occur. Outbreaks of gingivostomatitis have resulted from transmission by infected healthcare workers (Manzella et al., 1984), and the disease has been demonstrated in newborns exposed to the virus during childbirth (Nahmias, Alford, & Korones, 1970).

Although HSV-1 is most commonly involved in oral and pharyngeal infections, while HSV-2 is more common in infections of the genitalia, HSV-2 has played an increasingly important role in oral disease in young adults as sexual practices have changed. Both viruses are capable of primary, secondary, or recurrent infection of either site.

Humans are the primary host for HSV, and the virus has been demonstrated in populations throughout the world. Although HSV-2 is more common among newborns, HSV-1 predominates among older children. HSV-1 incidence varies with socioeconomic status; 90% of individuals from lower socioeconomic backgrounds are seropositive, and 40–60% have antibodies by age 5 (Kohl, 1992). In contrast, only 30% of university students exhibit serologic evidence of HSV-1 exposure (Wu, Sayre, Wiesmeier, Bernstein, Visscher, & Bryson, 1984). HSV-2 seropositivity is relatively rare among children, but the incidence begins to increase during adolescence. Risk factors associated with recurrent HSV include exposure to ultraviolet light, febrile illnesses, immunosuppression, and stress.

Pathogenesis

HSV has a predilection for cells of ectodermal origin, including those of the skin, mucous membranes, and central nervous system. Glycoproteins within the lipid envelope serve to attach and transport the virus within the cell membrane. The incubation period in most HSV infections is between 2 and 14 days, during which the virus multiplies and impairs normal cellular function. Cellular edema results, correlating clinically with vesicle formation. Subsequent degeneration results in ulceration, particularly in mucous membranes. Following initial infection, the virus is transported from mucosal or cutaneous nerve endings to ganglia where the virus remains latent, periodically emerging to cause recurrent disease throughout life.

Individuals exposed to HSV for the first time initially mount a nonspecific host response, including recruitment of polymorphonuclear and mononuclear leukocytes, activation of macrophages and natural killer cells, and release of lymphokines. Virus-specific antibody is produced several days later, while specific cellular immunity takes several weeks. Children born to mothers with antibody titers are protected by placentally transferred antibodies for the first 6 months of life; however, those contracting the disease during infancy are at high risk for viremia and disseminated infection. Immunosuppressed and immunodeficient patients also may face significant morbidity or mortality due to HSV.

HSV in the Mouth and Pharynx

Although many individuals with primary HSV infection never display signs or symptoms of infection, the mouth and pharynx are the most common areas involved when clinical manifestations are present. Symptoms of herpetic gingivostomatitis usually begin during the incubation period with the onset of fever and malaise. Within several days, vesicles begin to appear on and around the lips, on the gingiva, and on the mucosa of the anterior tongue and palate. These lesions usually rupture quite easily, resulting in small, shallow ulcers, that subsequently bleed and crust (Figure 6–2). Likewise, the gingival tissues become erythematous, swollen, and ulcerated. The pharynx is typically inflamed and cervical adenopathy is often present. Children will often refuse to eat or drink, and their reduced oral clearance and oral hygiene results in foul-smelling breath. Intravenous fluids may be required to prevent dehydration. Occasionally, the disease will spread to areas of the face and hands (herpetic whitlow). After 4 to 5 days, the lesions begin to resolve, and the mucosa returns to its baseline appearance 7 to 10 days later.

Latency and recurrence are the hallmarks of HSV infection. In most cases, the symptoms of recurrent infection are milder than those of the primary illness, although recurrent lesions have been found in patients with no history of primary infection. Symptoms of HSV-1 may also be less severe when the patient already has a history of exposure to HSV-2, most likely due to cross-immunity.

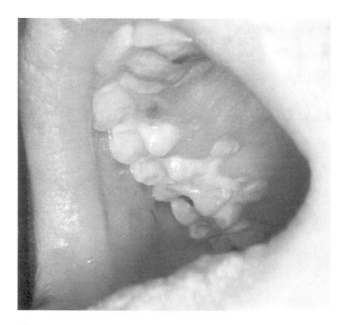

Figure 6–2. Ulceration of the palatal mucosa in primary herpetic gingivostomatitis. (Photo courtesy of Dr. John Svirsky)

Herpes labialis, also known as "cold sores" or "fever blisters," is the most common presentation of recurrent HSV infection. The lesions appear in 25–50% of patients with HSV-1 primary oral infection, and about 25% of those with HSV-2 primary oral infection (Kohl, 1992). Mean rate of recurrence after primary infection with HSV-1 is about 0.1 per month. Recurrent genital lesions occur in 25–55% of individuals with primary genital infection by HSV-1.

Most children with herpes labialis experience a prodrome of burning, tingling, or itching of the lips, which may last several days. Papules then appear at the site, which progress to vesicles (Figure 6–3), and finally to ulcers and crust. Intraoral lesions rarely occur and usually appear on the attached gingiva, distinguishing them from aphthous ulcers, which affect the mobile mucosa. Viral titers in the lesions peak by the 2nd day, but may be detected in the lesions for as long as 5 days, and in the saliva as well.

Diagnosis

The traditional methods used in diagnosing infection by HSV are cytologic examination by Giemsa, Wright's, or Papanicolaou staining (Tzanck preparation), and electron microscopy. Although neither modality is specific for HSV, the presence of a herpes virus can usually be confirmed. The techniques require vigorous scraping of the base of the lesion to obtain an adequate specimen. Typical findings include giant cells, ballooning degeneration of the nucleus, and Cowdry type A intranuclear inclusions. Sensitivity of cytologic examination is 50–60%, but may be greater than 80% with fluorescent staining (Kohl, 1992).

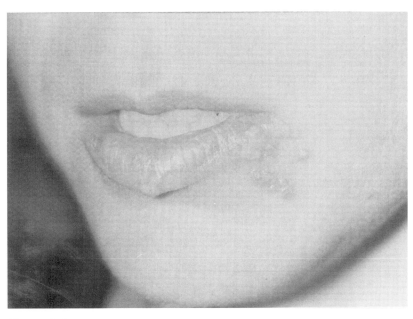

Figure 6–3. Vesicles of the lower lip typical of recurrent herpes labialis. (Photo courtesy of Dr. John Svirsky)

Tests that employ immunologic identification of antigen or antibody are more specific than microscopic study. Antigen identification studies such as enzyme-linked immunosorbent assays (ELISA) use specific hyperimmune serum to HSV or monoclonal antibodies to HSV glycoproteins. Sensitivity and specificity of the newer antigen identification kits is 90–95% (Kohl, 1994). Antibody testing includes ELISA, radioimmunoassays, and Western blot analysis.

Tissue culture remains the gold standard for diagnosis of HSV; however growth of the virus takes an average of 2 to 3 days, and up to a week when low titers are present. The virus may be grown in a variety of host cells and diagnosis is confirmed by the typical cytopathogenic effect.

Newer testing methods primarily employ molecular biologic techniques including endonuclease restriction analysis, nucleic acid hybridization, and polymerase chain reaction. Drug susceptibility testing with acyclovir is also used in some centers.

Treatment

Traditional treatment of primary oral infection by HSV is symptomatic; antipyretics, oral hydration, and topical anesthetics may be useful as the disease runs its course. However, case reports suggest that systemic use of acyclovir, a drug that inhibits DNA replication in HSV-infected cells, may accelerate resolution of primary gingivostomatitis in patients with severe disease. It is unknown whether this therapy may protect against recurrent herpetic infection. Use of topical and systemic steroid medications is contraindicated.

In recurrent cases, systemic acyclovir given at adequate doses (400 mg five times daily) during the prodromal period may hasten healing of the lesions and the duration of pain (Spruance, Stewart, Rowe, McKeough, Wenerstrom, & Freeman, 1990), but is generally not used in routine cases. Topical acyclovir has been demonstrated to decrease the period of viral shedding, but has little effect on symptomatology (Spruance et al., 1982). In contrast, topical use of penciclovir, a newer nucleoside analog, has demonstrated efficacy in hastening resolution of lesions and pain, and in reduction of viral shedding (Raborn, 1996; Spruance, Rea, Thoming, Tucker, Saltzman, & Boon, 1997).

Prevention

Prevention against HSV infection begins with reducing the potential for transmission. HSV is sensitive to heat, light, soaps, and solvents, which will readily sterilize surfaces contacted by infected individuals. Cleansing open lesions with soap and hot water also reduces contagion.

Prophylaxis of HSV infection in HSV-seropositive immunocompromised children, particularly those undergoing transplantation or chemotherapy, has been accomplished using both intravenous and oral acyclovir. Among patients undergoing bone marrow transplantation, acyclovir has reduced the incidence of symptomatic HSV infection from about 70% to 5–20% (Saral, Burns, Laskin, Santos, & Lietman, 1981; Wade, Newton, Flournoy, & Meyers, 1984). A regimen of intravenous followed by oral acyclovir for 3 to 6 months is commonly employed in these patients.

Vaccination against HSV has shown promise in animal studies, but has yet to demonstrate efficacy in humans. Potential vaccines have been developed using subunit glycoproteins, genetically attenuated live HSV, and vaccinia/HSV recombinants. Active research continues in this area.

Varicella Zoster Virus

Varicella zoster virus (VZV) is another member of the herpes virus family with the capacity for latency and recurrence. Primary infection with the virus causes varicella or chickenpox, a disease most common during childhood. Recurrent infection results in zoster (shingles), which may occasionally be present in the pediatric population.

Epidemiology

VZV is among the most prevalent diseases of childhood, with an incidence of 8.3 to 9.1% per year among children 1 to 9 years of age (Weibel et al., 1984). Most patients contract the disease in the late winter and early spring, and the duration of illness is somewhat longer among patients residing in colder climates.

Although VZV is labile under normal conditions, close contact during the prodrome facilitates transmission via the respiratory route. Infection rates as high as 87% have been reported among susceptible household contacts (Ross, 1962).

Pathogenesis

VZV is a herpes virus similar in structure and function to HSV. It therefore shares the tendency to affect cells of ectodermal origin, ultimately resulting in the formation of vesicles and ulcers. The incubation period is between 11 and 20 days in 99% of cases (Ross, 1962). Microscopic appearance is also similar to that of HSV.

VZV also has the ability to lie dormant in cells of the nervous system. Reactivation resulting in zoster occurs in 3 to 5 individuals per 1000 with VZV (Juel-Jensen, 1973). Children with no prior exposure to VZV may develop chickenpox following contact with a patient with zoster.

VZV in the mouth and pharynx

In immunocompetent children, chickenpox is characterized by a generalized pruritic vesicular eruption accompanied by mild systemic symptoms. Lesions usually first appear on the scalp or trunk; however, the oral cavity and mucous membranes of the eye are also frequently involved. Vesicles commonly rupture into ulcers that may be quite similar in appearance to aphthous ulcers; however, primary involvement of the trunk and centrifugal spread of lesions readily distinguishes infection by VZV. Oral involvement may be more dramatic in immunosuppressed children, and in those with leukemia, lymphoma, or HIV disease. The disease generally runs its course in 7 to 10 days.

Zoster is rare among children, but does occur, particularly in immunocompromised states. In contrast to adults, there is commonly no prodrome of pain and paresthesia. Rather, unilateral vesicles spontaneously appear in clusters along the course of the affected nerve. In most cases affecting the oral cavity, intraoral lesions appear at the same time as facial lesions, corresponding to a trigeminal distribution (Figure 6–4). Postherpetic neuralgia may persist several weeks following the infection.

Diagnosis

Diagnosis of VZV infection can usually be made on the basis of history and physical examination. Serologic testing such as complement-fixation, ELISA, and fixed-cell fluorescent microscopy may be useful in equivocal cases. Cell culture is rarely necessary for diagnosis alone.

Treatment

Varicella and zoster usually require no specific therapy. The pruritis associated with facial lesions may be managed with drying agents such as calamine. Aspirin is to be avoided due to the risk of Reye's syndrome, and acetaminophen has little effect on symptomatology. Topical anesthetics may be useful for oral lesions. Oral acyclovir may diminish febrile episodes and number of lesions, but has no effect on itching, incidence of complications, or spread to household contacts (Dunkle et al., 1991). Systemic acyclovir given early in the course of the illness may be useful in severe cases and in immunocompromised patients (Prober, Kirk, & Keeney, 1982; Shepp, Dandliker, & Meyers, 1986). Most physicians also recommend trimming fingernails and bathing regularly to reduce the risk of secondary infection.

Prevention

The development and licensure of a vaccine against VZV represents a major advance in control of the disease. Varivax, a live, attenuated VZV preparation, was licensed in 1995 for use in the United States. Clinical trials have demonstrated efficacy, long-term persistence of antibody, and cost-effectiveness (Asano et al., 1994, Lieu et al., 1994; White et al., 1991). Current recommendations of the Advisory Council on Immunization Practices include routine immunization for all children over 12 months of age with no history of exposure to VZV (ACIP, 1995). Susceptible individuals over 13 years of age who are at high risk of exposure should also be vaccinated. The varicella vaccine has now largely replaced the use of varicella-zoster immune globulin (VZIG).

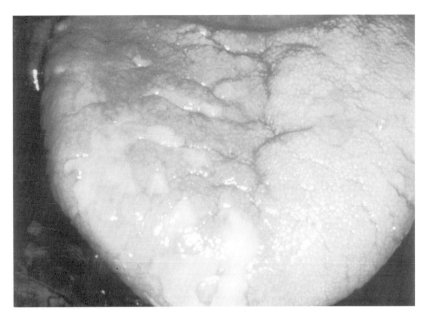

Figure 6–4. Zoster involving the dorsum of the tongue in a patient infected with HIV. Note the unilateral distribution of lesions. (Photo courtesy of Dr. John Svirsky)

Precautions against VZV infection should be taken whenever susceptible immunosuppressed patients may potentially be exposed to the virus. Children electively admitted to the hospital who are found to have varicella should be discharged, and inpatients with the disease must be isolated. Cleansing of open lesions reduces the risk of direct transmission.

Cytomegalovirus

Over the last two decades, cytomegalovirus (CMV) has emerged as a significant oral pathogen, largely due to its prevalence in HIV infection. CMV, originally named for the swollen cells it causes in salivary gland infection, is the largest member of the herpes virus family. No distinct serotypes are recognized.

Epidemiologic studies have demonstrated CMV antibodies in 40–60% of adults of middle and upper socioeconomic status, and 80% in those of lower socioeconomic status. In developing counties, 80% of children have antibodies by age 3, and most of the population is infected by the adult years. Transmission may occur by intrauterine infection resulting from maternal virus reactivation during pregnancy, intentional or unintentional exchange of body fluids or tissues, or direct contact.

Primary infection by CMV is usually inapparent, but often involves low-grade infection of the salivary glands and kidneys. More severe infections may affect the brain, causing a characteristic sensorineural hearing loss, as well as the eye, liver, pancreas, adrenal glands, and a number of other organs. Intact T-cell function is critical in the immune response to CMV and appears to regulate the virulence of the disease.

In the oral cavity, CMV infection is characterized by large ulcers of the oral mucosa, occurring almost exclusively in immunosuppressed and immunodeficient patients (Langford, Kunze, Timm, Ruf, & Reichart, 1990). Since these children also have a propensity to develop aphthous ulcers, periodontal disease, and gingival hyperplasia, it is often unclear whether CMV is causing these lesions or is merely present due to reactivation of the virus. However, the increased incidence of ocular and gastrointestinal ulceration due to CMV suggests a pathogenic role. In addition, serologic studies suggest a correlation between CMV and atypical gingivitis in HIV-positive hemophiliacs (Brightman, 1994a).

Unlike HSV and VZV, cellular infection by CMV produces minimal virus-specific thymidine kinase, the enzyme with which acyclovir and vidarabine interfere. Ganciclovir, a structural relative of acyclovir, has excellent virostatic activity against CMV, but is usually reserved for cases when sight or life are in jeopardy. Use of foscarnet has similar restrictions, and there is little experience with the drug in children. As a result, treatment of oral ulcers associated with CMV is largely symptomatic, unless a variety of organ systems are affected.

Coxsackievirus (Herpangina; Hand, Foot, and Mouth Disease)

Coxsackie viruses are RNA enteroviruses known to cause a wide variety of inflammatory processes. Named for the New York town in which they were discovered, coxsackie viruses are divided into two groups, A and B, within which there are 24 and 6 subtypes, respectively.

Epidemiology

Coxsackie virus is spread by fecal-oral and oral-oral routes. Children tend to transmit the virus from feces-to-mouth via the skin or from mouth-to-mouth via fomites, and are considered more susceptible than adults due to their immunologic immaturity. Incidence peaks between the ages of 5 and 14 years.

Coxsackie virus is found among populations throughout the world. In temperate climates, incidence is greatest during the summer and fall, while tropical areas experience coxsackie virus infection throughout the year. Regions of lower socioeconomic status with less efficient sanitation may be more susceptible to coxsackie virus epidemics.

Pathogenesis

Penetration of the pharyngeal mucosa by coxsackie virus occurs shortly after its acquisition by the oral route. Spread to regional lymph nodes generally occurs within 24 hours. Mild viremia follows within 72 hours, resulting in spread of the disease to a variety of organ systems. The virus multiplies in these affected areas, causing major viremia and associated symptomatology. Clinical improvement usually coincides with a decrease in viral concentration on about day seven.

Coxsackie Virus in the Mouth and Pharynx

Infection by coxsackie virus is generally associated with mild symptomatology. It is estimated that 50% of infections by group A coxsackie viruses and 20% by group B coxsackie viruses are completely asymptomatic (Cherry, 1992c). Furthermore, a large percentage of symptomatic patients experience nothing more than a nonspecific febrile episode that clears within about a week.

Although most enteroviruses are capable of causing some degree of pharyngitis, two clinically distinct disorders of the oral cavity are commonly associated with infection by coxsackie virus: herpangina and hand-foot-mouth disease. It should be noted that despite the differences in their clinical presentation, each of these illnesses may be caused by any one of a number of coxsackie viruses of both the A and B groups.

Herpangina was first described in the 1920s, and its association with infection by group A coxsackie viruses was established in the 1950s. Nevertheless, recent data suggest that the disorder is caused by a wide variety of enteroviruses, and that group B coxsackie viruses has been a more common etiology in recent years (Cherry, 1992a).

Herpangina begins with an acute febrile illness typical of enterovirus infection, usually less severe than that associated with HSV. Associated symptoms frequently include coryza, headache, and vomiting. Oral lesions develop 1 to 2 days following the onset of fever,

initially presenting as 1 to 2 mm papules. The lesions progress to somewhat larger vesicles over the next 2 to 3 days, most ultimately ulcerating. Typically, three to seven lesions will be present on the mucosa of the anterior tonsillar pillars, soft palate, uvula, tonsils, and posterior pharyngeal wall, surrounded by an erythematous halo (Figure 6–5). Lesions of herpangina are distinguished from those of HSV infection by their smaller size and more posterior location, and gingivitis is not seen. The disorder generally runs its course within 1 week, and no specific therapy is required.

Hand, foot, and mouth disease is primarily associated with infection by coxsackie viruses A16 and A10. Following a 4–6 day incubation period, most patients experience a prodrome of fever, malaise, and oral irritation. Oral lesions develop within 48 hours of the onset of symptoms, usually appearing as ulcers 0.5 to 1 cm in diameter on the buccal mucosa and tongue. These ulcerations are somewhat larger than those of herpangina and may be mistaken for aphthous ulcers prior to the appearance of skin lesions. Skin involvement occurs 1 to 2 days later, generally presenting as small vesicles over the dorsal surfaces of the hands and feet, and as macular lesions on the buttocks. Lesions of both the mouth and skin generally clear without treatment within 1 week.

Diagnosis, Treatment, and Prevention

Given the benign nature and short duration of coxsackie virus infections, diagnosis is usually made on clinical grounds. Occasionally, cytologic examination is useful to differentiate coxsackie virus infection from other viral illnesses and is remarkable for the absence of ballooning degeneration and multinucleated giant cell. Cell culture and techniques employing molecular biological methods may be useful when accurate diagnosis is critical.

Coxsackie virus infection is treated symptomatically; specific therapy is neither available nor desirable in most cases. Strict attention to handwashing and hygiene may reduce the risk of epidemics of coxsackie virus infection. Vaccination against the disease is not yet available.

Hairy leukoplakia

Hairy leukoplakia is an adherent white patch that commonly appears on the lateral border of the anterior two-thirds of the tongue in immunosuppressed patients. This lesion results from hyperplasia of the epithelium, and has been shown to contain latent Epstein-Barr virus (EBV) (Greenspan & Greenspan, 1992). Local replication of EBV is believed to take place within the parakeratinized mucosa.

Hairy leukoplakia has been recognized with greater regularity in recent years, coinciding with the rapid rise in prevalence of HIV around the world. As a result, when the clinical picture is suggestive, no addi-

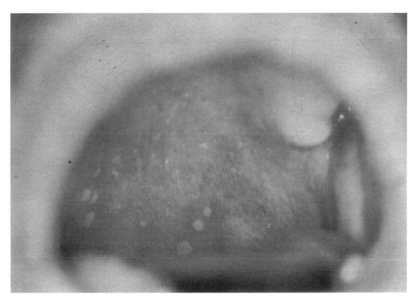

Figure 6–5. Posterior palatal vesicles in a patient with herpangina. (Photo courtesy of Dr. John Svirsky)

tional testing is usually necessary (Figure 6–6). In equivocal cases, microscopy will reveal intranuclear inclusions in keratinocytes with ballooned or ground glass cytoplasm (Fernandez, Benito, Lizaldez, & Montanes, 1990). EBV may be demonstrated by electron microscopy, immunocytochemistry, or Southern blot hybridization for EBV DNA (Cubie, Felix, Southam, & Wray, 1991; Greenspan et al., 1992).

Hairy leukoplakia is usually asymptomatic and does not undergo malignant transformation. The lesion is significant primarily for its diagnostic value in HIV-positive patients; over 60% of individuals with hairy leukoplakia develop AIDS within 2 years, and over 80% within 3 years (Greenspan et al., 1992; Moniaci, Greco, Flecchia, Raiteri, & Sinicco, 1990).

Treatment is usually for cosmesis only, since the lesions tend to recur. Good results have been obtained with systemic acyclovir and topical retinoids (Resnick et al., 1988; Schofer, Ochsendorf, Helm, & Milbradt, 1987).

Trauma, Idiopathic Diseases, and Other Etiologies

Trauma

A wide variety of traumatic lesions may be observed in the mouth and pharynx of children. Most common among these are lesions due to physical trauma. Such injuries may result from accidental laceration of the oral soft tissues by an object placed in the mouth, or from repeated injury due to habitual biting of the cheek or lip. Superficial oral ulceration is the most common manifestation; however, deep lacerations, crenations in the lateral tongue, and a white streak across the buccal mucosa (linea alba) may also result from physical trauma to the mouth. It has been suggested that children suffering impalement injuries of the tonsil and soft palate be observed for possible thromboembolic events (Hengerer, DeGroot, Rivers, & Pettee, 1984); however, this protocol has not been supported in more recent literature (Radkowski, McGill, Healy, & Jones, 1993; Schoem, Choi, Zalzal, & Grundfast, 1997).

Traumatic oral ulcerations are also seen in adolescents engaging in sexual activity involving the oral cavity. The primary affected site is the lingual frenulum, which may be irritated when protruded, particularly if the frenulum is short or the lower incisors have rough edges. Ulceration of the central portion of the palate has also been observed in patients engaging in fellatio.

Chemical injury of the oral mucosa is also common in the pediatric age group. Such injuries are frequently associated with accidental caustic ingestions. Historically, alkaline household cleaning products have been responsible for the majority of these events; however, bleach ingestion is also common, and ingestion of alkaline hair relaxer products has risen sharply in recent years. While esophageal injury due to bleach and hair relaxer products may be rare, oral burns are seen frequently and may be severe (Cox & Eisenbeis, 1997; Holinger, 1997). Chemical injury to the mucosa may also result in children whose parents inappropriately treat orodental pain using analgesics held in the oral vestibule (Figure 6–7).

Thermal injury to the oral tissues in children may result from the consumption of excessively hot food or liquids. The affected site depends on the texture of the food and the child's stage of oromotor development. Thermal injury to the lips most often occurs due to chewing of electrical wires, and may result in severe scarring of the oral commissure.

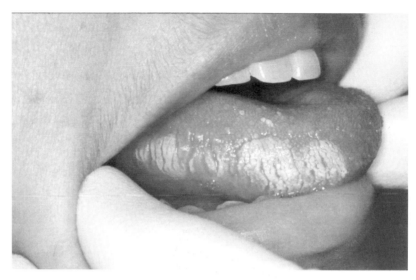

Figure 6–6. Hairy leukoplakia of the lateral border of the tongue is often the presenting symptom in patients infected with HIV. (Photo courtesy of Dr. John Svirsky)

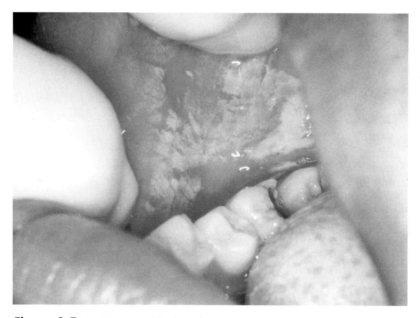

Figure 6–7. Aspirin burn of the buccal mucosa. Note lesion is adjacent to a carious molar tooth. (Photo courtesy of Dr. John Svirsky)

Most episodes of oral trauma are mild and require no specific intervention. In some cases, emollients and analgesics may be useful. In severe burns involving the oral commissures, patients often benefit from early intervention with stents to prevent extensive fibrosis at the affected site.

Recurrent Aphthous Stomatitis

Recurrent aphthous stomatitis (RAS) is generally recognized as the most common disease affecting the oral mucosa. First described over a century ago (von Mikulicz & Kummel, cited in Ship, 1996), the disease re-

mains poorly understood and unpreventable, and treatment remains largely symptomatic. However, recent research has linked the disorder with genetic and immunologic defects, and the high incidence of RAS among the growing population of immunodeficient patients may serve to hasten the development of strategies for treatment and prevention of the disease.

Epidemiology and Pathogenesis

Most patients with RAS develop their first episode of the disease during adolescence and experience multiple recurrences throughout their lifetime. RAS is the most common cause of oral ulcers among children (Field, Brookes, & Tyldesley, 1992), with a peak age of onset between 10 and 19 years. Prevalence in the general population is estimated at 5–25% (Ship, 1996).

Heredity is perhaps the best-documented risk factor for RAS. In one study, patients whose parents had a history of RAS had a 90% chance of developing the disease, compared to 20% among those with no parental history (Ship, 1972). Association of RAS with specific HLA subtypes has also been demonstrated (Gallina, Cumbo, Messina, & Caruso, 1985). Other well-documented risk factors for RAS include deficiencies of iron, folate, and vitamin B-12. Trauma, stress, allergy, and high socioeconomic status may also play some role in the development of RAS. It has been suggested that cessation of smoking causes an increase in frequency and severity of the disease (Axell & Henricsson, 1985).

Despite these findings, most current research implicates underlying immunologic disorders as the primary etiology of RAS. Increased antibody-dependent cell-mediated cytotoxicity and serum immunoglobulin levels have been found in RAS patients. These individuals also have increased numbers of T-helper lymphocytes, and decreased numbers of T-suppressor lymphocytes. It is widely believed that RAS represents an activated cell-mediated immune response, and the high prevalence of RAS among HIV-positive patients seems to support this etiology. Ship (1996) has suggested that RAS occurs in individuals genetically predisposed to RAS as a result of antibody-dependent cellular cytotoxicity and local immune complex-related reactions; however, there is currently no uniformly accepted theory of pathogenesis based on immunologic factors.

Clinical Features and Diagnosis

Mucosal ulcerations due to RAS are categorized as minor aphthous ulcers, major aphthous ulcers, and herpetiform ulcers, based on the number, size, location, and duration of the lesions. Minor aphthous stomatitis accounts for approximately 80% of cases. These lesions are usually associated with a prodrome ranging from several hours to several days, during which a localized burning sensation and erythema develop. Subsequently, a small, white papule forms and then ulcerates, gradually expanding over 2 to 3 days. The resulting lesion is round to ovoid and less than 1 cm in diameter, with a surrounding raised, erythematous border and a gray-white pseudomembrane. The lesions occur primarily on nonkeratinized oral mucosa, such as the mucosa of the cheek, lip, and floor of mouth (Figure 6–8). They are further distinguished by their lack of tissue tags from ruptured vesicles, the absence of systemic illness, and the normal appearance of adjacent tissues. Lesions generally heal in 10 to 14 days without scarring.

Some patients with RAS develop major aphthous ulceration, also known as periadenitis mucosa necrotica recurrens. This disorder is characterized by single lesions that are generally larger than are those of the minor variety, and appear more posteriorly along the floor of mouth, soft palate, or peritonsillar areas (Figure 6–9). The associated pain is typically greater than that with minor RAS. Lesions of major RAS may take as long as 6 weeks to heal, ultimately resulting in scarring at the affected site. These lesions have commonly been reported in HIV-infected patients, likely due to impaired immune regulation in these individuals.

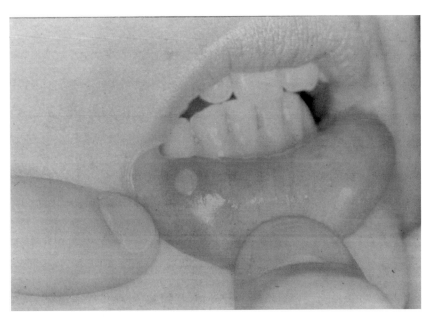

Figure 6–8. Aphthous ulcers are typically found on the moveable, nonkeratinized mucosa of the lip, cheek, and floor of mouth. (Photo courtesy of Dr. Jeffrey Powell)

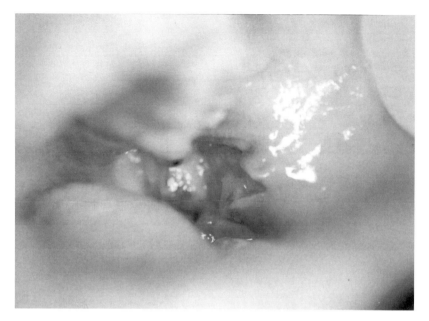

Figure 6–9. Major aphthous ulcer of the posterior buccal mucosa. (Photo courtesy of Dr. John Svirsky)

Herpetiform ulcers are the least common lesions of RAS. These occur as groups of pinpoint ulcerations resembling those of herpes simplex, which coalesce into larger, irregular lesions. Any site within the oral cavity may be affected. The process usually persists for 7 to 10 days.

In Behcet disease, a relatively rare disorder in children, patients classically present with aphthous stomatitis, iritis, and genital ulcers. Recent literature suggests that the diagnosis should be made in the presence of RAS and some combination of the following: synovitis, cutaneous vasculitis, uveitis, genital ulcers, and meningoencephalitis (Rakover, Adar, Tal, Lang, & Fedar, 1989). Behcet disease is most common among individuals of Mediterranean extraction. Involvement of the oral cavity is the presenting symptom in 50-70% of patients, and is eventually seen in 98%. A positive "pathergy test" is pathognomonic of the disease, consisting of needle puncture of the skin followed by erythematous induration and pustule formation. The etiology and appropriate treatment of this disorder have yet to be firmly established.

Aphthouslike ulcerations have also been reported in up to 20% of patients with Crohn's disease (regional enteritis). It is unknown whether the lesions represent a manifestation of the disease or are coincidental. The areas most frequently involved are the buccal mucosa, where cobblestoning is usually present, and the vestibule, where linear hyperplastic folds may also be evident (Bernstein & McDonald, 1978). In patients with oral involvement, acute attacks of RAS often herald exacerbation of the enteritis.

Diagnosis of RAS is usually made on clinical grounds, although culture and/or biopsy may be use-

ful when other etiologies are suspected. Medical evaluation should include serum levels of iron, B vitamins, folate, and ferritin. HIV testing should be considered when the history is suggestive.

Treatment

There is presently no specific treatment for RAS. As a result, management of the disorder focuses on control of local pain and inflammation, and on elimination of potential risk factors.

In mild cases of RAS, control of pain has been obtained with emollients such as orabase, Maalox, and sucralfate, and with topical anesthetic agents. Medical therapy is usually advocated only in more severe cases, due to the self-limited nature of the disease. The simplest forms of therapy usually involve oral rinses with commercial mouthwashes or antibiotic solutions such as tetracycline and chlorhexidine, although the mechanisms by which these agents work are unclear.

Topical application of corticosteroid preparations is commonly used in the management of RAS. Triamcinolone, fluocinolone, and clobetasol have demonstrated efficacy, often in combination with emollients and adhesive pastes for improved pain control and duration of application. Systemic and intralesional steroid use has also been advocated. In HIV infected patients, topical therapy with steroids was enhanced by use of the immunosuppressant drug azathioprine (Brown & Bottomley, 1990). Other immunosuppressive agents have been used with some success, including colchicine (Katz, Langevitz, Shemer, Barak, & Livneh, 1994), cyclosporin (Eisen & Ellis, 1990), and thalidomide (Revuz et al., 1990). Levamisole, immunocyte extract, and gammaglobulin are immunopotentiating agents which have demonstrated some efficacy in treatment of RAS (Ship, 1996). Pentoxifylline, a hemorrheologic agent, has shown some anti-inflammatory effect and hastened recovery in patients with RAS (Pizarro, Navarro, Fonseca, Vidaurrazaga, & Herranz, 1995; Wahba-Yahav, 1995).

Sustained relief of pain associated with RAS has recently been demonstrated in a randomized, double blinded clinical trial using topical diclofenac in hyaluronan (Saxen, Ambrosius, Rehemtula, Russell, & Eckert, 1997). Hyaluronic acid is an endogenous polysaccharide elicited in the presence of inflammation, which may work by binding to adhesion molecules in aphthous ulcers. Diclofenac is a non-steroidal antiinflammatory agent. The two together produced a 35–52% reduction of pain 2 to 6 hours after application of the medication.

The use of antiviral agents such as interferon and acyclovir has been advocated based on the theory that RAS may represent reactivation of a herpes virus; however, results have been equivocal (Hutchinson, Angenend, Mok, Cummins, & Richards, 1990; Pedersen, 1992; Wormser et al., 1988), and there is little support for this etiology. Prostaglandin E-2, a mediator of inflammation, and azelastine, which stabilizes cell membranes, have also effectively controlled lesions of RAS (Taylor, Walker, & Bagg, 1993; Ueta, Osaki, Yoneda, Yamamoto, & Kato, 1994).

Erythema Multiforme

Erythema multiforme (EM) is a mucocutaneous disorder manifested by well-defined erythematous plaques on the trunk and extremities and erosive lesions on the mucosal surfaces of the oral cavity, eyes, and genitalia. Two forms of the disease are generally recognized: erythema multiforme minor, which is a mild syndrome affecting primarily cutaneous surfaces, and erythema multiforme major, or Stevens-Johnson syndrome, which is distinguished by marked mucosal damage. The precise mechanism by which EM occurs has not been fully elucidated; however, the disorder is triggered by a wide variety of infectious and pharmacologic agents.

Epidemiology

Although EM is typically a disease of young adults, children and adolescents may account for up to 20% of cases (Huff, Weston, & Tonnesen, 1983). The annual incidence has been estimated at 0.01–1% (Huff et al., 1983). EM is slightly more common in males, and there is no racial predilection. Cases may occur sporadically throughout the year; however, recurrences during the spring and fall are well documented.

Pathogenesis

EM is an inflammatory disorder resulting from a host-specific immune response. Both immune complex (Type III) and cell-mediated (Type IV) hypersensitivity reactions have been implicated; immune complexes have been isolated from skin lesions and serum, while a cellular infiltrate of macrophages and T-lymphocytes is typically seen.

Literally hundreds of precipitating factors have been proposed, however three are considered well documented: infection by HSV, infection by mycoplasma, and reactions to drugs. While the former is generally associated with EM minor, the latter two causes are more commonly followed by the Stevens-Johnson syndrome.

Infection by HSV-1 or HSV-2 may precede signs and symptoms of EM in 60-70% of cases (Brice, Huff, & Weston, 1991). Although HSV is rarely identified by viral culture or electron microscopic study of EM lesions, advances in molecular biology have been used to demonstrate HSV-specific nucleic acids and antigens. The lesions of EM minor usually appear some 10 days following the initial herpes infection. In contrast, mucosal and skin lesions may erupt as long as 3 weeks following infection by mycoplasma.

Drug-induced EM has classically been associated with the use of antibiotics, such as penicillin and sulfa drugs, and chemotherapeutic agents such as methotrexate. A number of vaccines including hepatitis B and diphtheria-pertussis-tetanus (DPT) have also been implicated. EM lesions develop hours to months after exposure, with cases of prior sensitization occurring more rapidly.

Genetic factors may also play some role in the development of EM. Patients with human leukocyte antigens (HLA) B15, Dr w53, AW 33, and DQw3 have demonstrated an increased risk of acquiring the disorder (Brice et al., 1991). In addition, genetic differences may explain why a minority of HSV-exposed individuals develops EM.

Clinical features and diagnosis

Prodromal symptoms of fever, headache, myalgia, cough, and sore throat may precede the diagnosis of EM by 1 to 2 weeks, but may be associated with an inciting infectious process rather than the developing mucocutaneous disorder. A prodrome is more commonly associated with EM major than with EM minor.

Skin lesions in EM are round, erythematous macules that progress to papules with central blistering or epidermal necrosis. The dusky center and erythematous periphery constitute the so-called "target" or "iris" lesion. Merging of the lesions may result in a "geographic" appearance. The lesions typically spread in a symmetrical fashion over the extremities, particularly on the extensor surfaces of the arms. Lesions also frequently appear at sites of previous skin trauma. Large bullae and desquamation may be present in EM major.

Oral lesions are present in 25–60% of cases of EM (Huff et al., 1983). They usually appear simultaneously with the skin lesions, but may precede or follow skin involvement by several days. Oral lesions of EM begin as small bullae, and then rapidly become discrete erosions as the roof of the bulla separates (Figure 6–10). Extent of involvement may vary from a handful of small lesions in EM minor to severe oral necrosis, hemorrhagic crusting, and halitosis in EM major. Cervical adenopathy is common in cases with oral involvement.

Skin lesions in EM are associated with itching and burning. Mucosal lesions, which may involve the eyes and genitalia as well as the oral cavity, may be quite painful. Most patients complain of malaise, but those with EM major may also have high fevers, myalgia, and headache. Symptoms and lesions in cases of EM minor generally dissipate within 4 weeks, while those in EM major may last as long as 6 weeks. In patients with EM major, prolonged, severe mucosal involvement may result in ocular, pharyngoesophageal, gastrointestinal, and laryngotracheobronchial complications.

Diagnosis of EM is usually made on the basis of clinical criteria. Histologic findings include necrotic keratinocytes and subepidermal blistering. Immunofluorescence is mainly useful in ruling out other mucocutaneous bullous disorders, but will often demonstrate C3 or IgM in the blood vessels of the superficial dermis.

Treatment

There is no specific treatment for EM. Episodes of EM minor are generally mild and require minimal intervention. Oral antihistamines may be useful in reducing skin symptoms, and mouth rinses containing antacids, topical anesthetics, and steroid suspensions may alleviate pain due to mucosal ulcerations. Topical antibiotics may prevent secondary infection of skin lesions. Use of systemic steroids is controversial, but should not be necessary in mild cases. Systemic acyclovir may be useful in recurrent cases associated with HSV infection.

Candidiasis

Candida is an opportunistic organism that produces oral pathosis in debilitated patients. The organism has become increasingly prevalent as the population with HIV has grown, and therapy for candidiasis has rapidly evolved in an effort to keep pace with this epidemic.

Epidemiology

Candida sp. are considered a component of the normal oral flora, although they are typically present in low concentrations. Carriage rates cited in the literature

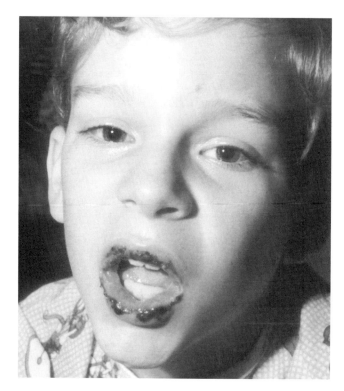

Figure 6–10. Erosive, crusty lesions of the lips in a patient with Stevens-Johnson syndrome resulting from use of a sulfa-containing drug. (Photo courtesy of Dr. Douglas Mitchell)

are quite diverse, depending on the age group tested and the culture technique used (Brightman, 1994b).

Children at risk for infection with *Candida* include neonates, in whom the immune system has not yet matured, and those with altered immunity due to congenital or acquired immune compromise, immune suppression, diabetes, or prolonged antibiotic therapy. Candidiasis has become quite common among HIV-infected children, with reported prevalence rates ranging from 20–72% (Kline, 1996).

Transmission is dependent on direct exposure of susceptible oral mucosa to a colonized site. Intrauterine infection of the fetus is rare, and infant-to-infant transmission in hospital nurseries is uncommon (Hughes, 1992). *Candida* may, however, be acquired by other nosocomial means in debilitated patients.

Pathogenesis

Candida is a dimorphic organism, appearing as round to oval cells in a yeast form (blastospore) or as pseudohyphae. *Candida* sp. do not possess a capsule.

Because *Candida* is an organism of low virulence, infection primarily depends on the size of the inoculum and on host resistance. Studies suggest that, in immunocompetent hosts, all components of the immune system will respond to the organism (Hughes, 1992). In the oral cavity, lysozyme and secretory IgA supplement circulating antibodies in response to the presence of *Candida*; a robust cellular response is also typical.

Candida attaches in its yeast form to receptor sites on the cells of mucosal epithelium. Pseudohyphae develop during the infection process, depending on the local microenvironment. As the mucosa is invaded, a pseudomembrane is usually produced, consisting of organisms, epithelial cells, leukocytes, and food debris. Progression of the infection results in ulceration, granulation tissue, and occasionally microabscesses beneath the pseudomembrane.

Superficial candidiasis may involve a number of body orifices such as the mouth and anogenital area, as well as the intertriginous areas of the skin. In rare cases, deep invasion may lead to hematogenous spread and systemic disease. Chronic candidiasis is usually associated with deficient T lymphocyte function.

Candida in the mouth and pharynx

Although six forms of the disease are recognized (see Table 6–3), only three are commonly seen among children:

Acute pseudomembranous candidiasis is the most common type of candidiasis in children. In this disorder, the mucosal lesions have a white spotted appearance, owing to the formation of the pseudomembrane. The lesions may easily be mistaken for curds of milk or food debris (Figure 6–11). Removal of the pseudomembrane exposes the underlying ulceration and granulation, and may cause bleeding. The sites most commonly involved are the buccal mucosa, dorsal tongue, lateral tongue, gingivae, and pharynx.

Acute atrophic candidiasis is far less common, and occurs almost exclusively as a result of antibiotic therapy. The pseudomembrane is usually absent in this form, and an erythematous and ulcerated mucosa is seen. Depapillation of the tongue is also common. Children will typically complain of oral burning, foul taste, or sore throat.

Angular cheilitis (perleche) is associated with pain, erythema, and fissuring in the corners of the mouth (Figure 6–12). Progression of the lesions may result in erosions of the skin and desquamation of the epithelium surrounded by hyperkeratosis. This diagnosis should be made only after other causes such as trauma,

environmental exposure, or herpes labialis have been ruled out. In many children, use of a pacifier and habitual sucking or licking of the lips may predispose to this disorder.

Diagnosis

In most cases, the diagnosis of *Candida* may be based on the appearance of the oral lesions and the medical status of the patient. Microscopic identification may occasionally be necessary, and surface scrapings may be mounted in 10–20% potassium hydroxide to

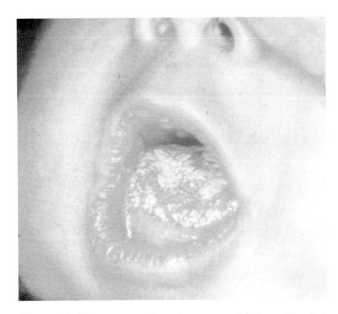

Figure 6–11. Acute pseudomembranous candidiasis, or "thrush," involving the tongue in an infant.

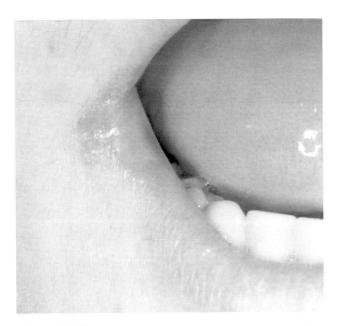

Figure 6–12. Angular cheilitis affecting the commissure of the lips is often the result of infection with *Candida*.

Table 6–3. Classification of oral candidiasis.

Acute
    Acute pseudomembranous candidiasis (thrush)
    Acute atrophic candidiasis (antibiotic sore mouth)
Chronic
    Chronic atrophic candidiasis
        Denture stomatitis
        Angular cheilitis (perleche)
        Median rhomboid glossitis
    Chronic hyperplastic candidiasis

demonstrate budding yeast or pseudohyphae. Culture serves to definitively distinguish *Candida* from other yeast and fungi. Incubated at room temperature on Sabouraud's agar, the organism grows as soft, cream-colored colonies with a yeasty odor. Septated extensions known as germ tubes may aid in identification of *C. albicans*. *C. albicans* is also the only *Candida* species which will ferment glucose and maltose. Serologic tests for *Candida* have yet to be perfected.

Treatment

Oral candidiasis in children is usually treated with topical agents. For infants and young children, nystatin oral suspension is applied to the oral mucosa via syringe in a dose of 50,000 to 200,000 units administered four times a day. Older children may prefer nystatin pastilles or clotrimazole troches dissolved slowly in the mouth five times a day. Therapy is usually continued for 2 weeks. Patients in whom predisposing conditions cannot be corrected may experience frequent recurrences, and may be candidates for prophylactic therapy.

Systemic therapy may be considered in children who fail to respond to topical agents after 5 to 7 days, or in children whose lesions are interfering with normal alimentation. Ketoconazole or fluconazole administered once daily for 5 to 7 days is a typical regimen, often used in conjunction with topical therapy.

Inflammatory Bullous Diseases

Inflammatory bullous diseases are relatively rare in the pediatric population. However, these dermatologic disorders frequently involve the mucosa of the oral cavity and upper airway, and therefore should be familiar to the practicing pediatric otolaryngologist. The bullae in these disorders result from blistering either within the epidermis or below the epidermis. The subepidermal bullous diseases include linear IgA dermatosis of childhood (LADC), bullous pemphigoid (BP), cicatricial pemphigoid (CP), dermatitis herpetiformis (DH), epidermolysis bullosa acquisita (EB), and erosive and bullous forms of lichen planus (LP), while pemphigus vulgaris (PV) is the primary intradermal blistering disease.

In all bullous diseases affecting the oral cavity, the lesions frequently rupture, resulting in denuded, painful ulcerations (Figure 6–13). Diminished oral intake in severely affected patients may lead to dehydration and weight loss. Sloughing of mucosa may also lead to airway compromise. Healing of the lesions by secondary intention may result in intraoral scarring and microstomia.

Approximately 50% of patients with subepidermal bullous diseases develop oral lesions (Rabinowitz & Esterly, 1993). LADC, a chronic but self-limiting disease of early childhood, is probably the most common bullous disease in children. This disorder is characterized

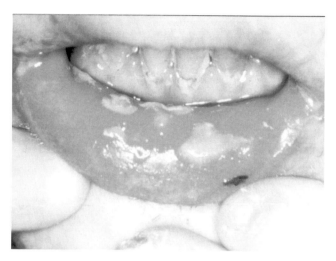

Figure 6–13. Sloughing of the labial mucosa in a patient with EB. (Photo courtesy of Dr. John Svirsky)

by irregularly shaped bullae, herpetiform clustering of blisters, and "rosettes" of new blisters encircling healing lesions. Sites of involvement include the groin, thighs, and trunk. Remission is typically seen within 3–5 years. In BP, the flexural creases are sites of predilection, and involvement of the face and buttocks is uncommon. Lesions of the palms and soles, rarely seen in the adult form of the disease, are common in infants. Remission often occurs within 1 year. CP primarily involves the mucous membranes of the eye, mouth, and genitalia. This disease has a more prolonged course and results in more scarring than does BP. DH causes intensely pruritic bullous lesions that readily excoriate when scratched. The disorder may occur in association with gluten-sensitive enteropathy. In EB, tissue-bound and circulating antibodies to type VII collagen are present in addition to the subepidermal bullae. Like CP, head and neck structures are commonly involved, particularly the mucous membranes of the oropharynx, nasopharynx, esophagus, and conjunctiva. Even mild intraoral trauma may cause sloughing of mucosa; therefore dental, otolaryngologic, and anesthetic procedures in children with EB must be performed delicately. Erosive and bullous forms of lichen planus are usually accompanied by the more typical white lesions (Wickham's striae) and are distinguished on biopsy by hydropic degeneration of the basal epithelial layer.

PV is a chronic disease that primarily affects the oral cavity, with frequent involvement of the glabrous skin as well. The bullae expand with gentle pressure on the blister or surrounding normal tissue (Nikolsky's sign) and may coalesce. Involvement of the oral cavity is seen in nearly all patients with PV. In neonates, PV may occur as a result of passive transfer of maternal antibodies to the fetus, but usually resolves spontaneously within several weeks.

Because many of the inflammatory bullous diseases present with similar features, direct and indirect immunofluorescence and other investigations of autoimmune etiology may be necessary to establish a diagnosis. These studies often identify deposits of specific immunoglobulins and/or complement at the affected site within the epidermis or dermal-epidermal junction. Assays of circulating antibodies are also occasionally useful for diagnostic purposes.

Treatment of the inflammatory bullous diseases typically includes steroids, dapsone, or sulfapyridine. Immunosuppressant therapy may be used in severe and recalcitrant cases. Management of oral lesions includes topical steroids and rinses of immunosuppressant drugs, as well as a variety of emollients.

Geographic Tongue

Geographic tongue (GT) is characterized by patchy depapillation of the epithelium of the dorsal tongue. The lesions are typically reddish in color, surrounded by a sharply contrasting white ring of regenerating papillae. Also known as migratory glossitis, the pattern may change every few days.

GT has been identified in 1–2% of the normal adult population. Estimates of the incidence among children are approximately ten times lower (Brightman, 1994c). The disorder may be associated with Reiter's syndrome, which is characterized by similar lesions of the eyes and urethra, as well as generalized arthritis.

Microscopically, the epithelium is spongiotic and infiltrated with clusters of polymorphonuclear leukocytes. The lesions are generally asymptomatic, but may occasionally be associated with burning or stinging.

The cause of GT remains unknown. Studies have implicated immune (Fenerli, Papanicolaou, Papanicolaou, & Laskaris, 1993), allergic (Marks & Czarny, 1984), and psychosomatic (Redman, Vance, Gorlin, Peagler, & Meskin, 1966) factors. Chronic bacterial and fungal etiologies have also been suggested.

Symptomatic GT is best treated with topical anesthetics and aqueous antihistamines. Topical tretinoin (Retin-A) has also been used successfully in severe cases (Helfman, 1979).

Drug-induced and Allergic Stomatitis

Stomatitis may result either directly or indirectly from use of a variety of medications and materials. Oral allergic reactions to drugs taken systemically are usually manifest as inflammation, ulceration, and vesicle formation, similar to that seen in erythema multiforme. Lesions may be noted over the skin as well as the oral mucosa. In patients with contact allergic stomatitis, lesions may be noted in areas of oral mucosa which have contacted specific topical antigens. In these cases, erythema and edema are noted at the site of contact, occasionally associated with ulceration and/or burning. Comprehensive history-taking and skin testing are usu-

ally adequate to establish the diagnosis, and the offending medication should be avoided.

In patients receiving chemotherapy, direct ulceration of the oral mucosa frequently results from impairment of epithelial regeneration by drugs which interfere with DNA synthesis, protein synthesis, or mitosis. Indirect oral ulceration is also seen in chemotherapy patients, as well as in those with drug-induced aplastic anemia or idiosyncratic drug reactions resulting in neutropenia. In these individuals, suppression of the bone marrow and systemic immunity lead to ulceration due to secondary infection. Biopsy of ulcers in these individuals will frequently demonstrate organisms in the absence of a significant inflammatory response, making such infections severe and potentially fatal. Mouthwashes combining topical emollients or analgesics with antibiotics are often useful, but may require additional systemic antibiotic therapy.

Leukemia

In leukemia, malignant leukocytes replace the normal bone marrow cells, resulting in anemia, thrombocytopenia, and impaired cellular immunity. The malignant cells may also infiltrate other normal organs as the disease progresses.

In the oral cavity, depressed platelet and red blood cell counts result in a pale-appearing mucosa, petechiae or ecchymoses, and gingival bleeding. As previously discussed, oral ulceration may result due to neutropenia complicated by secondary infection. In most children with leukemia, the offending organism is HSV (Greenberg & Garfunkel, 1994), which responds well to acyclovir. Other more serious infections may also occur, however, and the clinician must maintain a low threshold for biopsy and culture of oral ulcerations in these patients. Direct ulceration due to chemotherapeutic agents is also common (see above).

Orodental management of leukemic patients includes preventive measures such as meticulous oral hygiene and correction of potentially traumatic tooth surfaces or restorations. Combination mouthwashes with topical emollients or analgesics and antibiotics are useful in patients who have already developed stomatitis.

Lupus Erythematosis

Systemic lupus erythematosis (SLE) is a disorder characterized by immune complex deposition in a variety of organ systems. Its cause remains elusive, but immune, endocrine, viral, and genetic etiologies have been suggested. SLE rarely affects young children, but may be seen among adolescents and, more commonly, in young adults.

In patients with SLE, autoantibodies cause hemolytic anemia, thrombocytopenia, and lymphopenia. Antinuclear antibody is present in virtually all patients with the disease. Scaling skin lesions with inflammation are common, and a malar or "butterfly rash" often suggests the diagnosis. Other skin manifestations include Raynaud's phenomenon and alopecia. Arthritis, pericarditis, pulmonary infiltrates, and muscle atrophy are common. Renal involvement occurs in 50% of patients and results in glomerulonephritis and nephrotic syndrome. Involvement of the central nervous system signals a poor prognosis.

Over 75% of patients with SLE have oral manifestations, including burning mouth or xerostomia; ulcerations of the oral mucosa and lips are demonstrable in 25–50% of these individuals (Greenberg, 1994b). Immunofluorescence performed on oral biopsy tissues will usually detect deposits of immunoglobulin and C3 in the basement membrane zone, distinguishing the disease from LP or leukoplakia, and occasionally making the diagnosis for the first time.

Management of SLE relies heavily on chronic use of systemic steroids and cytotoxic agents. Topical mouthwashes containing emollients and steroids may be useful in controlling intraoral symptoms.

Malnutrition

Malnourished children may develop a variety of inflammatory disorders of the oral cavity. Studies have suggested that RAS and ANUG may be associated with malnutrition. In third world countries, ANUG is known to progress in severely malnourished individuals to noma, a severely disfiguring necrosis of orofacial tissues. Vitamin C deficiency, also seen primarily in these nations, may be associated with scurvy and severe gingival disease. In contrast, deficiencies of B vitamins and iron are far more common among the developed countries. Affected children occasionally have malabsorption syndromes and must therefore be carefully evaluated. Oral inflammatory changes include atrophic glossitis or "bald tongue," which primarily affects the filiform papillae, and angular cheilitis. Generalized oral ulceration may also be seen.

PHARYNGITIS

Common Bacterial and Viral Infections

Pharyngitis is a general term used to describe any inflammation of structures of the nasopharynx and oropharynx. Typically, the disorder will present with symptoms of odynophagia; however, objective signs of inflammation must be present in order to make the diagnosis.

Pharyngitis may be classified based on duration of symptoms as acute, subacute, or chronic; most patients present with acute illness. Alternatively, pharyngitis may also be characterized as either nasopharyngitis, in which common symptoms include rhinorrhea, nasal congestion, sneezing, and cough, or pharyngotonsillitis, in which nasal symptomatology is usually absent. In most cases, nasopharyngitis is associated with viral illness; pharyngotonsillitis, on the other hand, may have a wide variety of causes.

Nasopharyngitis typically occurs during the cold weather months among young children during their initial exposure to respiratory viruses. Adenoviruses, influenza viruses, parainfluenza viruses, and enteroviruses are the most common etiologic agents. Rhinovirus and respiratory syncytial virus occur almost exclusively in preschool children and are rarely associated with overt signs of pharyngeal inflammation. Adenoviruses are more common among older children and adolescents. Nonviral agents rarely associated with nasopharyngitis include *C. diphtheriae*, *N. meningitidis*, *H. influenzae*, and *Coxiella burnetii*. Nasopharyngitis of viral etiology is most commonly acute and self-limited, with symptoms resolving within 10 days.

The etiologic agents responsible for pharyngotonsillitis are far more diverse than are those in nasopharyngitis. Nevertheless, Group A beta-hemolytic *Streptococcus*, adenoviruses, influenza viruses, parainfluenza viruses, enteroviruses, EBV, and *Mycoplasma* account for over 90% of these infections (Cherry, 1992b). Treatment of these illnesses varies depending on the etiology; therefore throat culture for treatable bacterial etiologies is usually indicated. As in nasopharyngitis, most viral pharyngotonsillitis requires no specific therapy. In the remainder of this chapter, we address other causes of pharyngotonsillitis that may require more aggressive diagnosis and treatment.

Group A Beta-hemolytic and Other Streptococci

The group A beta-hemolytic streptococcus (GABHS) is the most common bacterium associated with pharyngitis in children. In the half-century since the advent of antibiotics, most pharyngeal infections by GABHS have been benign, self-limited, and uncomplicated processes. In fact, in many patients symptoms improve without any medical intervention whatsoever. However, a small number of affected individuals continue to develop severe renal and cardiac complications following GABHS infection. In addition, there is evidence that early antibiotic therapy may be useful in the treatment of GABHS. As a result, appropriate diagnosis and treatment of these infections is imperative.

Epidemiology

The incidence of GABHS pharyngitis has not been estimated on the basis of population-based data (Markowitz, 1994). Nevertheless, "strep throat" is well recognized as a common disease among children and adolescents. The incidence peaks during the winter and spring seasons, and it is more common in cooler, temperate climates. Close interpersonal contact in schools, military quarters, dormitories, and families with several children appears to be a risk factor for the disease.

Transmission of GABHS is believed to occur through droplet spread. The risk of contagion most likely depends on the inoculum size and the virulence of the infecting strain. As a result, individuals are most infectious early in the course of the disease. The incubation period is usually between 1 and 4 days. Following initiation of antimicrobial therapy, most physicians will allow affected children to return to school within 36 to 48 hours (Kaplan, 1992). The role of individuals colonized with GABHS in the spread of the disease is uncertain, although data suggest that carriers rarely spread the disease to close contacts (Kaplan, 1992).

Pathogenesis

The streptococci are gram-positive, catalase-negative cocci, characterized by their growth in long chains or pairs in culture. These organisms are traditionally classified into 18 groups with letter designations (Lancefield groups) on the basis of the antigenic carbohydrate component of their cell walls. While the group A beta-hemolytic streptococcus is isolated from most patients with streptococcal pharyngitis, group C, G, and B streptococci may also occasionally cause this disorder. Further subclassification of streptococci is made based on their ability to lyse sheep red blood cells in culture; the beta-hemolytic strains cause hemolysis associated with a clear zone surrounding their colonies, whereas alpha-hemolytic strains cause partial hemolysis and gamma-hemolytic strains cause no hemolysis.

The primary determinant of streptococcal pathogenicity is an antigenically distinct protein known as the M protein. Among the more pathogenic bacteria, this molecule is found within the fimbriae, which are fingerlike projections from the cell wall of the organism that facilitate adherence to pharyngeal and tonsillar epithelium. Over 80 M serotypes are known. The M protein allows a streptococcus to resist phagocytosis in the absence of type-specific antibody. In the immunocompetent host, the synthesis of type-specific anti-M and other antibodies, which belong primarily to the IgG class of immunoglobulins, confers long-term serotype-specific immunity to the particular strain in question. In laboratory-produced penicillin-resistant strains of GABHS, the M protein is absent, thereby rendering these strains more vulnerable to phagocytosis (Gerber, 1996). This finding may help to explain why there have been no naturally occurring penicillin resistant GABHS isolated in over 40 years of penicillin use.

GABHS are capable of elaborating at least 20 extracellular substances that affect host tissue; the interested reader may find a complete discussion of these substances elsewhere. Among the most important are streptolysin O, an oxygen-labile hemolysin, and streptolysin S, an oxygen-stable hemolysin, which lyse erythrocytes and damage other cells such as myocardial cells. Streptolysin O is antigenic, while streptolysin S is not. GABHS also produce three erythrogenic or pyrogenic toxins (A, B, and C) whose activity is similar to that of bacterial endotoxin. Other agents of significance include exotoxin A, which may be associated with toxic shock syndrome, and bacteriocins, which destroy other gram-positive organisms. Spread of infection may be facilitated by a variety of enzymes elaborated by GABHS that attack fibrin and hyaluronic acid.

Clinical Features

Signs and symptoms of GABHS pharyngotonsillitis vary from mild sore throat and malaise (30–50% of cases) to high fever, nausea and vomiting, and dehydration (10%) (Kaplan, 1992). The disorder is acute in onset, usually characterized by high fever, odynophagia, headache, and abdominal pain. The mucosal surfaces of the pharynx and tonsillar fossae are typically erythematous and occasionally edematous, with exudate present in 50–90% of cases. Cervical adenopathy is also common, seen in 30–60% of cases. Most patients spontaneously improve in 3–5 days, unless otitis media, sinusitis, or peritonsillar abscess occur as secondary illnesses.

Sequelae

The risk of rheumatic fever following GABHS infection of the pharynx is approximately 0.3% in endemic situations and 3% under epidemic circumstances (Kaplan, 1992). A single episode of rheumatic fever places an individual at high risk for recurrence following additional episodes of GABHS pharyngitis (Kaplan, 1992). Acute glomerulonephritis occurs as a sequela in 10–15% of those infected with nephritogenic strains (Kaplan, 1992). In patients who develop these sequelae, there is usually a latent period of 1–3 weeks.

The Carrier State

Carriers of GABHS are individuals who demonstrate a positive culture for the organism but no rise in antistreptolysin O (ASO) convalescent titer. This condition is not associated with particular subtypes of the organism, although there is a high posttreatment concentration of penicillinase-producing organisms. There are no pharyngeal conditions that are specific to the carrier state. The prevalence of GABHS carriers has been estimated at 10–50%; however this figure may be overestimated due to the use of antibiotics that interfere with the rise in ASO titer.

Carriers appear to be at little risk to transmit GABHS or to develop sequelae of the disease. It is unknown whether these individuals are at increased risk for recurrent pharyngitis. The importance of this condition is in the diagnosis of true acute streptococcal pharyngitis; when this disorder must be distinguished from nonstreptococcal disease in a carrier, a convalescent ASO titer should be considered.

Diagnosis

Early diagnosis of streptococcal pharyngitis has been a priority in management of the disease, primarily due to the risk of renal and cardiac sequelae. A number of authors have studied the predictive value of various combinations of signs and symptoms in an effort to distinguish streptococcal from nonstreptococcal pharyngitis; however, none of these has been particularly reliable (Kaplan, 1992). Taken together, these studies demonstrate a false negative rate of about 50% and a false positive rate of 75% (Kline & Runge, 1994). Adenopathy, fever, and pharyngeal exudate have the highest predictive value for a positive culture. Rise in ASO titer, and absence of these findings in the presence of cough, rhinorrhea, hoarseness, or conjunctivitis, most reliably predicts a negative culture or a positive culture without rise in ASO (Kline et al., 1994).

Although the cost-effectiveness of throat culture has been questioned (Tompkins, Burnes, & Cable, 1977), most clinicians still advocate this procedure as the gold standard to determine appropriate treatment for GABHS. However, the tonsils, tonsillar crypts, or posterior pharyngeal wall must be swabbed for greatest accuracy. The decision whether to treat pending culture results or to delay treatment until the results are available remains controversial, although some studies suggest that early treatment hastens the clinical response to antibiotics (Randolph, Gerber, DeMeo, & Wright, 1985).

In the mid-1980s, tests for rapid detection of the group-specific carbohydrate became available. Such assays have simplified the decision to treat at the time of the office visit and have eliminated the need for additional postvisit communication. However, while these tests have demonstrated a specificity of greater than 90%, their sensitivity is generally in the 60–90% range. As a result, many clinicians advocate throat culture for children with suspected streptococcal disease and negative rapid strep tests. Rapid antigen detection is usually more expensive than throat culture, and this technique must still be interpreted with care, given the high incidence of posttreatment carriers. Studies also suggest a "learning curve effect" associated with this diagnostic modality.

Serologic tests for ASO are recognized as the definitive means for diagnosing acute streptococcal infection. A positive test is defined as a twofold dilution increase in titer between acute and convalescent serum, or any single value above 333 Todd units in children (Kline et al., 1994). Response to treatment does not predict a rise in antibody titer (Kline et al., 1994).

Treatment

Although most upper respiratory infections by GABHS resolve without treatment, studies suggest that antimicrobial therapy prevents suppurative and nonsuppurative sequelae including rheumatic fever, and may also hasten clinical improvement. Treatment is therefore indicated for all patients with positive rapid tests for the group A antigen. When the test is negative or not available, one may treat empirically for a full course, assuming the test was falsely negative or that another penicillin-sensitive organism may be the etiology, or for a few days while formal throat cultures are incubating. Given the low sensitivity of rapid strep testing, a decision not to treat based on a negative test may not be the best choice.

GABHS is sensitive to a number of antibiotics, however penicillin remains the drug of choice in nearly all cases. To date, no strains of GABHS acquired *in vivo* have demonstrated penicillin resistance *in vitro*. During the 1980s, several authors reported a decrease in bacteriologic control rates, attributed primarily to inoculum effects and to increased tolerance to penicillin. However, relapses and failure to eradicate were not associated with significant symptomatology or with suppurative or nonsuppurative sequelae. In addition, a 1993 metaanalysis found no increase in the bacteriologic failure rate with penicillin over the last 40 years (Markowitz, Gerber, & Kaplan, 1993).

Depot benzathine penicillin G is still advocated by the American Heart Association for primary treatment of GABHS pharyngitis; however, a 10-day course of penicillin administered orally is the most widely prescribed regimen. Twice daily dosing by the enteral route yields results similar to those obtained with four times a day dosing (Gerber, Spadaccini, Wright, Deutsch, & Kaplan, 1985). Courses of shorter duration are associated with bacteriologic relapse and are less efficacious in the prevention of rheumatic fever. When poor compliance is anticipated, azithromycin dosed once daily for 5 days may be a reasonable alternative. Erythromycin remains the drug of choice for patients with penicillin allergy.

Most patients with positive cultures following treatment are GABHS carriers; these individuals need not be retreated if their symptoms have resolved. For patients in whom complete bacteriologic clearance is desirable, such as those with a family member with a history of rheumatic fever, a course of clindamycin or a second course of penicillin combined with rifampin may yield increased success. In patients with recurrent symptoms, serotyping may aid in distinguishing bacterial persistence from recurrence. There are no data available regarding the use of antibiotic prophylaxis in these patients, and in such cases tonsillectomy may be most advantageous.

During antimicrobial therapy, patients must be carefully monitored for fluid intake, pain control, and impending suppurative complications such as peritonsillar abscess. Small children may become rapidly dehydrated, and may require hospitalization for intravenous administration of fluids intravenously.

Recurrent Pharyngotonsillitis and Tonsillectomy

Removal of the tonsils as prevention against infection has been a popular concept for decades. During the 1960s and 1970s, the procedure finally came under attack for its lack of scientific basis. A recent resurgence of interest in the procedure has resulted from a series of trials by Paradise and colleagues at the University of Pittsburgh supporting the use of tonsillectomy in cases of recurrent pharyngitis. However, the results of these studies must be interpreted with caution, and the procedure offered only to those patients who meet their strict entrance criteria.

The first two trials (Paradise et al., 1984) were parallel studies with identical design, except that assignment to surgical or nonsurgical treatment was random in one and according to parental preference in the other. Throat infection was defined to include one of the following features: temperature greater than 38.5° C, cervical adenopathy greater than 1 cm, tonsillar exudate, or positive culture for GABHS. No other attempt was made to determine the etiology of the infection. Patients were entered into the study if they had physician documentation of seven episodes in 1 year, five episodes per year for 2 years, or three episodes per year for 3 years. Tonsillectomized patients in the trial with random assignment had 1.85, 1.05, and 0.43 fewer episodes of throat infection than did control patients for each of the first 3 postoperative years, respectively. Those in the parallel nonrandom trial had 1.32, 1.32, and 1.58 fewer episodes. In each trial, the differences were statistically significant in the first 2 years. However, the mean rate of infection in the control groups in both trials during the first 3 years of the study dropped to only two to three episodes per year. Based on these studies, one may conclude that tonsillectomy offers a definite, albeit small, advantage in the treatment of severely affected children in whom a pattern of recurrent pharyngotonsillitis has been well documented. The authors themselves state, however, that a decision whether or not to perform tonsillectomy should consider risks, preferences, and anxieties of parent and child; school absences due to illness; accessibility to health care services; cost; and availability of surgical facilities.

In a third trial, Paradise and colleagues established three arms, in which the entrance criteria from the first two studies were relaxed for frequency, severity, or documentation, respectively (Paradise et al., 1992). In this study, control subjects developed less than one episode of moderate or severe pharyngitis per year. The authors concluded that surgery was not justifiable under these circumstances.

Infectious Mononucleosis

Pharyngitis is one of the hallmarks of infectious mononucleosis, a disorder associated with primary infection by EBV. A member of the herpes virus family, this virus was initially discovered by workers studying cells cultured from patients with Burkitt's lymphoma (Epstein, Achong, & Barr, 1964). The development of infectious mononucleosis in one of these individuals subsequently led to a series of studies definitively linking the disease with seroconversion to EBV antigens (Evans, Niederman, & McCollum, 1968; Niederman, McCollum, Henle, & Henle, 1968)

Epidemiology

Among populations studied around the world, serologic reactivity to EBV antigens has been demonstrated in 80–95% of adults (Henle & Henle, 1980). However, although primary infection by EBV occurs during the second and third decade in developed nations and regions of high socioeconomic status, young children are more commonly affected in developing countries and regions of low socioeconomic status. When the virus is acquired at a younger age, symptoms are generally less severe. The incidence of infectious mononucleosis in the United States is approximately 1 in 50–100,000 per year, but increases to about 100 in 100,000 among adolescents and young adults (Plotkin, 1992). Infected individuals transmit EBV by way of saliva exchanged during kissing or other close contact.

Pathogenesis

EBV preferentially infects and transforms human B-lymphocytes. The virus enters the cell by attaching to a receptor designed for proteins of the complement chain, and its genetic material is transported by vesicles to the nucleus, where it dwells as a plasmid and maintains a "latent" state of replication.

An incubation period of 2–7 weeks follows initial exposure, during which EBV induces a proliferation of infected B-cells. This process is subsequently countered by a potent cellular immune response, characterized by the appearance of atypical lymphocytes (most likely T-lymphocytes responding to the B-cell infection) in the blood. The number of infected circulating B-cells is reduced during this 4–6 week period from approximately 1:100 to 1:1,000,000.

Clinical Features and Diagnosis

Infectious mononucleosis is characterized by a prodrome of malaise and fatigue, followed by the acute onset of fever and sore throat. Physical examination typically reveals enlarged, erythematous palatine tonsils, in most cases with yellow-white exudate on the surface and within the crypts (Figure 6–14A). Cervical adenopathy is present in nearly all patients (Figure 6–14B), and involvement of the posterior cervical nodes often helps distinguish EBV infection from that by streptococcus or other organisms. Between the 2nd and 4th weeks of illness, approximately 50% of patients de-

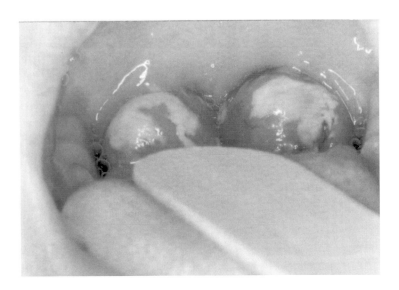

A

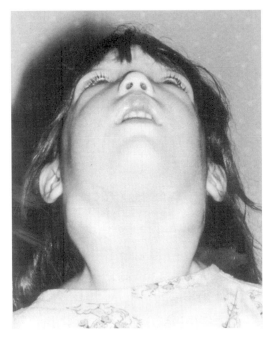

B

Figure 6–14. Tonsillar swelling, erythema, and exudate (**A**) and massive lymphadenopathy (**B**) due to infectious mononucleosis. (Photos courtesy of Dr. Craig Derkay)

velop splenomegaly, and 30–50% develop hepatomegaly (Sumaya, 1992). Rash, palatal petechiae, and abdominal pain may also be present in some cases. The fever and pharyngitis generally subside within about 2 weeks, while adenopathy, organomegaly, and malaise may last as long as 6 weeks.

Diagnosis of infectious mononucleosis can usually be made on the basis of clinical presentation, absolute lymphocytosis, the presence of atypical lymphocytes in the peripheral smear, and detection of Paul-Bunnell heterophil antibodies. The latter is the basis of the Mono-Spot, Mono-Diff, and Mono-Test assays, which test for agglutination of horse erythrocytes. Children under 5 years of age may not develop a detectable heterophil antibody titer; in these patients, it is possible to determine titers of IgG antibodies to the viral capsid antigen, as well as antibodies to the "early antigen" complex. Antibodies to EBV nuclear antigen appear late in the course of the disease.

Treatment

In most cases, rest, fluids, and analgesics are adequate to manage the symptoms of infectious mononucleosis. In more symptomatic patients, particularly those with respiratory compromise due to severe tonsillar enlargement and those with hematologic or neurologic complications, a course of systemic steroids may hasten resolution of the acute symptoms. Placement of a nasopharyngeal trumpet or endotracheal intubation may be necessary on rare occasions when complete air-

way obstruction is imminent. Antibiotics may be useful in cases of concomitant group A beta-hemolytic pharyngotonsillitis; however, ampicillin use is known to induce a rash in this setting.

The use of antiviral agents in infectious mononucleosis has yielded disappointing results. In clinical trials, acyclovir reduced viral shedding in the pharynx but demonstrated little efficacy in the treatment of symptoms (Andersson et al., 1986; van der Horst et al., 1991). Other agents have exhibited greater *in vitro* effect than acyclovir but have yet to be tested clinically (Sumaya, 1992).

Other Bacterial and Viral Infections

Gonorrhea

Infection by *Neisseria gonorrhea* is a rare source of pharyngitis in children, occurring almost exclusively among those who are sexually abused. In one series of such children, oropharyngeal gonorrhea was reported in 4–6% (White, Loda, Ingram, & Pearson, 1983), while another reported pharyngeal involvement in 3 of 11 children infected by sexual abuse (De Jong, 1986).

Gonococcal pharyngitis most commonly presents as an exudative pharyngitis accompanied by fever and adenopathy, not unlike that associated with a number of other organisms. The physician must therefore remain cognizant of other possible manifestations of gonococcal infection, and of signs and symptoms of other sexually transmitted diseases. Cultures should be obtained to confirm the diagnosis in suspicious cases, and to direct antibiotic therapy.

In most cases, gonococcal pharyngitis may be adequately treated with a single parenteral administration of ceftriaxone, although some physicians prefer to continue the injections daily for 7 to 10 days. Treatment should also be offered to the offending individual, and the infections must be reported to the appropriate local and national authorities.

Diphtheria

Diphtheria pharyngitis, caused by the gram-positive bacillus *Corynebacterium diphtheria*, remains a rare but serious cause of airway obstruction in children. This disorder frequently progresses to involve the larynx and trachea, and is therefore addressed in more detail in Chapter 7 of this volume.

Idiopathic and Other Causes

Kawasaki Disease (Mucocutaneous Lymph Node Syndrome)

Kawasaki disease (KD) is a disorder of unknown etiology characterized by fever, rash, pharyngitis, conjunctival inflammation, edema of the extremities, and cervical adenopathy. Initially reported in the Japanese literature in 1967 as a benign disorder of childhood, KD has been linked over the last three decades to serious cardiac complications, arthritis, and a number of other manifestations.

Epidemiology and Pathogenesis

KD is a disease of young children, with 80% of cases occurring in children less than 5 years of age (American Academy of Pediatrics, 1994). Fatalities are most common during infancy. The disease is slightly more common in males and among individuals of Asian extraction. Between 2000 and 4000 cases occur annually in the United States of America (American Academy of Pediatrics, 1994).

Most investigators believe KD to be the result of an infectious agent or an immune response to an infectious agent. A number of organisms have been implicated, but none is yet confirmed as the definitive cause. Epidemic occurrence of KD supports the theory of an infectious etiology, and has been reported in several countries with most outbreaks observed during the winter and spring months. The mode of transmission is not known.

Clinical Features and Diagnosis

KD occurs in three distinct clinical phases. The acute phase lasts 1 to 2 weeks, and is characterized by prolonged high spiking fever, oral and oropharyngeal changes (see below), rash, erythema of the bulbar conjunctiva, swelling and erythema of the extremities, and adenopathy. Each of these findings is observed in over 90% of patients, except for adenopathy >1.5 cm which is seen in 50–75% (Rowley & Shulman, 1995). In the subacute phase, days 10–25, most of these signs and symptoms resolve; however, conjunctival changes usually persist and the child remains irritable. The toes and fingers begin to desquamate and joint pain is present in about 30% of patients. Cardiac dysfunction, including coronary arteritis, vascular dilatation and aneurysm formation, myocarditis, arrhythmia, and coronary insufficiency, typically become evident during this period, affecting about 20% of patients. The third or convalescent stage begins when clinical signs of KD have completely resolved and ends when the sedimentation rate returns to normal. KD disease may also be associated with sterile pyuria, aseptic meningitis, hepatic dysfunction, distension of the gallbladder, diarrhea, uveitis, otitis media, and pneumonitis.

Diagnosis of KD is based on the clinical presentation. Patients must have a history of persistent fever, as well as four of the five other acute signs listed above. Laboratory evaluation is nonspecific; however, elevation of the sedimentation rate in the acute phase aids in excluding other etiologies, and thrombocytosis and anemia are common in the subacute phase.

KD in the Mouth and Pharynx

The oral cavity and oropharynx are both commonly involved in KD. The lips are usually swollen, fissured, and bleeding. The appearance of "strawberry tongue" resulting from diffuse erythema and prominent papillae is also common. The oropharyngeal mucosa is erythematous; however, there is not usually evidence of abscess, exudate, or ulceration.

Treatment

Therapy for KD in the acute phase is directed at prevention of cardiac complications. High-dose aspirin is usually administered with a watchful eye for signs of Reye's syndrome to decrease myocardial inflammation and prevent thrombosis. Addition of intravenous immune globulin (IVIG) to the protocol results in a more rapid anti-inflammatory effect than that seen with aspirin alone. IVIG also appears to lessen the risk of long-term coronary artery abnormalities. Other manifestations of KD are treated symptomatically. Once the convalescent phase is reached, patients are generally monitored at regular intervals for evidence of cardiac complications.

No specific therapy for the oral and oropharyngeal manifestations is necessary, although use of anesthetic and antacid mouthwashes may alleviate odynophagia. Lubrication of the lips may reduce fissuring and bleeding. Systemic antibiotic are indicated only if the diagnosis remains in doubt.

References

Advisory Council on Immunization Practices. (1995). Varicella vaccine recommendations. *Immunization Action News, 2,* 1.

American Academy of Pediatrics. (1994). Kawasaki disease. In G. Peter (Ed.), *1994 Red book: Report of the committee on infectious diseases.* (23rd ed., pp. 284–287). Elk Grove Village, IL: American Academy of Pediatrics.

Andersson, J., Britton, S., Ernberg, I., Andersson, U., Henle W., Skoldenberg B., & Tisell, A. (1986). Effect of acyclovir on infectious mononucleosis: A double-blind, placebo controlled study. *Journal of Infectious Diseases, 153,* 283–290.

Asano, Y., Suga, S., Yoshikawa, T., Kobayashi, I., Yazaki, T., Shibata, M., Tsuzuki, K., & Ito, S. (1994). Experience and reason: twenty year follow-up of protective immunity of the Oka strain live varicella vaccine. *Pediatrics, 94,* 524–526.

Axell, T., & Henricsson, V. (1985). Association between recurrent aphthous ulcers and tobacco habits. *Scandinavian Journal of Dental Research, 93,* 239–242.

Bernstein, M. L., & McDonald, J.S. (1978). Oral lesions in Crohn's disease: Report of two cases and update. *Oral Surgery, Oral Medicine, Oral Pathology, 46,* 234–245.

Brice, S. L., Huff, J. C., & Weston, W. L. (1991). Erythema multiforme minor in children. *Pediatrician, 18,* 188–194.

Brightman, V. J. (1994a). Sexually transmitted and bloodborne infections. In M. A. Lynch, V. J. Brightman, & M. S. Greenberg (Eds.), *Burket's oral medicine—diagnosis and treatment* (9th ed., pp. 629–725). Philadelphia: J. B. Lippincott.

Brightman, V. J. (1994b). Diseases of the tongue. In M. A. Lynch, V. J. Brightman, & M. S. Greenberg (Eds.). *Burket's oral medicine—diagnosis and treatment* (9th ed., pp. 240–298). Philadelphia: J. B. Lippincott.

Brown, R. S., & Bottomley, W. K. (1990). Combination immunosuppressant and topical steroid therapy for treatment of recurrent major aphthae. *Oral Surgery, Oral Medicine, Oral Pathology, 69,* 42–44.

Cherry, J. D. (1992a). Herpangina. In R. L. Feigin & J. D. Cherry (Eds.), *Textbook of pediatric infectious diseases* (3rd ed., pp. 230–231). Philadelphia: W. B. Saunders.

Cherry, J. D. (1992b). Pharyngitis. In R. D. Feigin & J. D. Cherry (Eds.), *Textbook of pediatric infectious diseases* (3rd ed., pp. 1705–1753). Philadelphia: W. B. Saunders.

Cherry, J. D. (1992c). Enteroviruses: Poliovirus, coxsackie viruses, echovirus, and enterovirus. In R. D. Feigin & J. D. Cherry (Eds.), *Textbook of pediatric infectious diseases* (3rd ed., pp. 159–166). Philadelphia: W. B. Saunders.

Cox, A. J. III, & Eisenbeis, J. F. (1997). Ingestion of caustic hair relaxer: is endoscopy necessary? *Laryngoscope, 107,* 897–902.

Cubie, H. S., Felix, D. H., Southam, J. C., & Wray, D. (1991). Application of molecular techniques in the rapid diagnosis of EBV-associated oral hairy leukoplakia. *Journal of Oral Pathology and Medicine, 20,* 271–274.

DeJong, A. R. (1986). Sexually transmitted diseases in sexually abused children. *Sexually Transmitted Diseases, 13,* 123–126.

Dunkle, L. M., Arvin, A. M., Whitley, R. J., Rotbart, H. A., Feder, H. M. Jr., Feldman, S., Gershon, A. A., Levy, M. L., Hayden, G. F., & McGuirt, P. V. (1991). A controlled trial of acyclovir for chickenpox in normal children. *New England Journal of Medicine, 325,* 1539–1544.

Eisen, D., & Ellis, C. N. (1990). Topical cyclosporin for oral mucosal disorders. *Journal of the American Academy of Dermatology, 23,* 1259–1263.

Epstein, M. A., Achong, B. G., & Barr, Y. M. (1964). Virus particles in cultured lymphoblasts from Burkitt's lymphoma. *Lancet, 1,* 702–703.

Evans, A. S., Niederman, J. C., & McCollum, R. W. (1968). Seroepidemiologic studies of infectious mononucleosis with EB virus. *New England Journal of Medicine, 129,* 1121–1127.

Fenerli, A., Papanicolaou, S., Papanicolaou, M., & Laskaris, G. (1993). Histocompatibility antigens and geographic tongue. *Oral Surgery, Oral Medicine, Oral Pathology, 76,* 476–479.

Fernandez, J. F., Benito, M. A., Lizaldez, E. B., & Montanes, M. A. (1990). Oral hairy leukoplakia: a histopathologic study of 32 cases. *American Journal of Dermatopathology, 12,* 571–578.

Field, E. A., Brookes, V., & Tyldesley, W. R. (1992). Recurrent aphthous ulceration in children: a review. *International Journal of Pediatric Dentistry, 2,* 1–10.

Gallina, G., Cumbo, V., Messina, P., & Caruso, C. (1985). HLA-A, B, C, DR, MT, and MB antigens in recurrent aphthous stomatitis. *Oral Surgery, Oral Medicine, Oral Pathology, 59,* 364–370.

Gerber, M. A. (1996). Antibiotic resistance: relationship to persistence of group A streptococci in the upper respiratory tract. *Pediatrics, 97,* 971–975.

Gerber, M. A., Spadaccini, L. J., Wright, L. L., Deutsch, L., & Kaplan, E. L. (1985). Twice-daily penicillin the treatment of streptococcal pharyngitis. *American Journal of Diseases of Children, 139,* 1145–1148.

Greenberg, M. S. (1994a). Ulcerative, vesicular, and bullous lesions. In M. A. Lynch, V. J. Brightman, & M. S. Greenberg (Eds.), *Burket's oral medicine—diagnosis and treatment,* (9th ed., pp. 11–50). Philadelphia: J. B. Lippincott.

Greenberg, M. S. (1994b). Immunologic diseases. In M. A. Lynch, V. J. Brightman, & M. S. Greenberg (Eds.), *Burket's oral medicine—diagnosis and treatment,* (pp. 563–591). Philadelphia: J. B. Lippincott.

Greenberg, M. S., & Garfunkel, A. (1994). In M. A. Lynch, V. J. Brightman & M. S. Greenberg (Eds.), *Burket's oral medicine—diagnosis and treatment,* (pp. 510–543). Philadelphia: J. B. Lippincott.

Greenspan, D., & Greenspan, J. S. (1992). Significance of oral hairy leukoplakia. *Oral Surgery, Oral Medicine, Oral Pathology, 73,* 151–154.

Helfman, R. J. (1979). The treatment of geographic tongue with topical Retin-A solution. *Cutis, 24,* 179–180.

Hengerer, A. S., DeGroot, T. R., Rivers, R. J. Jr., & Pettee, D. S. (1984). Internal carotid artery thrombosis following soft palate injuries: a case report and review of 16 cases. *Laryngoscope, 94,* 1571–1575.

Henle, W., & Henle, G. (1980). Epidemiologic aspects of Epstein-Barr virus (EBV)-associated diseases. *Annals of the New York Academy of Sciences, 354,* 326–331.

Holinger, L. D. (1997). Caustic ingestion, esophageal injury, and stricture. In L. D. Holinger, R. P. Lusk, & C. G. Green (Eds.), *Pediatric laryngology and bronchoesophagology* (pp. 295–303). Philadelphia: Lippincott-Raven Co.

Huff, J. C., Weston, W. L., & Tonnesen, M. G., (1983). Erythema multiforme: a critical review of characteristics, diagnostic criteria, and causes. *Journal of the American Academy of Dermatology, 8,* 763–775.

Hughes, W. T. (1997). In R. D. Feigin & J. D. Cherry (Eds.), *Textbook of pediatric infectious diseases* (3rd ed., pp. 1907–1916). Philadelphia: W. B. Saunders.

Hutchinson, V. A., Angenend, J. L., Mok, W. L., Cummins, J. M., & Richards, A. B. (1990). Chronic recurrent aphthous stomatitis: Oral treatment with low dose interferon alpha. *Molecular Biotherapy, 2,* 160–164.

Juel-Jensen, B. E. (1973). Herpes simplex and zoster. *British Medical Journal, 1,* 406–410.

Kaplan, E. L. (1992). Group A streptococcal infections. In R. D. Feigin & J. D. Cherry (Eds.), *Textbook of pediatric infectious diseases* (3rd ed., pp. 1296–1305). Philadelphia: W. B. Saunders.

Katz, J., Langevitz, P., Shemer, J., Barak, S., & Livneh, A. (1994). Prevention of recurrent aphthous stomatitis with colchicine: An open trial. *Journal of the American Academy of Dermatology, 31,* 459–461.

Kline, J. A. & Runge, J. W. (1994). Streptococcal pharyngitis: A review of pathophysiology, diagnosis, and management. *Journal of Emergency Medicine, 12,* 665–680.

Kline, M. W. (1996). Oral manifestations of pediatric immunodeficiency virus infection: A review of the literature. *Pediatrics, 97,* 380–388.

Kohl, S. (1992). Postnatal herpes simplex virus infection. In R. D. Feigin & J. D. Cherry (Eds.). *Textbook of pediatric infectious diseases,* (3rd ed., pp. 1558–1583). Philadelphia: W. B. Saunders.

Kohl, S. (1994). Herpes simplex virus infection—the neonate to the adolescent. *Israel Journal of Medical Sciences, 30,* 392–398.

Langford, A., Kunze, R., Timm, H., Ruf, B., & Reichart, P. (1990). Cytomegalovirus associated oral ulcerations in HIV-infected patients. *Journal of Oral Pathology and Medicine, 19,* 71–76.

Lieu, T. A., Cochi, S. L., Black, S. B., Halloran, M. E., Shinefield, H. R., Holmes, S. J., Wharton, M., & Washington, A. E. (1994). Cost-effectiveness of a routine varicella vaccination program for US children. *JAMA, 271,* 375–381.

Loesche, W. J., Syed, S. A., Laughon, B. E., & Stoll, J. (1982). The bacteriology of acute necrotizing ulcerative gingivitis. *Journal of Periodontology, 53,* 223–230.

Manzella, J. P., McConville, J. H., Valenti, W., Menegus, M. A., Swierkosz, E. M., & Arens, M. (1984). An outbreak of herpes simplex virus type 1 gingivostomatitis in a dental hygiene practice. *JAMA, 252,* 2019–2022.

Markowitz, M., Gerber, M. A., & Kaplan, E. L. (1993). Treatment of streptococcal pharyngotonsillitis: reports of penicillin's demise are premature. *Journal of Pediatrics, 123,* 679–685.

Markowitz, M. (1994). Changing epidemiology of group A streptococcal infections. *Pediatric Infectious Disease Journal, 13,* 557–560.

Marks, R., & Czarny, D. (1984). Geographic tongue: sensitivity to the environment. *Oral Surgery, Oral Medicine, Oral Pathology, 58,* 156–159.

Moniaci, D., Greco, D., Flecchia, G., Raiteri, R., & Sinicco, A. (1990). Epidemiology, clinical features, and prognostic value of HIV-1 related oral lesions. *Journal of Oral Pathology and Medicine, 19,* 477–481.

Nahmias, A. J., Alford, C. A., & Korones, S. B. (1970). Infection of the newborn with herpes virus hominis. *Advances in Pediatrics, 17,* 185–226.

Niederman, J. C., McCollum, R. W., Henle, G., & Henle, W. (1968). Infectious mononucleosis: clinical manifestations in relation to EB virus antibodies. *JAMA, 203,* 205–209.

Paradise, J. L., Bluestone, C. D., Bachman, R. Z., Colborn, D. K., Bernard, B. S., Taylor, F. H., Rogers, K. D., Schwarzbach, R. H., Stool, S. E., & Friday, G. A. (1984). Efficacy of tonsillectomy for recurrent throat infection in severely affected children. *New England Journal of Medicine, 310,* 674–683.

Paradise, J. L., Bluestone, C. D., Rogers, K. D., Taylor, F. H., Colborn, D. K., Bernard, B. S., & Bachman, R. Z. (1992). Comparative efficacy of tonsillectomy for recurrent throat infection in more vs. less severely affected children. *Pediatric Research, 31,* 126A.

Pedersen, A. (1992). Acyclovir in the prevention of severe aphthous ulcers. *Archives of Dermatology, 128,* 119–20.

Pizarro, A., Navarro, A., Fonseca, E., Vidaurrazaga, C., & Herranz, P. (1995). Treatment of recurrent stomatitis with pentoxifylline. *British Journal of Dermatology, 133,* 659–660.

Plotkin, S. A. (1992). Infectious mononucleosis. In R. E. Behrman, R. M. Kliegman, & W. E. Nelson (Eds.), *Nelson's textbook of pediatrics,* (14th ed., (pp. 805–808). Philadelphia: W. B. Saunders.

Prober, C. G., Kirk, L. E., & Keeney, R. E. (1982). Acyclovir therapy of chickenpox in immunocompromised children: a collaborative study. *Journal of Pediatrics, 101,* 622–625.

Rabinowitz, L. G., & Esterly, N. B. (1993). Inflammatory bullous diseases in children. *Dermatology Clinics, 11,* 565–581.

Raborn, G. W., for the Penciclovir Topical Collaborative Study Group. (1996). Penciclovir cream for recurrent herpes simplex labialis: an effective new treatment. Cited in Spruance, S. L., Rea, T. L., Thoming, C., Tucker, R., Saltzman, R., & Boon, R. Penciclovir cream for the treatment of herpes simplex labialis. *JAMA, 277,* 1374–1379.

Radkowski, D., McGill, T. J., Healy, G. B., & Jones, D. T. (1993). Penetrating trauma of the oropharynx in children. *Laryngoscope, 103,* 991–994.

Rakover, Y., Adar, H., Tal, I., Lang, Y., & Kedar, A. (1989). Behcet disease: Long-term follow-up of three children and review of the literature. *Pediatrics, 83,* 986–992.

Randolph, M. F., Gerber, M. A., DeMeo, K. K., & Wright, L. (1985). Effect of antibiotic therapy on the clinical course of streptococcal pharyngitis. *Journal of Pediatrics, 106,* 870–875.

Redman, R. S., Vance, F. L., Gorlin, R. J., Peagler, F. D., & Meskin, L. H. (1966). Psychological component in the etiology of geographic tongue. *Journal of Dental Research, 45,* 1403–1408.

Resnick, L., Herbst, J. S., Ablashi, D. V., Atherton, S., Frank, B., Rosen, L., & Horwitz, S. N. (1988). Regression of oral hairy leukoplakia after orally administered acyclovir therapy. *JAMA, 259,* 384–388.

Revuz, J., Guillaume, J. C., Janier, M., Hans, P., Marchand, C., Souteyrand, P., Bonnetblanc, J. M., Claudy, A., Dallac, S., & Klene, C. (1990). Crossover study of thalidomide vs. placebo in severe recurrent aphthous stomatitis. *Archives of Dermatology, 126,* 923–927.

Ross, A. H. (1962). Modification of chickenpox in family contacts by administration of gamma globulin. *New England Journal of Medicine, 267,* 369–376.

Rowley, A. H. & Shulman, S. T. (1995). Kawasaki syndrome. In H. B. Jenson & R. S. Baltimore (Eds.), *Pediatric infectious diseases: principles and practice* (pp. 629–638). Norwalk, CT: Appleton and Lange.

Saral, R., Burns, W. H., Laskin, O. L., Santos, G. W., & Lietman, P. S. (1981). Acyclovir prophylaxis of herpes-simplex-virus infections: A randomized, double-blind, controlled trial in bone-marrow-transplant recipients. *New England Journal of Medicine, 305,* 63–67.

Saxen, M. A., Ambrosius, W. T., Rehemtula, al-K. F., Russell, A. L., & Eckert, G. J. (1997). Sustained relief of oral aphthous ulcer pain from topical diclofenac in hyaluronan. *Oral Surgery, Oral Medicine, Oral Pathology, Oral Radiology, and Endodontics, 84,* 356–361.

Schoem, S. R., Choi, S. S., Zalzal, G. H., & Grundfast, K. M. (1997). Management of oropharyngeal trauma in children. *Archives of Otolaryngology—Head and Neck Surgery, 123,* 1267–1270.

Schofer, H., Ochsendorf, F. R., Helm, E. B., & Milbradt, R. (1987). Treatment of oral hairy leukoplakia in AIDS patients with vitamin A acid (topically) or acyclovir (systemically). *Dermatologica, 174,* 150–151.

Shepp, D. H., Dandliker, P. S., & Meyers, J. D. (1986). Treatment of varicella-zoster virus infection in severely immunocompromised patients: A randomized comparison of acyclovir and vidarabine. *New England Journal of Medicine, 314,* 208–212.

Ship, I. I. (1972). Epidemiologic aspects of recurrent aphthous ulcerations. *Oral Surgery, Oral Medicine, Oral Pathology, 33,* 400–406.

Ship, J. A. (1996). Recurrent aphthous stomatitis: An update. *Oral Surgery, Oral Medicine, Oral Pathology, Oral Radiology, and Endodontics, 81,* 141–147.

Spruance, S. L., Rea, T. L., Thoming, C., Tucker, R., Saltzman, R. & Boon, R. (1997). Penciclovir cream for the treatment of herpes simplex labialis. *JAMA, 277,* 1374–1379.

Spruance, S. L., Schnipper, L. E., Overall, J. C. Jr., Kern, E. R., Wester, B., Modlin, J., Wenerstrom, G., Burton, C., Arndt, K. A., Chiu, G. L., & Crumpacker, C. S. (1982). Treatment of herpes simplex labialis with topical acyclovir in polyethylene glycol. *Journal of Infectious Diseases, 146,* 85–90.

Spruance, S. L., Stewart, J. C., Rowe, N. H., McKeough, M. B., Wenerstrom, G., & Freeman, D. J. (1990). Treatment of recurrent herpes simplex labialis with oral acyclovir. *Journal of Infectious Diseases, 161,* 185–190.

Sumaya, C. V. (1992). Epstein-Barr virus. In R. D. Feigin & J. D. Cherry (Eds.), *Textbook of pediatric infectious diseases* (3rd ed., pp. 1547–1557). Philadelphia: W. B. Saunders.

Taylor, L. J., Walker, D. M., & Bagg, J. (1993). A clinical trial of prostaglandin E2 in recurrent aphthous ulceration. *British Dental Journal, 175,* 125–129.

Tompkins, R. K., Burnes, D. C., & Cable, W. E. (1977). An analysis of the cost-effectiveness of pharyngitis management and acute rheumatic fever prevention. *Annals of Internal Medicine, 86,* 481–492.

Ueta, E., Osaki, T., Yoneda, K., Yamamoto, T., & Kato, I. (1994). A clinical trial of azelastine in recurrent aphthous ulceration, with an analysis of its actions on leukocytes. *Journal of Oral Pathology and Medicine, 23,* 123–129.

van der Horst, C., Joncas, J., Ahronheim, G., Gustafson, N., Stein, G., Gurwith, M., Fleisher, G., Sullivan, J., Sixbey, J., & Roland, S. (1991). Lack of effect of peroral acyclovir for the treatment of acute infectious mononucleosis. *Journal of Infectious Diseases, 164,* 788–792.

Wade, J. C., Newton, B., Flournoy, N., & Meyers, J. D. (1984). Oral acyclovir for prevention of herpes simplex virus reactivation after marrow transplantation. *Annals of Internal Medicine, 100,* 823–838.

Wahba-Yahav, A. V. (1995). Pentoxiphylline in intractable aphthous stomatitis: An open trial. *Journal of the American Academy of Dermatology, 33,* 680–682.

Weibel, R. E., Neff, B. J., Kuter, B. J., Guess, H. A., Rothenberger, C. A., Fitzgerald, A. J., Connor, K. A., McLean, A. A., Hilleman, M. R., & Buynak, E. B. (1984). Live attenuated varicella virus vaccine, *New England Journal of Medicine, 310,* 1409–1415.

White, C. J., Kuter, B. J., Hildebrand, C. S., Isganitis, K. L., Matthews, H., Miller, W. J., Provost, P. J., Ellis, R. W., Gerety, R. J., & Calandra, G. B. (1991). Varicella vaccine (Varivax) in healthy children and adolescents: Results from clinical trials, 1987–1989. *Pediatrics, 87,* 604–610.

White, S. T., Loda, F. A., Ingram, D. L., & Pearson, A. (1983). Sexually transmitted diseases in sexually abused children. *Pediatrics, 72,* 16–21.

Wormser, G. P., Mack, L., Lenox, T., Hewlett, D., Goldfarb, J., Yarrish, R. L. & Reitano, M. (1988). Lack of effect of oral acyclovir on the prevention of aphthous stomatitis. *Otolaryngology Head and Neck Surgery, 98,* 14–17.

Wu, E., Sayre, J., Wiesmeier, E., Bernstein, D., Visscher, B., & Bryson, Y. (1984). A prospective seroepidemiological survey of herpes simplex (HSV) infections in a college population. *Pediatric Research, 18,* 289A.

7

Infectious and Inflammatory Illness of the Larynx, Trachea, and Bronchi

David H. Darrow, M.D., D.D.S.,
and Gregory C. Zwack, M.D.

Infectious and inflammatory diseases in children frequently involve one or more components of the airway. When such illnesses cause even mild swelling, respiratory distress may result and rapidly progress to complete obstruction. As a result, rapid recognition of the disorder is imperative, and prompt institution of therapy may spare the child significant morbidity or mortality.

HISTORY

Prior to the 20th century, diphtheria infection was most often implicated as the cause of infection in the airway, and nearly all cases ended fatally. As techniques of examination improved, however, other disorders were identified in which physical findings differed from those of diphtheritic croup. Mainwaring [cited in Wurtele 1992] in 1791 presented the first unequivocal description of epiglottitis, in which the epiglottis was found on transoral examination to be "thickened and standing erect." He stated, "this disease had a strong resemblance to croup, but it is still to be considered as different from it." In 1928, Baum first described laryngotracheobronchitis as a separate entity using the term "croup," and proposed an underlying viral etiology. Tracheitis due to organisms other than diphtheria, *Haemophilus influenzae* type b (Hib), and viruses was initially reported in the early 1940s but downplayed (Rabe, 1948a, 1948b, 1948c) until 1979, when Han, Dunbar, and Striker and Jones, Santos, and Overall reported two series of cases.

Early treatment for disorders of the airway included bloodletting, leeches, and topical herbs and ointments (Stool, 1988). Although intubation and tracheotomy were recognized even by the ancients as potential life-saving procedures, their use had fallen into disfavor due to associated complications.

In the late 1800s, Joseph O'Dwyer, a New York physician, introduced an intubation system for cases of diphtheria laryngotracheitis (Stool, 1988), and with the addition of diphtheria antitoxin in the 1880s, the disease became survivable. By the early part of this century, tracheotomy had also become popular in managing cases of diphtheria, as the principles taught by surgeons such as Chevalier Jackson brought the risk of complications down to acceptable levels. The advent of diphtheria immunization in 1924 ushered in a new era in the treatment of inflammatory airway disease, as the incidence of diphtheria declined precipitously and emphasis shifted to diseases of other etiologies.

The treatment of epiglottitis was advanced by the first report of this disease in a child in 1926 (Daily & Allen, cited in Wurtele 1992), and by the report of epiglottitis associated with *H. influenzae* bacteremia in 1936 (Lemiere, cited in Wurtele 1992). These reports were followed by the landmark paper of Sinclair (1941) that described a series of 10 children with acute laryngitis associated with *H. influenzae* bacteremia. The 6 patients in the series who received sulfa antibiotics were the only to survive; 4 of the 6 survivors initially underwent tracheotomy to establish an airway.

Over the last 25 years, antibiotics have become the mainstay of therapy for bacterial infections of the pediatric airway, while supportive care is used in viral illnesses. Recent controversies in treatment have focused on the use of racemic epinephrine and steroids in viral croup and on the choice between intubation and tracheotomy in securing the airway in acute supraglottitis. These issues, as well as the development of late-generation antibiotics and the Hib vaccine, will be discussed in detail.

CLASSIFICATION

A classification of inflammatory disorders of the pediatric airway is presented in Table 7–1. In the remainder of this chapter, we will consider individually the common infectious and inflammatory processes of the lower pediatric airway for which the otolaryngologist is commonly consulted. The interested reader is referred to other sources for a more complete discussion of tracheobronchial foreign bodies, bronchitis, caustic ingestion, and intubation trauma of the larynx and trachea.

VIRAL CROUP (LARYNGITIS, LARYNGOTRACHEITIS, LARYNGOTRACHEOBRONCHITIS)

Viral croup refers to a group of viral infections that may affect any or all segments of the pediatric airway. This disorder is usually accompanied by low-grade fever, hoarseness, and barky cough with mild stridor. Croup is the most common illness affecting the airway in children and is the most common cause of airway obstruction in children.

Epidemiology

The incidence of viral croup over all ages has been estimated at 1–2% (Denny et al., 1983). Three to 5% of children have at least one episode of croup (Denny et al., 1983; Walker & Crysdale, 1992), and the disease will recur in 5% of these cases (Walker & Crysdale 1992). Most authors cite a peak incidence of the disease in the late fall and early winter months (Denny et al., 1983; Sendi, Crysdale, & Yoo, 1992; Skolnik, 1989). Boys are affected more commonly than girls, in a ratio of approximately 2:1 (Denny et al., 1983; Walker & Crysdale 1992). The majority of patients are between the ages of 6 months and 4 years, with few cases occurring after age 6 (Denny et al., 1983; Skolnik, 1989; Walker & Crysdale, 1992).

Etiology and Pathophysiology

Various organisms have been implicated in croup, each with a predilection for a specific portion of the airway. Laryngitis is most commonly associated with adenoviruses, particularly types 4 and 7, and with influenza virus types A and B (Cherry, 1992). Parainfluenza virus, rhinovirus, and respiratory syncytial virus are also seen. Laryngotracheitis and spasmodic croup are typically caused by parainfluenza virus types 1, 2, and 3; by respiratory syncytial virus; and by influenza virus type A, which causes the most severe symptomatology (Cherry, 1992). Laryngotracheobronchitis frequently begins as an extension of laryngotracheal infection by

Table 7–1. Classification of inflammatory disease of the pediatric airway.

Infectious
Viral croup
Laryngitis
Laryngotracheitis
Laryngotracheobronchitis
Spasmodic croup
Acute supraglottitis
Bacterial tracheitis (pseudomembranous croup, membranous laryngotracheobronchitis)
Diphtheria laryngotracheitis

Chemical
Gastroesophageal reflux
Caustic ingestion

Traumatic
Intubation trauma
Foreign body

Other
Angioedema

parainfluenza or influenza viruses, but is often complicated by secondary bacterial infection of the lower airways. The disorder is then more appropriately termed bacterial tracheitis, membranous laryngotracheobronchitis, or pseudomembranous croup, and will be discussed later in this chapter.

Other factors may predispose a child to develop croup. Cold temperatures and low humidity appear to correlate with an increase in admissions for croup (Fielder, 1989). Pollution (Sprem & Branica, 1993; Zach, 1990) and passive smoking (Salzman, Biller, & Schechter, 1987) have also been implicated, but definitive epidemiologic studies are lacking. Patients with a history of croup and associated gastroesophageal reflux (GER) may be at increased risk for recurrence (Burton, Pransky, Katz, Kearns, & Said, 1992), and have been shown to present at an earlier age and have more rapid recurrence than those without GER (Waki, Madgy, Belenky, & Gower, 1995).

Viral croup begins when the offending virus is acquired via the nasal or pharyngeal passages, causing symptoms of nasal congestion and sore throat. The incubation period is 2 to 6 days. Spread to the larynx and trachea follows, facilitated by inhibition of ciliary function and impairment of local cellular defenses. Edema and inflammatory cell infiltration result, producing intensely erythematous folds in the subglottic larynx and a narrowed trachea. Hoarseness results when the vocal folds are affected, but the glottis is usually less severely affected than the subglottis. Thick secretions may further compromise the airway; however, purulence is unusual in the absence of secondary bacterial infection. As the disease progresses, atelectasis and mucous plugging of the airways result in hypoxia, and abnormalities of gas exchange may develop. With involvement of the bronchi and lungs, secondary bacterial infection may result and is frequently associated with a fibrinous exudate.

Spasmodic croup is frequently associated with the same viruses seen in laryngotracheitis. However, in this disorder, edema of the airway is seen in the absence of inflammation. The underlying pathophysiology is poorly understood; however, organisms of lower virulence and allergic mechanisms are thought to play a role.

Clinical Features

When hoarseness is the only symptom of lower airway involvement, children are commonly given a diagnosis of laryngitis. However, systemic illness may be present as well, depending on the infecting organism. Laryngitis associated with parainfluenza virus and respiratory syncytial virus may cause nasal congestion, but otherwise few constitutional symptoms. In contrast, adenovirus and influenza infections tend to be severe and may be accompanied by headache, myalgia, and odynophagia.

Involvement of the trachea and larynx, or laryngotracheitis, may be seen 1 to 3 days following the onset of upper respiratory illness. Typically, the child develops a cough, which in most cases assumes a characteristic "barking" quality. Inspiratory stridor follows in about 60% of cases (Walker & Crysdale, 1992). Fever is common, but temperatures are usually low grade. The voice is frequently hoarse but not muffled.

Less severe cases of laryngotracheitis begin to resolve after 3 or 4 days. However, many patients have a more protracted course, involving a greater degree of airway obstruction and toxicity. In such cases, it is important to distinguish the disorder from more severe infections of the airway. In contrast to supraglottitis, children with laryngotracheitis are willing to assume a supine position and can adequately manage their oral secretions. Tachycardia, sternal retraction, cyanosis, and lethargy are less common in croup than in supraglottitis, but when they are present, assisted ventilation may be necessary. As the disease spreads to the bronchi and lungs, rales, air trapping, and wheezing may also be noted.

Symptoms of spasmodic croup are usually similar to those of mild laryngotracheitis. This disorder is distinguished by its nighttime onset, absence of fever, and rapid recovery. Recurrent attacks are the rule and may be noted over several days or even during the same evening. The etiology is unclear and may vary.

Laboratory studies add little to the diagnosis of croup. Elevated blood leukocyte counts are common, especially in cases of secondary bacterial infection, and therefore do not distinguish croup from supraglottitis. Throat culture may help exclude a bacterial pharyngitis or mononucleosis, but viral typing is of little therapeutic value.

Management

Viral croup is a self-limited disease. As a result, adequacy of the airway during the course of the disease is the primary management consideration. However, despite decades of study, considerable controversy regarding pharmacologic and supportive therapy for airway maintenance in croup remains.

Diagnosis

The diagnosis of croup is based primarily on clinical evaluation of the child. In severe cases, it may be difficult to differentiate between croup and supraglottitis. When the diagnosis is in doubt, the patient should be managed with a presumptive diagnosis of supraglottitis. More commonly, however, the patient with croup is significantly less toxic, allowing ample time for radiographic confirmation of the diagnosis. Anteroposterior view of the airway will typically reveal subglottic swelling, which changes the appearance of the square-shouldered space below the vocal folds to that of a steeple or pencil (Figure 7–1). The hypopharynx and proximal larynx appear distended, most likely due to increased pharyngeal pressure or to an active muscle reflex designed to reduce airway resistance (Currarino & Williams, 1982). Ballooning of the cervical trachea on expiration radiographs has also been noted (Currarino & Williams, 1982). Radiographs may also aid in excluding supraglottitis, congenital anomalies of the airway, and foreign body aspiration as diagnostic possibilities.

Airway Management

Few patients with croup develop airway obstruction or respiratory fatigue severe enough to require hospitalization, and most of these respond well to medical and supportive therapy. Elective intubation is required in 1.6 to 6.7% of patients admitted with a diagnosis of tracheitis (Freezer, Butt, & Phelan, 1990; Sendi, Crysdale, & Yoo, 1992; Sofer, Dagan, & Tal, 1991; Tan & Manoukian, 1992), which represents less than 1% of all patients evaluated in the emergency room for the same diagnosis. Indications for intubation include progressive fatigue, poor respiratory effort, hypoxemia, hypercapnia, acidosis, presence of a chronic medical or surgical condition, and poor response to frequent treatments with racemic epinephrine.

Intubation is performed in the OR when the history is atypical or the diagnosis is in doubt, but otherwise can be managed by the intensive care team. Rapid sequence induction techniques may be necessary if the child's stomach is full. Nasotracheal intubation is preferred for the comfort of the patient, and an endotracheal tube at least one size smaller than normal for age is generally employed (normal tube size = [age of patient/4] + 4). Infants may be at risk for developing subglottic stenosis following endotracheal intubation for croup and should therefore be intubated with the smallest tube adequate for ventilation and clearance of secretions. Restraints, sedation, and paralysis are used as necessary.

Elective extubation may be attempted when the fever has dissipated and the airway is relatively free of secretions. Many clinicians use the presence of an air leak around the tube with positive pressure ventilation as an additional criterion. This test should be interpreted with caution, as the presence of a leak varies with the pressure used (anywhere from 25 to 40 cm of water) and with the size of the endotracheal tube.

Most patients are ready for extubation within 5 to 7 days whether or not a leak is present, and steroids may improve the chances of successful extubation (Freezer, Butt, and Phelan 1990; Tibbals, Shann, & Landau, 1992). However, the risk of extubation failure is 16–34% (Freezer, Butt, & Phelan, 1990; McEniery, et al., 1991; Tibbals, Shann, & Landau 1992). Should extubation fail, a second trial is reasonable, but two failures are an indication for endoscopic evaluation. Endoscopy should also be considered for patients with an increased risk for subglottic stenosis (history of stridor,

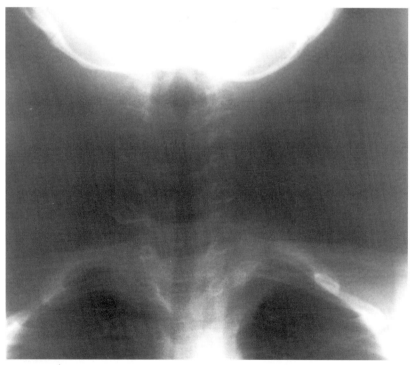

A

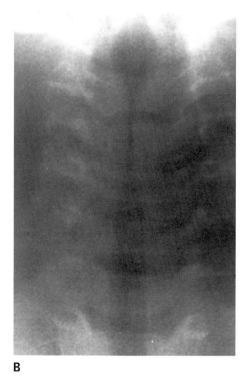

B

Figure 7–1. Anterior radiographic view of the airway in a child with croup (**A**), with magnification of the subglottic larynx and upper trachea (**B**). The classic "steeple sign" is present.

prior intubation for croup, intubation during infancy, or Down syndrome), a history of endotracheal tube trauma, or an atypical presentation (patients younger than 6 months or older than 6 years). The procedure should be performed 3 to 4 weeks following the acute event to allow the acute inflammatory changes time to resolve.

Urgent tracheotomy is reserved for cases in which intensive care personnel are not readily available. In patients found to have other subglottic pathology (i.e., stenosis or hemangioma), early elective tracheotomy or alternative surgical management (such as laser laryngoscopy) may be indicated. Tracheotomy following intubation may be necessary in patients who fail extubation.

Acquired subglottic stenosis can occur as a complication of intubation for croup. The condition likely results from prolonged contact of the endotracheal tube with the inflamed tracheal wall. Mucosal injury results in annular scarring and airway compromise. Studies of subglottic stenosis following intubation for croup report a mean incidence of 5% (McEniery et al., 1991), but when small tubes are used for shorter periods of time, the risk may be considerably lower.

Medical Management

Medical and supportive therapy in croup are directed at maintenance of the airway while the infection runs its course. Laryngitis and spasmodic croup are mild, short-lived disorders and usually require no specific treatment. In contrast, most clinicians do intervene medically in cases of laryngotracheitis and laryngotracheobronchitis in order to arrest the progression toward airway obstruction. Sedation is often used to decrease the child's work of breathing; however, the primary modalities used to treat the airway itself are humidification, nebulized racemic epinephrine, and systemic glucocorticoids.

Humidification is the most frequently prescribed remedy in croup. Because the majority of patients with croup do not require hospitalization, home vaporizer therapy is usually recommended. In the hospital, mist hoods or "croup tents" are commonly used to deliver humidification. In theory, humidification helps prevent drying of the epithelial surfaces and reduces the viscosity of secretions and exudate, facilitating their clearance. It has also been suggested that mist therapy serves to reduce the anxiety of the patient and, therefore, his or her oxygen demand and risk of obstruction (Henry, 1983). Temperature of the mist is not critical and should be adjusted to keep the child comfortable. Supplemental oxygen may be administered as necessary; alternatively, inhaled helium-oxygen mixtures may increase gas flow at the subglottis and decrease the work of respiration.

Unfortunately, hospital studies have failed to demonstrate the efficacy of humidification in croup (Bourchier, Dawson, & Fergusson, 1984), and it is ques-

tionable whether home vaporizers deliver enough mist to be effective in the lower airways. Furthermore, home humidification equipment is known to become colonized with bacteria and environmental allergens, which may aggravate the airway infection (Szilagyi, 1991). Despite these reservations, and given the preponderance of anecdotal evidence, it seems reasonable to employ a vaporizer or mist tent for most children with croup. Proper maintenance of these devices and close observation of the patient are mandatory when humidification is used.

The use of racemic epinephrine in patients with croup was introduced in 1966 by Jordan (cited in Cherry, 1992), and advanced in 1971 by Adair's report of his 10-year experience with this therapy (Adair, Ring, Jordan, et al 1971). The α-adrenergic effect of the drug, attributed to the L-isomer, causes vasoconstriction in the mucosa within 10 to 30 minutes, thereby reducing edema in the inflamed tissues. Some bronchodilation may also be obtained from the β-adrenergic activity of the D-isomer, although several authors advocate use of the L-isomer alone, citing its efficacy, low cost, availability, and reduced cardiac side effects (De Boeck, 1995; Waisman et al., 1992). Improvement is generally short-lived (approximately 2 hours), and the presence of a rebound effect may demand frequent treatments. Nevertheless, of five double-blind, placebo-controlled trials performed since 1973, four have convincingly demonstrated the efficacy of aerosolized epinephrine, whether delivered by nebulizer or by intermittent positive pressure breathing (Skolnik, 1989). Additional studies demonstrate the efficacy of nebulized epinephrine in outpatients monitored for 2 hours for evidence of rebound edema (Kelly & Simon, 1992; Prendergast, Jones, & Hartman, 1994). The recommended dose is 0.25–0.5 ml of 2.25% racemic epinephrine in 1.5–3.5 ml of normal saline. Frequency of administration is restricted only by the development of tachycardia, although caution should also be exercised in treating patients with a history of left ventricular outflow obstruction (Cressman & Myer, 1994).

The efficacy of corticosteroids in croup is the subject of an ongoing debate, which spans 4 decades in the pediatric literature. Proponents believe that steroids reduce subglottic edema by inhibiting local inflammation, lymphoid swelling, and capillary permeability. However, results from clinical trials have been conflicting. Skolnik (1989), in a review of the major clinical trials performed between 1960 and 1988, highlighted the methodologic flaws in these studies and attributed the inconsistency of results to the use of differing doses of steroids. He concluded, "Since the adverse effect of a short course of corticosteroids is very small, . . . it seems that the evidence is overwhelmingly in favor of recommending intramuscular administration of dexamethasone phosphate in a dose of 0.6 mg/kg to be given on admission to any child admitted to the hospital with a diagnosis of viral croup." In a meta-analysis of these clinical trials (Kairys, Olmstead, & O'Connor, 1989), a statistically significant difference in clinical improvement was documented in steroid-treated patients at 12 and 24 hours following treatment. Further support for parenteral use of steroids comes from prospective randomized double-blind trials in which these results were duplicated using a single dose of dexamethasone (Cruz, Stewart, & Rosenberg, 1995; Super et al., 1989). Other studies have demonstrated a reduction in the duration of intubation (Tibbals, Shann, & Landau, 1992) as well as the risk of reintubation in patients receiving steroids (Freezer, Butt, & Phelan, 1990; Tibbals, Shann, & Landau, 1992). As a result, the early use of a single dose of dexamethasone is recommended by the Canadian Paediatric Society (1992) and the Thoracic Society of Australia and New Zealand (Dawson, et al., 1992).

Several recent trials support the use of alternative routes of steroid administration in the treatment of mild to moderate croup in outpatients. Dexamethasone given orally (Ledwith, Shea, & Mauro, 1995) and nebulized budesonide (Fitzgerald, et al., 1996; Husby, Agertoft, Mortensen, & Pederson, 1993; Klassen, Feldman, Watters, Sutcliffe, & Rowe, 1994) have demonstrated efficacy and avoid the pain associated with intramuscular therapy. In a study of patients with mild to moderate croup, cohorts treated with oral dexamethasone, nebulized budesonide, or both, demonstrated similar degrees of improvement (Klassen et al., 1998). The authors concluded that oral dexamethasone is the preferred intervention, given its ease of administration, lower cost, and widespread availability. Nebulized steroids, on the other hand, decrease the risk of gastrointestinal hemorrhage associated with systemic therapy.

Prognosis

Short-term prognosis is excellent, as viral croup is a self-limited disease. However, studies suggest that some adolescents and adults with a history of croup in childhood may suffer increased bronchial reactivity or asthma (Friedman, Reilly, & Kenna, 1985; Litmanovitch, Kivity, Soferman, & Toplisky, 1990; Pearlman 1989). Acute inflammation secondary to croup during periods of rapid lung growth is thought to be the mechanism responsible (Friedman, Reilly, & Kenna 1985). As a result, infants with croup may be more likely to develop pulmonary disease later in life than are toddlers and older children.

SUPRAGLOTTITIS

Acute supraglottitis is an infection of the epiglottis, aryepiglottic folds, and soft tissues of the arytenoid cartilages. This term, first used by Camps in 1952 (Camps, 1970), has largely replaced the term "acute epiglottitis," which permeated the literature after first appearing in 1900. Supraglottitis, although certainly less common than other inflammatory diseases of the airway, is the most serious and carries the highest risk of morbidity and mortality.

Epidemiology

The incidence of supraglottitis in the years preceding vaccination for Hib has been estimated at 3.2 to 8.6 cases per 10,000 pediatric hospital admissions (Andreassen, Baer, Mielsen, Dahm, & Arndahl, 1992; Bass, Steel, & Wiebe, 1974), and 0.4 to 0.6 cases per 10,000 pediatric population (Frantz & Rasgon, 1993; Wurtele, 1990). Temperate climates and warmer weather may increase the risk of risk of the disease (Daum & Smith, 1992). Supraglottitis has been shown to have a slight male preponderance (Daum & Smith, 1992). Mean age of onset is approximately 3.5 years (Daum & Smith, 1992), but cases affecting all ages have been reported.

Etiology and Pathophysiology

Among pediatric patients, supraglottitis has been a disease almost uniformly attributable to Hib. Blood cultures are positive for Hib in 80% of cases; however, throat culture has been shown to correlate poorly with disease (Daum & Smith, 1992). Other organisms associated with supraglottitis in the pediatric population include *Streptococcus pneumoniae*; *Streptococcus* Group A, B, and C; *Staphylococcus aureus*; *Pseudomonas aeruginosa*; *Candida*; and herpes simplex virus. These organisms cause less than 1% of cases in this age group and are usually isolated from patients with immunodeficiency. Rarely, thermal injury, trauma, or caustic ingestion may also cause severe supraglottic inflammation.

Infection is thought to begin with transmucosal invasion of the supraglottic structures by the organism, resulting in diffuse infiltration of the tissues by polymorphonuclear leukocytes, blood, and edema, and occasionally in microabscess formation. As the epiglottis enlarges, a ball-valve effect is created, resulting in mild hypoxia without a significant rise in CO_2. Increased inspiratory effort only serves to worsen the mechanical obstruction. In addition, the airway is often compromised by thick secretions, which are poorly handled by the patient due to odynophagia and the rigidity of the supraglottic structures. Spread of the process to the glottis, however, is limited by the close adherence of the epithelium of the vocal cords.

Clinical Features

Symptoms in supraglottitis develop rapidly, usually leading to emergency evaluation within 24 hours. Occasionally, symptoms of viral upper respiratory infection will precede the disease. The single most distinctive feature of supraglottitis is odynophagia. The exquisite pain associated with swallowing results secondarily in dysphagia and drooling, each of which is present in about 50% of patients (Daum & Smith, 1992). Typically, the physician will encounter a pale, anxious, and irritable child who insists on sitting to be examined. The patient holds the head forward and in extension with the jaw protruded to maximize the lumen of the airway. Breathing may be shallow to minimize the painful movement of the supraglottic structures. The voice may be of a muffled, "hot potato" quality, but is generally not hoarse.

Temperatures above 38.5°C are common, but low-grade or normal temperatures may be encountered. White blood cell counts are usually elevated; however, phlebotomy is likely to agitate the child and increase the risk of sudden airway obstruction. Additional laboratory studies are rarely useful.

Management

Over the last 50 years, advances in antibiotics and technology have made treatment of supraglottitis safer, and the recent development of the Hib vaccine has led to a dramatic reduction in the incidence of the disease. Still, many treatment issues remain controversial.

Despite the absence of uniformity in the management of supraglottitis, the concept of the management protocol has been widely embraced. Such protocols streamline the process of confirming the diagnosis and instituting appropriate therapy. All hospitals treating patients with supraglottitis should develop protocols tailored to the ability and availability of personnel capable of urgently establishing an airway. These facilities must also cooperate with their referring physicians to establish appropriate care criteria for the management and transport of patients diagnosed with supraglottitis in the primary care setting.

Diagnosis

Initial evaluation of the patient with suspected supraglottitis usually takes place in the hospital emergency room. As in croup, presumptive diagnosis is usually based on the physical appearance of the child. Direct examination of the pharynx and larynx is usually avoided due to the risk of sudden airway obstruction, although some authors (Andreassen et al., 1992; Mauro, Poole, & Lockhart, 1988; Sendi & Crysdale, 1987) advocate such an examination in the older child with a relatively stable airway when personnel capable of urgent intubation are present. The epiglottitis may be visualized using a tongue depressor, mirror, or fiberscope, and will typically appear beefy red and swollen, surrounding a slitlike entrance to the glottis (Figure 7–2).

Once a tentative diagnosis is made, a predetermined supraglottitis protocol is activated, and further

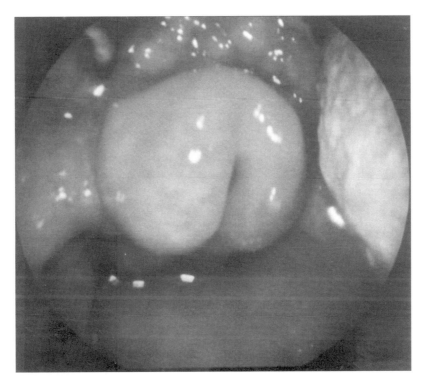

Figure 7–2. Endoscopic view of the epiglottis in a patient with acute supraglottitis. Inflammation of the epiglottis results in slitlike narrowing of the laryngeal inlet. (Courtesy of Laruen D. Holinger, M.D.)

management is based on the stability of the patient. In patients with severe respiratory distress, positive pressure ventilation by mask will invariably buy enough time to transport the patient to the operating room for controlled intubation. Urgent intubation in the emergency room is rarely necessary. When personnel skilled in pediatric airway management are not available, urgent tracheotomy may be the treatment of choice. Equipment for tracheotomy should be available at all times.

In patients who are relatively stable and in whom the diagnosis is equivocal, lateral neck radiographs may be useful in differentiating supraglottitis from croup or foreign body aspiration. The films are taken either in the intensive care unit or in the emergency room in the presence of a physician. In most cases the diagnosis is suggested by the presence of the characteristic "thumb" sign, indicating a swollen epiglottis (Figure 7–3). A more objective criterion has been employed by Rothrock, Pignatiello, and Howard (1990), using the ratio of the aryepiglottic width to the width of the third cervical vertebra. Based on their series of cases, a ratio greater than 0.35 is 100% sensitive and 96% specific in the diagnosis of supraglottitis. In another study, John, Swischuk, Hayden, and Freeman (1994) assessed the width at the upper half of the aryepiglottic folds and found that measurements taken where the folds overlie the arytenoid cartilages were inaccurate. Although data from a large university hospital suggest a sensitivity of only 50% for radiographs in supraglottitis (Stankiewicz & Bowes, 1985), other studies from children's hospitals

(Butt et al., 1988; Kimmons & Peterson, 1986; Sendi & Crysdale 1987; Vernon & Sarnaik, 1986) have documented an average sensitivity of 94%. Such studies underscore the importance of experience with children in radiographic technique and interpretation.

The combination of physical and radiographic examination should be sufficient to make the diagnosis of supraglottitis. Though phlebotomy for white cell count and culture are useful in the medical management of supraglottitis, these are deferred until the airway has been secured.

Airway Management

Management of the airway in supraglottitis is controversial. Some clinicians believe mild cases may be managed by observation (Vernon & Sarnaik, 1986), although 24–60% of such cases eventually require intubation (Arndal & Andreassen, 1988; Sendi & Crysdale, 1987). The authors maintain that the risk of sudden airway obstruction significantly outweighs the risk and discomfort of endotracheal intubation and that a secure airway is the cornerstone of treatment in supraglottitis.

Prolonged endotracheal intubation, first described by Allen and Steven (1965), has replaced tracheotomy at most centers as the procedure of choice in securing the airway in cases of supraglottitis. Although tracheotomy avoids the risk of additional irritation of the airway that accompanies endotracheal intubation, no significant long-term sequelae have resulted from short-term intubation (Schuller & Birch, 1975). In addi-

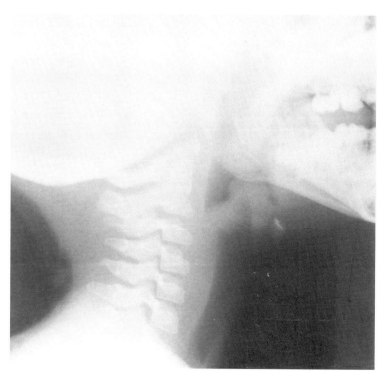

Figure 7–3. Lateral neck radiograph of a patient with acute supraglottitis. A "thumb sign" due to epiglottic swelling can be appreciated.

tion, intubation is associated with lower morbidity and mortality compared to tracheotomy (Mjeon, Dahl, Swensen, and Westheim, 1979) and requires shorter hospitalization (Oh & Motoyama, 1977). Sudden-onset pulmonary edema has been reported at a rate of 2.1% among patients intubated for supraglottitis (Bonadio & Kosek, 1991), but may occur following tracheotomy as well. Endotracheal intubation carries a risk of accidental extubation of 2–13% (Arndal & Andreassen, 1988; Butt et al., 1988; Crockett, Healy, McGill, & Friedman, 1988; Kimmons & Peterson, 1986; Sendi & Crysdale, 1987; Vernon & Sarnaik, 1986), but few patients require reintubation. This risk may be avoided by close observation and by the use of restraints, sedation, and paralysis as necessary.

Children with suspected supraglottitis are transferred from the intensive care unit or the emergency room to the OR following radiographic confirmation of the disease. A tracheotomy tray is opened and ventilating bronchoscopes of at least two sizes are assembled. As soon as the child arrives in the OR, halothane anesthesia is induced by mask in the sitting position. The child is placed supine and intravenous lines are started, while sufficient positive pressure is administered to ventilate past the supraglottic obstruction. With a laryngoscope designed for use in the vallecula, the larynx is visualized, and an endotracheal tube one size smaller than normal is passed through the glottis. In the event intubation is unsuccessful, a rigid ventilating bronchoscope may be passed, and after several minutes, compression of the supraglottic edema may allow the tube to pass more easily. Once orotracheal intubation has been accomplished, the child is oxygenated and the tube is cleared of secretions. The tube is then replaced with a nasotracheal tube, which is carefully secured to the nose or around the head. Blood is drawn for leukocyte count and culture, and antibiotics are started, prior to transfer back to the intensive care unit. Older patients may be permitted to emerge completely from anesthesia, while others are kept lightly sedated and restrained. Muscle relaxants are avoided if possible, but may occasionally be necessary to avoid accidental extubation.

Various criteria have been used to determine the appropriate time for extubation. Resolution of the supraglottic inflammation may be determined by direct visualization of the larynx in the intensive care unit or the OR, or by fiberoptic visualization of the larynx at the bedside. Some authors delay extubation until the fever has completely resolved (Gonzalez, Reilly, Kenna, & Thompson, 1986) or until an air leak around the tube can be obtained at pressures of 20 to 30 cm of water or less (Crockett et al., 1988). However, size of the epiglottis does not correlate with severity of obstruction, visual findings do not correlate with resolution of fever, and persistent fever does not preclude successful extubation (Holbrook, 1988). As a result, many clinicians prefer to extubate arbitrarily, anywhere from 12–48 hours after initiating therapy.

Medical Management

Traditionally, ampicillin has been the antimicrobial agent of choice in the treatment of supraglottitis, owing to its efficacy, safety, and low cost. However, resistance to ampicillin has risen steadily over the last 2 decades, now estimated at 20 to 40% among isolates of Hib (Vallejo, Kaplan, & Mason, 1991). The addition of chloramphenicol to the treatment regimen, pending the results of ampicillin sensitivity tests, has been advocated but carries the risk of severe bone marrow depression. Increasing resistance to chloramphenicol has also been reported (Knight, Harris, Parbari, O'Callaghan, & Masters, 1992).

As a result, in most centers, the late generation cephalosporins have replaced ampicillin and chloramphenicol as first line therapy for supraglottitis. Cefuroxime (75–100 mg/kg/day divided into three or four equal doses) was the first such antibiotic used, but is not recommended for cases of supraglottitis in which Hib meningitis is suspected. Cefotaxime (75-180 mg/kg/day divided into four doses) may be used when CNS involvement is a concern. Most recently, a single daily dose therapy with ceftriaxone (100 mg/kg/day) has emerged as the treatment of choice in a number of institutions (Frenkel 1988; Knight et al., 1992), including our own. Though the cost per dose of this antibiotic is somewhat higher, the lower cost of administration and smaller risk of resistance and side effects justify its use. Successful treatment without complications has been reported with as few as two doses of ceftriaxone (Sawyer et al., 1994); however, appropriate duration of therapy has not been studied in a controlled fashion. Three to 5 days of intravenous antibiotics followed by 5 to 7 days of cefuroxime or amoxicillin/clavulanic acid taken orally is a more typical treatment regimen. In cases of penicillin allergy, single-agent therapy with chloramphenicol (100 mg/kg/day divided into four doses) is most appropriate.

The use of steroids in supraglottitis has little support in the literature and may be contraindicated. In one study, 91 patients with supraglottitis received steroids, 4 of whom developed gastrointestinal hemorrhage; 2 of these patients required transfusion (DiTirro, Silver, & Hengerer, 1984). Similarly, racemic epinephrine is of little clinical use. Cool mist delivered by face mask may be of some benefit following extubation.

Prevention

Although not yet available in all parts of the world, vaccination against Hib in childhood is the key to contemporary management of supraglottitis. In the United States, the Hib polysaccharide vaccine was first licensed in 1985. Although this preparation was poorly immunogenic and of limited efficacy for younger children, licensure was granted for use in children 24 to 59 months of age based on results of Finnish efficacy trials. In the meantime, work continued on a polysaccharide-protein conjugate vaccine that would have greater immunogenicity and immunologic memory. The first such vaccine was licensed in 1987 for children over 18 months of age. In late 1990, two conjugate vaccines, HbOC (Hib oligosaccharide and diphtheria CRM197 protein conjugate) and PRP-OMP (Hib polysaccharide and *Neisseria meningitidis* outer-membrane protein complex), were approved for use in all children beginning at 2 months of age. A polysaccharide-tetanus toxoid conjugate and a combination vaccine using HbOC and DTP (diphtheria, tetanus toxoid, and pertussis) have also been approved.

Recent studies document a significant decrease in the incidence of supraglottitis in children since the start of routine vaccination. Broadhurst, Erickson, and Kelley (1993), in a review of children of American military personnel, demonstrated a significant downward trend in the incidence of supraglottitis from 1.8/10,000 in 1987 to 0.6/10,000 in 1991. Similarly, Frantz and Rasgon (1993) studied a northern California HMO population and found a decline in incidence from 0.35/10,000 in 1980 to 0.06/10,000 in 1990, the greatest change noted in the year 1985–1986 following the introduction of vaccination. This trend has been cited in other epidemiologic studies of supraglottitis (Alho, Jokinen, Pirila, et al., 1995; Kessler, Wetmore, & Marsh, 1993; Ryan, Hunt, & Snowberger, 1992; Takala et al., 1994) and of Hib disease in general (Adams et al., 1993; Broadhurst, et al., 1993; Murphy et al., 1993).

The effect of a reduced Hib colonization rate on the general population has not been fully assessed. Prior to vaccination, older children and adults developed antibodies to Hib as a result of pharyngeal colonization during early childhood, and were therefore less susceptible to supraglottitis. Recent studies have demonstrated a reduction in the Hib carriage rate (Takala et al., 1994), and it is unknown whether the immunity provided by the vaccination will be adequate to protect older patients as well as children. As a consequence, an increased incidence of Hib supraglottitis in the older population may be seen. Such a trend has already been suggested by several authors (Alho et al., 1995; Ryan et al., 1992; Senior, Radkowski, MacArthur, Sprecher, & Jones, 1994).

Additional prophylaxis against Hib disease has been recommended for household contacts of patients with Hib supraglottitis. The Committee on Infectious Diseases of the American Academy of Pediatrics has advised that in households with at least one unimmunized child 4 years of age or under, all contacts receive prophylaxis with a single daily dose of rifampin, 20 mg/kg, to a maximum of 600 mg (American Academy of Pediatrics, 1993). In homes with any child 12 months of age or younger, all contacts should be treated with rifampin, regardless of the immunization status of the child (American Academy of Pediatrics, 1993). Reports of secondary Hib infection in adults have led some authors to recommend rifampin prophylaxis for contacts regardless of age.

BACTERIAL TRACHEITIS

Bacterial tracheitis is a rare but aggressive infection affecting the lower pediatric airway. Also termed pseudomembranous croup and membranous laryngotracheobronchitis, this disorder was first recognized over 50 years ago. However, as most cases of croup were found to be of viral etiology, interest in the role of bacteria in this disorder waned.

In 1979, one month apart, reports by Han, Dunbar, and Striker and by Jones, Santos and Overall each described a group of patients who developed inflammatory disease of the lower airway accompanied by adherent mucopurulent tracheal membranes. These children responded poorly to routine supportive care, and usually required intubation. Culture of the membrane aspirated from the trachea often yielded bacteria, and clinical improvement was noted only after the institution of antimicrobial therapy.

Epidemiology

The incidence of bacterial tracheitis has been estimated at 4/10,000 hospital admissions (Gallagher & Myer, 1991). Males are affected more than females in a ratio of 2:1, and the mean age at onset is 4 years (Gallagher & Myer 1991).

Etiology and Pathophysiology

Although the etiology of bacterial tracheitis remains uncertain, studies suggest the disease likely results when bacteria superinfect a viral illness of the lower airway, most commonly associated with parainfluenza virus (Davidson, Barzilay, Yahav & Rubenstein, 1982; Lisston, Genrz, Siegel, & Tilelli, 1983). The viral infection causes changes seen in croup, such as impairment of mucociliary function and mucosal damage, but may also induce changes in the cells responsible for immune surveillance. A favorable environment is thus created for colonizing bacteria to adhere to the tracheal wall. As bacteria along the wall multiply, a mucopurulent collection results, and sloughing of the mucosa therefore forms a sticky membrane. Culture of this material obtained at endoscopy or through an endotracheal tube most commonly reveals *Staphylococcus aureus* (45%), *Streptococcus* sp. (22%), or *Haemophilus influenzae* (16%) (Gallagher & Myer, 1991). Preexisting immunodeficiency may be a risk factor for bacterial tracheitis (Donnelly, McMillan, & Weiner 1990), and the disease has been reported as a complication of tonsillectomy and adenoidectomy (Eid & Jones 1994).

Clinical Features

The initial clinical presentation of bacterial tracheitis is much the same as that in viral croup. However, after several days of symptoms, patients with bacterial tracheitis will become dramatically more ill, with higher fever and increased stridor as the tracheal accumulation grows. Cardiopulmonary arrest secondary to airway obstruction may occur if the airway is not examined and protected. Pneumonia develops in about 60% of patients (Donnelly et al., 1990), presumably by spread of the purulent material to the distal airway.

As in croup, laboratory studies are of little value in making the diagnosis. Leukocyte counts are inconsistent, and blood cultures are rarely positive. Organisms identified on throat culture, on the other hand, may often be a reflection of those in the trachea.

Management

As in all cases of laryngotracheal infection, stable patients undergo radiographic evaluation. Airway films typically demonstrate the subglottic narrowing characteristic of croup. The tracheal membrane may be seen as a vague radiodensity, suggestive of an airway foreign body (Figure 7–4). This finding is an indication for immediate endoscopic evaluation in the OR.

When bacterial tracheitis is suggested by history or physical examination and airway radiographs fail to demonstrate a membrane, flexible endoscopic examination of the subglottis may help to direct further therapy. The presence of purulent secretions should be considered an indication for rigid endoscopy. Alternatively, patients with purulent secretions may be followed clinically and later examined endoscopically if necessary. If endoscopy is performed, the membranes are thoroughly debrided and cultures obtained. An endotracheal tube is placed if needed.

Proper management of the airway in bacterial tracheitis has not been definitively established. Some authors believe an artificial airway is rarely needed when early, aggressive medical therapy is instituted and the patient is closely observed (Friedman 1988). On the other hand, support for intubation comes from a review of 161 patients with bacterial tracheitis, of whom 134 (83%) eventually required an artificial airway (Gallagher & Myer, 1991). Risk factors for airway support include younger age and pulmonary involvement (Friedman et al., 1985). Tracheotomy has also been advocated in bacterial tracheitis patients in order to facilitate suctioning of the airway and to avoid the risk of subglottic stenosis. A preferred management strategy may emerge as more large case series are reported.

Although most authors report a poor overall response to racemic epinephrine in bacterial tracheitis (Gallagher & Myer, 1991), a therapeutic trial may be indicated, especially when the diagnosis is in doubt. The efficacy of steroid use in bacterial tracheitis has not been studied, but a single dose is unlikely to cause immune suppression and may hasten resolution of the disease.

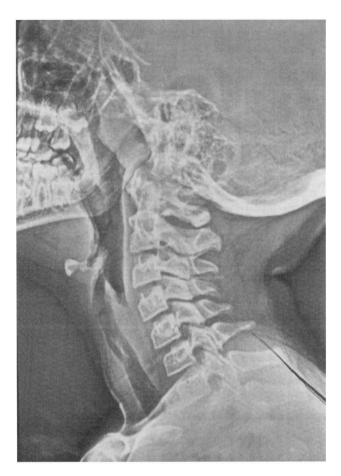

Figure 7–4. Radiopaque irregularity of the trachea demonstrated by xeroradiography in a child with bacterial tracheitis. This finding suggests the presence of a tracheal membrane, but may be mistaken for a tracheal foreign body. (Courtesy of Lauren D. Holinger, M.D.)

Broad spectrum antibiotic therapy should be started presumptively if bacterial tracheitis is suspected and altered as culture results return. Vancomycin (40 mg/kg/day, divided into four doses) is recommended for coverage of *Staphylococcus*, while ceftriaxone (100 mg/kg, one dose daily) is appropriate for streptococci and *H. influenzae*.

DIPHTHERIA LARYNGOTRACHEITIS

With the development of diphtheria toxoid and aggressive immunization programs, diphtheria laryngotracheitis has become all but extinct in the United States as the 21st century approaches. Over the 10-year period from 1982 to 1991, an average of 2.8 cases per year were reported to the U.S. Centers for Disease Control (Centers for Disease Control, 1992). Nevertheless, the disease remains endemic in many nations throughout the world.

Diphtheria laryngotracheitis is caused by *Corynebacterium diphtheriae*, a club-shaped, gram positive bacillus. The bacterium is usually acquired via the respiratory passages or, rarely, the mucous membranes. Nasal congestion, pharyngitis, anorexia, and low-grade fever may be present. Cervical lymphadenitis and edema of the soft tissues of the neck are also common.

Following an incubation period of 2 to 4 days, diphtheria exotoxin is released by the organism, initiating local tissue necrosis and exudate. As the affected area expands, the exudate turns fibrinous and develops into an adherent gray membrane also containing inflammatory cells, epithelial cells, and red blood cells. Enlargement of the membrane and progressive edema cause airway compromise and stridor, and dislodgement of the membrane may cause frank obstruction. Systemic effects of the toxin include myocarditis, peripheral neuritis, and acute tubular necrosis of the kidneys.

Definitive diagnosis is made on the basis of a culture of the membrane, but management should not be delayed for culture results. Severely compromised patients will require an artificial airway; because the membranes are generally more tenacious than those in bacterial tracheitis, tracheotomy is generally preferred. Once the airway is secure and a presumptive diagnosis is made, the patient is tested for sensitivity to horse serum and antitoxin is administered. Antibiotic therapy with penicillin or erythromycin is started subsequently, and nonimmune personal contacts are treated as well. Prognosis depends on the immunization status of the host, the promptness of medical therapy, and the virulence of the infecting organism. Prevention of diphtheria is achieved through immunization during infancy.

GASTROESOPHAGEAL REFLUX

Increasingly, gastroesophageal reflux (GER) has been recognized as a source of inflammation in the pediatric airway. This phenomenon, which bathes the mucosal lining of the esophagus and the airway in a mixture of acids and digestive enzymes, is common and considered normal during the first year of life, owing to the immaturity of the lower esophageal sphincter. However, excessive exposure, as defined by a pH less than 4 for greater than 7–10% of the time, may cause significant acute and chronic pathology both within and outside the esophagus.

GER is thought to affect the airway by two primary mechanisms (Burton et al., 1992). First, mucosal damage may result from prolonged direct contact with the refluxate. This type of injury is a common cause of hoarseness and chronic cough, and severe reflux may be associated with stridor. Reported mucosal findings include hypertrophy and edema within the larynx, vocal fold granulomas, "cobblestoning" and edema of the posterior tracheal wall, friable mucosa, and blunting of the carina. In addition, raw mucosal surfaces created by GER are thought to be associated with an in-

creased risk of postintubation subglottic stenosis. Alternatively, GER may induce laryngospasm, bronchospasm, or apnea by reflex mechanisms.

The classic symptomatology of postprandial epigastric pain is not generally seen in pediatric patients. Rather, children will present with a history of dysphagia, emesis, or choking and gagging, which can often be temporally related to feedings. Occasionally, reflux will first become manifest in the upper airway or in the lungs as recurrent bronchitis or pneumonia. An association of reflux with laryngomalacia and other disorders causing chronic airway obstruction has been suggested and is thought to result from changes in the normal thoracoabdominal pressure gradients.

All children undergoing surgical reconstruction of the laryngotracheal complex should be evaluated for evidence of silent reflux. In this group of patients, reflux is frequently associated with an abundance of granulation tissue and poor healing of the surgical site. This may be particularly troublesome in laryngotracheal reconstructions employing posterior cartilage grafts, and in the repair of cleft larynx.

Several studies may be used to confirm the diagnosis of GER including esophageal pH monitoring, esophagoscopy with biopsy, barium esophagram, nuclear medicine scintiscan, bronchoscopy with washings for fat-laden macrophages, and the modified Bernstein test. These tests are evaluated in detail elsewhere (Burton et al., 1992). It is generally accepted, however, that pH monitoring gives the most useful evaluation of the status of the esophagus over time. Biopsies and washings, on the other hand, serve primarily to localize the pathology caused by GER.

Consultation with a gastroenterologist is obtained for symptomatic patients with evidence of reflux and for all patients scheduled for laryngotracheal surgery. Most children with GER respond well to conservative therapy such as dietary changes and positioning. In some cases, pharmacologic agents such as antacids, prokinetic agents (metoclopramide, cisapride), salivary stimulators (bethanechol), H2 blockers (cimetidine, ranitidine, famotidine), and other antisecretory agents (omeprazole) may be necessary. Surgical correction by fundoplication or gastropexy is usually indicated only when medical management has failed.

Candidates for laryngotracheal reconstruction must have their reflux controlled medically or surgically prior to the airway procedure. For high-risk patients, such as those undergoing repair of cleft larynx, gastric division has occasionally been advocated. Prophylaxis against reflux following laryngotracheal reconstruction is advisable in asymptomatic patients.

ANGIOEDEMA

Angioedema is a localized, nonpitting edema most commonly affecting the face and mucosa of the upper aerodigestive tract. The swelling is of rapid onset and is short-lived, usually clearing within 24 to 72 hours. Inherited forms and some acquired forms of the disorder are associated with a deficiency of the C1-esterase inhibitor; however, in most affected patients the disorder is drug-induced, allergic, or idiopathic (Mergerian, Arnold, & Berger 1992). Association of the acquired type with the use of angiotensin-converting enzyme inhibitors is now well established (Greaves & Lawlor, 1991; Megerian et al., 1992). Acquired angioedema may also result in lymphoproliferative and autoimmune disorders in which excessive consumption of C1-esterase inhibitor occurs.

Patients with angioedema of the airway may present with a sensation of fullness in the throat, or may already have significant respiratory distress since the swelling spreads so rapidly. The history must be taken carefully to rule out supraglottitis, and the airway should be evaluated fiberoptically if no contraindications are present. Occasionally, endotracheal intubation is necessary prior to any other diagnostic studies. The keys to diagnosis are a meticulous medical history and a high index of suspicion. Low C4- and C1-esterase inhibitor levels are diagnostic of hereditary angioedema.

In most cases, no treatment is necessary because the swelling will improve with time. Antihistamines, corticosteroids, and adrenergic drugs are not useful in treating the hereditary form of this disorder but are occasionally used in the management of drug-induced and idiopathic angioedema. In cases of inherited angioedema, C1-esterase inhibitor concentrate is useful both for acute attacks and for prophylaxis. Alternative therapies include danazol which accelerates hepatic synthesis of C1-esterase inhibitor, and aminocaproic acid which reduces plasmin-induced complement activation by inhibiting the conversion of plasminogen to plasmin.

References

Adair, J. C., Ring, W. H, Jordan, W. S, & Elwyn, R. A. (1971) Ten-year experience with IPPB in the treatment of acute laryngotracheobronchitis. *Anesthesia Analgesia, 50,* 649–655.

Adams, W. G., Deaver, K. A., Cochi, S. L., Plikaytis, B. D., Zell, E. R., Broome, C. V., & Wenger, J. D. (1993). Decline of childhood *Haemophilus influenzae* type b (Hib) disease in the Hib vaccine era. *JAMA, 269,* 221–226.

Alho, O., Jokinen, K., Pirila, T., Ilo, A., & Oja, H. (1995). Acute epiglottitis and infant conjugate *Haemophilus influenzae* type b vaccination in northern Finland. *Archives of Otolaryngology—Head and Neck Surgery, 121,* 998–902.

Allen, T. H., & Steven, I. M. (1965). Prolonged nasotracheal intubation in infants and children. *British Journal of Anaesthesia, 37,* 566–571.

American Academy of Pediatrics, Committee on Infectious Diseases. (1993). *Haemophilus influenzae* type b conjugate vaccines: Recommendations for immunizations with recently and previously licensed vaccines. *Pediatrics, 92,* 480–487.

Andreassen, U. K, Baer, S., Nielsen, T. G., Dahm, S. L., & Arndal, H. (1992). Acute epiglottitis—25 years experience with nasotracheal intubation, current management policy and future trends. *Journal of Laryngology and Otolology, 106,* 1072–1075.

Arndal, H., & Andreassen, U. K. (1988). Acute epiglottitis in children and adults. Nasotracheal intubation, tracheostomy or careful observation? Current status in Scandinavia. *Journal of Laryngology and Otology, 102,* 1012–1016.

Bass, J. W., Steele, R. W., Wiebe, & R. A. (1974). Acute epiglottitis, a surgical emergency. *JAMA, 229,* 671–675.

Baum, H. L. (1928). Acute laryngotracheobronchitis. *JAMA, 91,* 1097–1102.

Bonadio, W. A., & Losek, J. D. (1991). The characteristics of children with epiglottitis who develop the complication of pulmonary edema. *Archives of Otolaryngology—Head and Neck Surgery, 117,* 205–207.

Bourchier, D., Dawson, K. P., & Fergusson, D. M. (1984) Humidification in viral croup: A controlled trial. *Australian Paediatric Journal, 20,* 289–291.

Broadhurst, L. E., Erickson, R. L., & Kelley, P. W. (1993). Decreases in invasive *Haemophilus influenzae* diseases in U.S. Army children, 1984 through 1991. *JAMA, 269,* 227–231.

Burton, D. M., Pransky, S. M., Katz, R. M., Kearns, D. B., & Seid, A. B. (1992). Pediatric airway manifestations of gastroesophageal reflux. *Annals of Otololaryngology, Rhinology and Laryngology, 101,* 742–749.

Butt, W., Shann, F., Walker C., Williams, J., Duncan, A., & Phelan, P. (1988). Acute epiglottitis: A different approach to management. *Critical Care Medicine, 16,* 43–47.

Camps, F. E. (1970). Acute epiglottitis (supraglottitis) due to *Haemophilus influenzae* type b. *Proceedings of the Royal Society of Medicine, 63,* 705–706.

Canadian Paediatric Society. (1992). Infectious Diseases and Immunization Committee: Steroid therapy for croup in children admitted to hospital. *Canadian Medical Association Journal, 147,* 429–430.

Centers for Disease Control. (1992). Notifiable diseases—Summary of reported cases, 1982–1991 (Table 1). *Morbidity and Mortality Weekly Report.* 40, 57.

Cherry, J. D. (1992). Croup (laryngitis, laryngotracheitis, spasmodic croup, and laryngotracheobronchitis). In R. D. Feigin & J. D. Cherry (Eds.), *Textbook of pediatric infectious diseases* (3rd ed., pp. 209–220). Philadelphia: W. B. Saunders.

Cressman, W. R., & Myer, C. M. (1994). Diagnosis and management of croup and epiglottitis. *Pediatric Clinics of North America, 41,* 265–276.

Crockett, D. M., Healy, G. B., McGill, T. J., & Friedman, E. M. (1988). Airway management of acute epiglottitis at the Children's Hospital, Boston: 1980–1985. *Annals of Otology, Rhinology and Laryngology, 97,* 114–119.

Cruz, M. N., Stewart, G., & Rosenberg, N. (1995). Use of dexamethasone in the outpatient management of acute laryngotracheitis. *Pediatrics, 96,* 220–223.

Currarino, G., & Williams B. (1982). Lateral inspiration and expiration radiographs of the neck in children with laryngotracheitis (croup). *Radiology, 145,* 365–366.

Daum, R. S., & Smith, A. L. Epiglottitis (supraglottitis). In R. D. Feigin & J. D. Cherry (Eds), *Textbook of pediatric infectious diseases* (3rd ed., pp. 197–208). Philadelphia: W. B. Saunders.

Davidson, S., Barzilay, Z., Yahav, J., & Rubinstein, J. (1982). Bacterial tracheitis—A true entity? *Journal of Laryngology and Otology, 92,* 173–175.

Dawson, K., Cooper, D., Cooper, P., Francis, P., Henry, R., Isles, A., Kemp, A., Landau, L., Martin, J., & Masters, B. (1992). The management of acute laryngo-tracheo-bronchitis (croup): A consensus view. *Journal of Paediatric Child Health, 28,* 223–224.

De Boeck, K. (1995). Croup: A review. *European Journal of Pediatrics, 154,* 432–436.

Denny, F. W., Murphy, T. F., Wallace, A. C., Clyde, W. A., Collier, A. M., & Henderson, F. W. (1983). Croup: An 11-year study in a pediatric practice. *Pediatrics, 71,* 871–876.

DiTirro, F. R., Silver, M. H., & Hengerer, A. S. (1984) Acute epiglottitis: Evolution of management in the community hospital. *International Journal of Pediatric Otorhinolaryngology, 7,* 145–152.

Eid, N. S., & Jones, V. F. (1994) Bacterial tracheitis as a complication of tonsillectomy and adenoidectomy. *Journal of Pediatrics, 125,* 401–402.

Eavey, R. D. (1985). The evolution of tracheotomy. In E. N. Myers, S. E. Stool, & J. T. Johnson (Eds.), *Tracheotomy* (pp. 1–11). New York: Churchill Livingstone.

Fielder, C. P. (1989). Effect of weather conditions on acute laryngotracheitis. *Journal of Laryngology and Otology, 103,* 187–190.

Fitzgerald, D., Mellis, C., Johnson, M., Cooper, P., & Van Asperen, P. (1996). Nebulized budesonide is as effective as nebulized adrenaline in moderately severe croup. *Pediatrics, 97,* 722–725.

Frantz, T. D., & Rasgon, B. M. (1993). Acute epiglottitis: Changing epidemiologic patterns. *Otolaryngology—Head and Neck Surgery, 109,* 457–460.

Freezer, N., Butt, W., & Phelan, P. (1990) Steroids in croup: Do they increase the incidence of successful extubation? *Anaesthia and Intensive Care, 18,* 224–228.

Frenkel, L. D., & Multicenter Ceftriaxone Pediatric Study Group. (1988). Once-daily administration of ceftriaxone for the treatment of selected serious bacterial infections in children. *Pediatrics, 82,* 486–491.

Friedman, E. M. (1988). Inflammatory illnesses of the pediatric airway. In M. P. Fried (Ed.), *The larynx: A multidisciplinary approach* (pp. 137–142). Boston: Little, Brown.

Friedman, E. M., Jorgensen, K., Healy, G. B., & McGill, T. J. (1985). Bacterial tracheitis—two-year experience. *Laryngoscope, 95,* 9–11.

Gallagher, P. G., & Myer, C. M. (1991) An approach to the diagnosis and treatment of membranous laryngotracheobronchitis in infants and children. *Pediatric Emergency Care, 7,* 337–342.

Gonzalez, C., Reilly, J. S., Kenna, M. A., & Thompson, D. E. (1986). Duration of intubation in children with acute epiglottitis. *Otolaryngology—Head and Neck Surgery, 95,* 477–481.

Greaves, M., & Lawlor, F. (1991). Angioedema: Manifestations and management. *Journal of the American Academy of Dermatology, 25,* 155–161.

Han, B. K., Dunbar, J. S., & Striker, T. W. (1979). Membranous laryngotracheobronchitis. *American Journal of Radiology, 133,* 53–58.

Henry, R. (1983). Moist air in the treatment of laryngotracheitis. *Archives of Disease in Childhood, 58,* 577.

Holbrook, P. R. (1988). Issues in airway management—1988. *Critical Care Clinics, 4,* 789–802.

Husby, S., Agertoft, L., Mortensen, S., & Pedersen, S. (1993). Treatment of croup with nebulized steroid (budesonide): A double-blind, placebo-controlled study. *Archives of Disease in Childhood, 68,* 352–355.

John, S. D., Swischuk, L. W., Hayden, C. K., & Freeman, J. H., Jr. (1994). Aryepiglottic fold width in patients with epiglottitis: Where should measurements be obtained? *Radiology, 190,* 123–125.

Jones, R., Santos, J. I., & Overall, J. C. (1979). Bacterial tracheitis. *JAMA, 242,* 721–726.

Kairys, S. W., Olmstead, E. M., & O'Connor, G. T. (1989). Steroid treatment of laryngotracheitis: A meta-analysis of the evidence from randomized trials. *Pediatrics, 83,* 683–693.

Kelley, P. B., & Simon, J. E. (1992). Racemic epinephrine use in croup and disposition. *American Journal of Emergency Medicine, 10,* 181–183.

Kessler, A., Wetmore, R. F., & Marsh, R. R. (1993). Childhood epiglottitis in recent years. *International Journal of Pediatric Otorhinolaryngology, 25,* 155–162.

Kimmons, H. C., & Peterson, B. M. (1986). Management of acute epiglottitis in pediatric patients. *Critical Care Medicine, 14,* 278–279.

Klassen, T. P., Craig, W. R., Moher, D., Osmond, M. H., Pasterkamp, H., Sutcliffe, T., Watters, L. K., & Rowe, P. C. (1998). Nebulized budesonide and oral dexamethasone for treatment of croup: A randomized controlled trial. *JAMA, 279,* 1629–1632.

Klassen, T. P., Feldman, M. D., Watters, L. K., Sutcliffe, T., & Rowe, P. C. (1994). Nebulized budesonide for children with mild-to-moderate croup. *New England Journal of Medicine, 331,* 285–289.

Knight, G. J., Harris, M. A., Parbari, M., O'Callaghan, M. J., & Masters, I. B. (1992). Single daily dose ceftriaxone therapy in epiglottitis. *Journal of Paediatric and Child Health, 28,* 220–222.

Ledwith, C. A., Shea, L. M., & Mauro, R. D. (1995) Safety and efficacy of nebulized racemic epinephrine in conjunction with oral dexamethasone and mist in the outpatient treatment of croup. *Pediatrics, 25,* 331–337.

Lisston, S. L., Genrz, R. C., Siegel, L. G., & Tilelli, J. (1983). Bacterial tracheitis. *American Journal of Diseases in Childhood, 13,* 764–767.

Litmanovitch, M., Kivity, S., Soferman, R., & Topilsky, M. (1990). Relationship between recurrent croup and airway hyperreactivity. *Annals of Allergy, 65,* 239–241.

Mauro, R. D., Poole, S. R., & Lockhart, C. H. (1988). Differentiation of epiglottitis from laryngotracheitis in the child with stridor. *American Journal of Diseases in Childhood, 142,* 679–682.

McEniery, J., Gillis, J., Kilhan, H., & Benjamin, B. (1991). Review of intubation in severe laryngotracheobronchitis. *Pediatrics, 87,* 847–853.

Megerian, C. A., Arnold, J. E., & Berger. M. (1992). Angioedema: 5 years' experience, with a review of the disorder's presentation and treatment. *Laryngoscope, 102,* 256–260.

Mjeon, S., Dahl, T., Swensen, T., & Westheim, A. (1979). Acute epiglottitis in children. An evaluation of the role of tracheostomy. *Journal of Laryngology and Otology, 93,* 995–1001.

Murphy, T. V., White, R. E., Pastor, P., Gabriel, L., Medley, F., Granoff, D. M., & Osterholm, M. T. (1993). Declining incidence of *Haemophilus influenzae* type b disease since introduction of vaccination. *JAMA, 269,* 246–248.

Oh, T. H., & Motoyama, E. D. (1977) Comparisons of nasotracheal intubation and tracheotomy in the management of acute epiglottitis. *Anaesthesiology, 46,* 214–220.

Pearlman, D. S. (1989). The relationship between allergy and croup. *Allergy Proceedings, 10,* 227–231.

Prendergast, M., Jones, J. S., & Hartman, D. (1994). Racemic epinephrine in the treatment of laryngotracheitis: Can we identify children for outpatient therapy? *American Journal of Emergency Medicine, 12,* 613–616.

Rabe, E. F. (1948a). Infectious croup: I. Etiology. *Pediatrics, 2,* 255–265.

Rabe, E. F. (1948b). Infectious croup: II. "Virus" croup. *Pediatrics, 2,* 415–427.

Rabe, E. F. (1948c). Infectious croup: III. *Haemophilus influenzae* type b croup. *Pediatrics, 2,* 559–566.

Rothrock, S. G., Pignatiello, G. A., & Howard, R. M. (1990). Radiologic diagnosis of epiglottitis: Objective criteria for all ages. *Annals of Emergency Medicine, 19,* 978–982.

Ryan, M., Hunt, M., & Snowberger, T. (1992). A changing pattern of epiglottitis. *Clinical Pediatrics, 31,* 532–535.

Salzman, M. B., Biller, H. F., & Schechter, C. B. (1987). Passive smoking and croup. *Archives of Otolaryngology, 113,* 844–849.

Sawyer, S. M., Johnson, P. D., Hogg, G. G., Robertson, C. F., Oppedisano, F., MacIness, S. J., & Gilbert, G. L. (1994). Successful treatment of epiglottitis with two doses of ceftriaxone. *Archives of Disease in Childhood, 70,* 129–132.

Schuller, D. E., & Birch, H. G. (1975). The safety of intubation in croup and epiglottitis: An eight year follow-up. *Laryngoscope, 85,* 33–46.

Sendi, K., & Crysdale, W. S. (1987). Acute epiglottitis: Decade of change—a 10-year experience with 242 children. *Journal of Otolaryngology, 16,* 196–202.

Sendi, K., Crysdale, W. S., & Yoo, J. (1992). Tracheitis: Outcome of 1,700 cases presenting to the emergency department during two years. *Journal of Otolaryngology, 41,* 20–24.

Senior, B. A., Radkowski, D., MacArthur, C., Sprecher, R. C., & Jones, D. (1994). Changing patterns in pediatric supraglottis: A multi-institutional review, 1980–1992. *Laryngoscope, 104,* 1314–1322.

Sinclair, S. E. (1941). *Haemophilus influenzae* type b in acute laryngitis with bacteremia. *JAMA, 117,* 170–173.

Skolnik, N. S. (1989). Treatment of croup—a critical review. *American Journal of Disease in Childhood, 143,* 1045–1049.

Sofer, S., Dagan, R., & Tal, A. (1991). The need for intubation in serious upper respiratory tract infection in pediatric patients (a retrospective study). *Infection, 19,* 131–134.

Sprem, N., & Branica, S. (1993). Effects of sulfur dioxide and smoke on the incidence of laryngotracheitis (croup). *International Journal of Pediatric Otorhinolaryngology, 26,* 245–250.

Stankiewicz, J. A., & Bowes, A. K. (1985). Croup and epiglottitis: A radiologic study. *Laryngoscope, 95,* 1159–1160.

Stool, S. E. (1988). Croup syndrome: Historical perspective. *Pediatric Infectious Disease Journal, 7,* S157–S161.

Super, D. M., Cartelli, N. A., Brooks, L. J., Lembo, R. M., & Kumar, M. L. (1989). A prospective randomized double-blind study to evaluate the effect of dexamethasone in acute laryngotracheitis. *Journal of Pediatrics, 115,* 323–329.

Szilagyi, P. G. (1991). Humidifiers and other symptomatic therapy for children with respiratory tract infections. *Pediatric Infectious Disease Journal, 10,* 478–479.

Takala, A. K., Peltola, H., & Eskola, J. (1994). Disappearance of epiglottitis during large-scale vaccinate with *Haemophilus influenzae* type b conjugate vaccine among children in Finland. *Laryngoscope, 104,* 731–735.

Tan, A. K. W., & Manoukian, J. J. (1990). Hospitalized croup (bacterial and viral): The role of rigid endoscopy. *Journal of Otolaryngology, 21,* 48–53.

Tibbals, J., Shann, F. A., & Landau, L. I. (1992). Placebo-controlled trial of prednisolone in children intubated for croup. *Lancet, 340,* 745–748.

Vallejo, J. G., Kaplan, S. L., & Mason, E. O. (1991). Treatment of meningitis and other infections due to ampicillin-resistant *Haemophilus influenzae* type b in children. *Reviews of Infectious Diseases, 13,* 197–200.

Vernon, D. D., & Sarnaik, A. P. (1986). Acute epiglottitis in children: A conservative approach to diagnosis and management. *Critical Care Medicine, 14,* 23–25.

Waisman, Y., Klein, B. L., Boenning, D. A., Young, G. M., Chamberlain, J. M., O'Donnell, R., & Ochsenschlager, D. W. (1982). Prospective randomized double-blind study comparing L-epinephrine and racemic epinephrine aerosols in the treatment of laryngotracheitis (croup). *Pediatrics, 89,* 302–306.

Waki, E. Y., Madgy, D. N., Belenky, W. M., & Gower, V. C. (1995). The incidence of gastroesophageal reflux in recurrent croup. *International Journal of Pediatric Otorhinolaryngology, 32,* 223–232.

Walker, P., & Crysdale, W. S. (1992). Croup, epiglottitis, retropharyngeal abscess, and bacterial tracheitis: Evolving patterns of occurrence and care. *International Anesthesiology Clinics, 30,* 57–70.

Wurtele, P. (1990). Acute epiglottitis in children and adults: A large scale incidence study. *Otolaryngology—Head and Neck Surgery, 103,* 902–908.

Wurtele, P. (1992). Acute epiglottitis: Historical highlights and perspectives for future research. *Journal of Otolaryngology, 21*(Suppl. 2), 1–15.

Zach, M. (1990). Air pollution and pediataric respiratory disease: Croup. *Lung 168*(Suppl), 353–357.

8

Tracheotomy

Chris de Souza, M.S., D.O.R.L., D.N.B., F.A.C.S., Cherie Ann Nathan, M.D., and Fred Stucker, M.D., F.A.C.S.

TRACHEOTOMY OR TRACHEOSTOMY?

Tracheotomy refers to an operative procedure that creates an artificial opening in the trachea that extends from the anterior aspect of the neck to the exterior aspect of the neck (Johnson, 1985). A tracheotomy is simply a tracheocutaneous fistula (de Souza & Ogale, 1995).

On the other hand, *tracheostomy* implies the creation of a permanent or semipermanent opening or stoma, as is created after laryngectomy. However, many physicians use these terms interchangeably, notwithstanding the etymological differences. For the purposes of clarity, we will use the term tracheotomy throughout this chapter in the context of the meaning given above.

Tracheotomy in Children Versus Tracheotomy in Adults

A tracheotomy in a child is much different than that done in an adult. Previously, the only difference was thought to be the obvious difference: the size and diameter of the pediatric airway as compared to the adult airway. It has recently been shown that tracheotomy in a child differs in several other ways as well. First, the child's larynx and trachea differ from the adult.

1. The pediatric larynx is situated high in the neck behind the mandible and is therefore well protected.
2. In children, and especially in infants, the neck is short and the pretracheal pad of fat obscures landmarks.
3. The trachea in infants is very flexible, rendering it difficult to palpate.

4. Hypertension of the infant neck causes the intrathoracic part of the trachea to be brought into the neck
5. The infantile cartilage is less susceptible to pressure necrosis.
6. The tracheal mucosa in children is more vascular and loosely attached to supporting structures than adult mucosa, making it more susceptible to accumulation of fluid, which results in edema. Thus, given the small caliber of the pediatric trachea, mucosal edema can quickly cause substantial obstruction.

Other anatomic differences that can contribute to respiratory failure in children are the following:

1. A soft bony thorax.
2. Horizontally placed ribs that do not allow for much expansion.
3. Small immature intercostal muscles leaving the work or respiration mainly to the diaphragm. Thus, any process that interferes with the diaphragm can cause a major problem.

Indications for Tracheotomy in Children

Tracheotomy in children is needed when one or a combination of these factors is present:

1. The upper airway is obstructed.
2. Mechanical ventilation is indicated.
3. Pulmonary toilet is needed on a regular and frequent basis.

The upper airway may be obstructed by nontraumatic lesions such as epiglottitis, severe peritonsillitis with peritonsillar abscess, large retropharyngeal abscess, or traumatic lesions, such as burns, maxillofacial trauma, or airway trauma. Trauma can readily compromise the pediatric airway for the following reasons: The small caliber of the pediatric airway can readily be compromised by edema and/or hemorrhage. The thinner intercartilaginous membranes in children can easily be ruptured. Airway injuries in children are likely to involve subglottic structures, often sparing higher levels. Since the subglottis is the narrowest part of the airway this area is rapidly compromised, leading to respiratory obstruction.

Tracheal tears, or even laryngotracheal disruptions, are more likely to occur in children. The loose attachment of the mucosa to cartilage predisposes it to ready separation from cartilage, especially in submucosal hemorrhage. This can cause rapid and significant airway compromise.

Mechanical ventilation is indicated when the child is in severe respiratory distress with signs of hypoxia not easily or readily reversed by medical measures and evidence of fatigue. The child is then considered to be at high risk for sudden complete airway obstruction (Mancuso, 1996). Thus, tracheotomy is indicated when respiratory insufficiency occurs with the real prospect that the child may need prolonged assisted mechanical ventilation (Pilmer, 1994).

In any case of airway distress, the child's airway patency must be evaluated and the child's respiratory pattern must be examined. Air movement, chest excursion, heart rate, quality of pulse, and perfusion need to be evaluated. It must be remembered that cyanosis is a late sign of hypoxia and is manifest when PO_2 has fallen below 400 mm Hg. Respiratory insufficiency requiring assisted mechanical ventilation may be presumed present when cyanosis persists despite administration of 100% oxygen or when the $PaCO_2$ continues to rise to 55 mm Hg.

Endotracheal Intubation

Endotracheal intubation is now a widely accepted practice as a means to overcome upper airway obstruction, assist mechanical ventilation, and perform pulmonary toilet. In short, endotracheal intubation may be used as an alternative to tracheotomy for the same indications that need tracheotomy (McDonald & Berkowitz, 1993). Endotracheal intubation is a much more efficient procedure in cases of dire emergencies, such as cardiac arrest, where the airway needs to be immediately secured and respiration maintained.

WHO SHOULD INTUBATE?

Anesthesiologists are usually better trained at making the intubation safe, atraumatic, and expeditious. They are usually able to judge the size of the tube

needed. Emergency room personnel are equally competent and adept at this procedure.

The Intubation Sequence

Awake intubation is indicated when physical examination demonstrates anatomy abnormalities that would make intubation under anesthesia difficult. These anatomic abnormalities include conditions such as limited neck mobility, temporomandibular joint disease, and trismus. The advantages of these techniques are (1) protective airway reflexes are preserved, and (2) if intubation is unsuccessful, the child can continue to spontaneously breathe as "no bridges have been burned" (Fanconi & Duc, 1987). The disadvantages of these techniques are that tracheal stimulation causes dynamic instability with wide fluctuations in heart rate and blood pressure and trauma to the teeth (Shribman, Smith, & Achola, 1987). Furthermore, the psychological sequelae to an awake intubation of an alert patient may be significant, although difficult to quantify.

Awake intubation requires a cooperative patient (Hancock & Pelenson, 1992). Unsedated nasal or oral intubation in the awake, alert pediatric patient can be attempted when the patient is small, easily overpowered, edentulous, and possesses normal atraumatized anatomy. Should awake intubation fail, intubation may be conducted with sedative-hypnotics or muscle relaxants.

Before attempting to intubate any child, the bedside should be **SOAP**ed (*S*uction, *O*xygen, *A*irway equipment, *P*harmacopeia). All the necessary personnel should be standing by.

The child's nasal cavity is anesthetized with a topical anesthetic. The posterior part of the tongue and pharynx are also anesthetized with viscous lidocaine.

Monitors are then applied to evaluate the child's vital parameters. The child should then be oxygenated with 100% oxygen for 15 minutes. This allows for a greater amount of time to perform the intubation before hypoxia sets in. The cricoid is then palpated to better stabilize and expose the laryngeal inlet. The endotracheal tube is then inserted. Auscultation and chest x-ray confirm tube placement. If awake intubation is not feasible, sedatives and/or muscle relaxants should be used when attempting to intubate.

Endotracheal Intubation Versus Tracheotomy

The advantage of endotracheal intubation is that it can be done rapidly in dire emergencies, and thus the airway can be immediately secured (McDonald & Berkowitz, 1993). The disadvantages are directly linked to the duration of time the endotracheal tube resides in the trachea. The longer the tube is in place, the greater the chance of a complication. It is not clear at this time how long an endotracheal tube may be kept in place without causing complications. In addition, the endotracheal tube does not eliminate dead space and the longer it is in place, the greater the possibility of it becoming blocked. If the child is conscious, the endotracheal tube can cause pain and discomfort, necessitating sedation and patient restraints.

In the absence of mitigating circumstances, short-term control of the airway is usually managed with endotracheal intubation; for the long-term tracheotomy is preferred. The difficulty lies in determining the duration of time an endotracheal tube may be kept without causing a complication.

CRICOTHYROIDOTOMY

Cricothroidotomy has been recommended only in dire situations to relieve acute upper airway obstruction when intubation or tracheotomy are not immediately available. Cricothyroidotomy can be performed much faster than tracheotomy and can be done by nonsurgeons (Brown & Sataloff, 1981).

The procedure itself is very simple. An incision is made directly through the skin overlying the thin and relatively avascular membrane that joins the thyroid cartilage. This incision can then be enlarged (Brantigan & Grow, 1980). Controversy still surrounds cricothyroidotomy. Chevalier Jackson was an opponent of cricothyroidotomy. He attributed many airway complications to cricothyroidotomy.

Advocates of cricothyroidotomy point to the ease with which it can be performed. They note that in Chevalier Jackson's era, cricothyroidotomies were done in an unscientific manner and the procedure fell into disrepute. However, when correctly done, cricothyroidotomy has few complications.

In their study, Weymuller and Cummings (1982) noted that prolonged endotracheal intubation is a contraindication to performing a cricothyroidotomy. They postulated that the endotracheal tube causes laryngeal inflammation, which in turn predisposes to complications if a cricothyroidotomy is performed. Another disadvantage is the absence of a cricothyroid tube, as standard tracheotomy tubes are not suited for this procedure. The art of tracheotomy and endotracheal intubation have recently been refined to a high level of sophistication while cricothyroidotomy has fallen into disuse. Generations of otolaryngologists and anesthesiologists have perfected the art of tracheotomy and endotracheal intubation. At this time there is no role for cricothyroidotomy as an elective procedure.

ANATOMY FOR TRACHEOTOMY IN CHILDREN

In very young children, the larynx is situated high in the neck and is well protected by the mandible. The cricoid cartilage lies at the level of the 2nd or 3rd cervical vertebra. The cricoid cartilage is the most prominent laryngeal cartilage at this age. These cartilaginous structures are very pliable in children and are difficult to define.

ELECTIVE TRACHEOTOMY

Tracheotomy may be performed under local or general anesthesia. Local anesthesia may be used in cooperative children (Hancock & Peterson, 1992). Elective tracheotomy should be performed in the operating room (OR) where facilities are available for resuscitation and endotracheal intubation (Myers, Stool, & Johnson, 1985). The OR also offers better asepsis. Monitors, suction, and trained OR personnel help make tracheotomy an efficient and safe procedure (Figure 8–1).

Technique of Tracheotomy

Position of the child

The child is kept warm and is laid supine on the operating table. The head is gently extended to increase the distance between the chin and the sternal notch, to smooth out the redundant folds of skin in the neck, and to bring the trachea closer to the surface. A roll of soft material is placed under the back to achieve this position. The head is stabilized by using a ring. The neck should not be overextended, as this serves to draw the lower trachea and mediastinal contents into the neck. Should a low tracheotomy be done under these circumstances, the tracheotomy would retreat into the chest when the extension is removed. This would likely result in complications (Myers, Stool, & Johnson, 1985).

The skin of the chest, chin, and neck are prepared. One percent xylocaine with 1:200,000 adrenaline is infiltrated under the skin. The local anesthetic reduces the postoperative discomfort as well as reduces bleeding during surgery.

Incision

Horizontal and vertical incisions have been described; the authors prefer to use the vertical incision. The main advantage of the vertical incision is that it runs in the same line as the trachea. This is important in children, as it is difficult to externally judge the precise level of the tracheotomy and the improved exposure helps determine a suitable site for making the stoma. The midline is also less vascular, making surgery more efficient.

Technique

Once the incision has been made the assistant retracts the edges of the incision with a retractor. It is important not to unnecessarily open up tissue planes. As

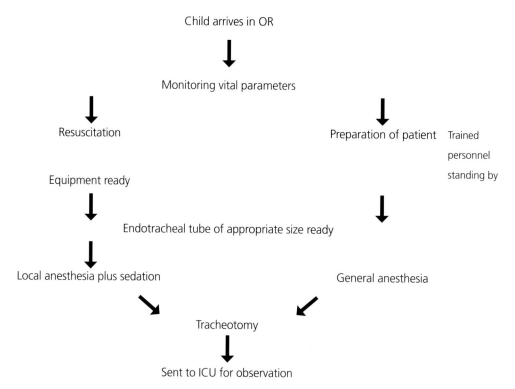

Figure 8–1. Sequence for performing a tracheotomy in a child.

the dissection progresses, the strap muscles are separated and retracted and the trachea is approached. If the surgeon stays in the midline, the tracheotomy can be efficiently completed. The surgeon should constantly palpate for the trachea to make sure he or she stays in the midline. The level of the cricoid should also be determined by palpation.

It is difficult to mistake the trachea, although in children the tracheal rings are softer and less obvious. Identifying the cricoid and then counting downward can help identify the tracheal rings. Identifying the thyroid isthmus is useful to identify the tracheal rings, as it consistently overlies the 2nd, 3rd, and 4th tracheal rings. Cutting the isthmus to provide better exposure is a matter of controversy. Good access to the trachea is obtained by clearing the fascia from the anterior surface of the trachea.

Tracheal Incision

In children, a vertical incision into the trachea is the best and the simplest procedure. However, the incision must be made at the correct level, which is one tracheal ring away from the cricoid. If it is made too near the cricoid, subglottic stenosis will likely result. If made too low, a tracheotomy can result in the tip of the tracheotomy tube entering the right main bronchus. The incision is made through the 2nd and 3rd tracheal rings. The incision should be made from below and upward to avoid damage to the mediastinum and its contents. Care should also be taken to avoid damage to the posterior wall of the trachea.

Some surgeons suture the tracheal incision and tape to the sutures to the child's chest. Should inadvertent decannulation take place, the sutures can be used to provide retraction to reinsert the tracheotomy tube. On the other hand, some surgeons consider this technique unnecessary as it weakens the trachea.

When incising the trachea, the secretions that emerge from the incision should be aspirated and cultured to identify bacteria and ascertain their sensitivity to various antimicrobial drugs.

A tracheotomy tube of suitable size and design is then inserted. The tracheotomy tube is then checked to see if it is indeed inserted into the tracheal lumen. The chest is auscultated to determine if the entry of air into both lungs is equal. The flanges of the tracheotomy tube are then securely taped. Although the tape should be secure, it should not be too tight or too loose.

A postoperative x-ray is taken to confirm that the tracheotomy tube is indeed in the trachea. Humidified air or humidified oxygen is supplied to prevent crusting. Regular suctioning of secretions in an aseptic manner is essential. The tracheotomy tract is usually well formed after 1 week. Regular aseptic suction and humidification are continued.

Complications

Commonly encountered complications are:

1. **Hemorrhage.** Transection of the anterior jugular veins or the thyroid isthmus is the cause of troublesome bleeding during the procedure. If the tra-

cheotomy is made low, there is a chance that the innominate artery can be traumatized. If pulsations are seen at the tracheotomy, they are likely to arise from the innominate artery. In this situation, the site of the tracheotomy should be changed to avoid hemorrhage from the innominate vessel, as there is a possibility that the tracheotomy tube can erode the artery.

2. **Intraoperative tracheoesophageal fistula (TEF).** To avoid creating a TEF the surgeon should avoid penetrating the posterior wall of the trachea. This is particularly important as the posterior wall of the trachea is devoid of cartilage. Should there be an accidental penetration, it should be immediately repaired at the time of tracheotomy. Repair consists of identifying the area of trauma with the interpositioning of tissue between the trachea and the esophagus. Drains should be put into the neck. A nasogastric tube should be inserted to feed patient until healing has occurred.

3. **Pneumothorax.** This is usually the result of damage to the apex of the lung. Timely diagnosis and timely treatment by inserting chest drains is critical.

Other complications that can occur are recurrent laryngeal nerve injury, injury to the cricoid cartilage, infection of the wound, blocked tracheotomy tube, and subcutaneous emphysema.

Antibiotics in Tracheotomy

Antibiotics are not indicated as a prophylactic measure in tracheotomy as they do not prevent bacterial colonization of the trachea (Johnson, 1985). Superinfection by resistant organisms often occurs following prophylactic administration of antibiotics. Pulmonary complications occur much more frequently in children receiving prophylactic antibiotic treatment following tracheotomy.

Physiologic Changes That Occur in Children Following Tracheotomy

Filtration, warming, and humidification of inspired air by the nose and nasopharynx are lost when air is inhaled through a tracheotomy. Normal mucociliary flow of secretions is disrupted. A tracheotomy acts as a foreign body and may harbor mucus and crusts, which in turn become a nidus of infection.

The cough effort is inefficient after tracheotomy. Glottic closure following tracheotomy becomes incomplete and this in turn leads to aspiration. Thus aspiration, ciliary dysfunction, and an ineffective cough lead to retention of secretions that in turn become colonized by bacteria, leading to pulmonary problems. Thus, following tracheotomy, the air passing through the tracheotomy should be warmed and humidified to maintain normal ciliary and mucosal integrity in the trachea and bronchi.

Choice of Tracheotomy Tube

Tracheotomy tubes for children are usually uncuffed and are miniature versions of adult uncuffed tracheotomy tubes. There are two types of tracheotomy tubes for children: plastic disposable and the silver tracheotomy tubes.

The advantages of the plastic tubes are:
1. They cause less of an inflammatory response.
2. The length of the tube can be shortened for neonates.
3. They conform well to the shape of the trachea and thus are less likely to cause ulceration of the trachea.

The primary disadvantage of the plastic tubes is that they get blocked more easily.

The advantages of silver tracheostomy tubes are:
1. The are reusable.
2. They have an inner valve that can be removed for cleaning and are less likely to get blocked.

The disadvantages include reactions to the metal tubes and a higher incidence of bleeding.

Angled pediatric tracheotomy tubes also have essentially the same design as angled adult tubes. It is important not to tie the neck straps too tightly in children fitted with tubes where the transmural limb is long.

Decannulation

The child can be decannulated only after the primary and secondary reasons that necessitated the tracheotomy have resolved (Rogers, 1988). Prior to decannulation the child should be assessed with regard to his or her ability to tolerate decannulation. The child's cough reflex should be robust. The chest should be normal. X-rays of the chest and neck should be normal. Oximetry should be normal (Mallory et al., 1983).

Some authors (e.g., Rogers, 1980) recommend that all children undergo endoscopic evaluation of the airway prior to decannulation. The endoscopic evaluation should reveal a normal airway as a necessary prerequisite for decannulation. Finally, psychological assessment of the child is carried out to determine if the child can tolerate decannulation.

The Decannulation Procedure

The only appropriate place to decannulate a child is a hospital and in the operating room in the presence of the appropriate staff. Two protocols for decannulating the child have been described. The first is to block the tracheotomy tube. The child should be observed for 48 hours. If the child tolerates the blocking well, the tube can be abruptly removed and the child is observed for another 24 hours. If this succeeds, the child is considered to be well and can be discharged from the hospital.

The other method consists of "weaning" the child off the tracheotomy tube by gradually decreasing the size of the tube in a graded manner. The smallest tube is inserted and is occluded and the child is observed to see how well she or he tolerates occlusion. The next morning the child is taken to the OR and the tracheotomy tube is removed. The stoma is dressed, and if the child continues to remain well, oral feeds are started. The child is observed for 48 hours following decannulation and is discharged from the hospital if no untoward complications arise.

Decannulation Failure

Should the child fail to tolerate decannulation, the tracheotomy tube is carefully reinserted. Great care is taken to avoid creating a false passage. After an aborted decannulation procedure, decannulation is not attempted for several months.

Causes for Failure of Decannulation

Stenosis

Tracheal narrowing is the more common cause for failure to decannulate. This is usually the result of a granuloma, in which case another endoscopic evaluation of the child is needed. The granuloma is then excised.

Dead Space

When the tracheotomy tube is removed, the dead space increases. This may initially cause the child increased respiratory effort. However, this usually gradually resolves without the child worsening.

Reduced vocal cord movement

The reflex adduction of the muscles of the vocal cord with inspiration is dependent on airway resistance, and this reflex is diminished in the presence of longstanding tracheotomy. However, with rehabilitation, this reflex gradually returns.

Nursing Management of the Child with a Tracheotomy

Nursing care of the child with a tracheotomy includes attention to the cardiorespiratory system, maintaining a patent airway, humidification of the airway, and regular suctioning and tube changes. Prevention of infection, ensuring safety, and providing emotional support and education for the child and the family are additional objectives.

Nursing Care in the Hospital

The child requires regular assessment of vital signs and blood pressure. Respiratory assessment includes examination of the child's color, respiratory rate and effort, and auscultation of breath sounds. Cardiopul-

monary monitoring and oxygen saturation are other parameters assessed. As a means to minimize or prevent infections in a hospital setting, aseptic techniques are employed when suctioning or changing the tracheotomy tube (Fitton, 1994).

Home Management

Before discharging the child with a tracheotomy from the hospital, both the child and the family need to be educated as to why the child was tracheotomized, the care required at home, and be provided with a list of do's and don'ts (Tym, 1988). Parents need to appreciate and understand why an artificial airway has been created and the extent to which normal laryngeal functions have been impaired.

The areas in which parents and family need to be educated include:
1. Stoma and skin care.
2. Regular, aseptic, and gentle suctioning.
3. Cleaning and changing the tracheotomy tube.
4. Chest physiotherapy.
5. Prevention, early detection, and management of complications.
6. Cardiopulmonary resuscitation.
7. Supplies and equipment necessary for the tracheotomized patient, such as suction machine, humidifier, etc.
8. Improving communication skills.
9. Availing themselves of help from the community.

Care of the Stoma and Skin

This should be carried out on a daily basis. Scabs and dried secretions should be gently cleaned. A dry pad of gauze should be placed between the skin and the tracheotomy tube to prevent excoriation of the skin.

Suction

This should be avoided as much as possible in the ambulatory patient by encouraging the child to cough out the secretions. If the secretions are tenacious and thick, the child is given mucolytics and other measures to liquefy secretions. Chest physiotherapy is also given to help expel mucous plugs. If the child is immobile and is unable to cough out mucus, suctioning is provided. This should be done in an aseptic, gentle manner.

Changing the Tracheotomy Tube

This should be done in the presence of trained nursing personnel. The new tube should be inserted in a gentle and aseptic manner to prevent creation of a false passage. The child and the parents should be educated regarding the dangers of aspiration when bathing. The tracheotomy should be guarded against insects.

Communication Development in Children

Tracheotomized children are at an increased risk for impairments in speech as there will be long periods of aphonia. The development of speech and language is related to the child's ability to vocalize.

Thus, the speech-language therapist plays an important role in the rehabilitation of the tracheotomized child. This therapist conducts language and articulation therapy, when possible, and augments verbalization with alternative methods of communication. Consistent audible vocalization, which allows for normal development of the spoken language in children, is difficult for children who have been tracheotomized in early infancy. The development of speech and spoken language needs to be attended to when a child is tracheotomized and when a child is decannulated.

Tracheotomized children also experience feeding difficulties. This may be a long-term or a chronic recurrent problem. Causes of feeding difficulties may include craniofacial anomalies such as cleft palate, choanal atresia, and tracheosophageal fistula. Other causes of feeding difficulties may result from the tracheotomy tube. The tracheotomy cannula makes flexion of the neck more difficult and can cause pain as the larynx is elevated during swallowing and the tracheotomy tube prevents complete glottic closure. Incomplete glottic closure can result in aspiration. The cough reflex is not effective in the presence of a tracheotomy, and thus aspirated material cannot be efficiently cleared from the trachea. In addition, in the presence of chronic respiratory disease, the child's caloric requirements increase; all of these issues need to be addressed in the tracheotomized child.

References

Brantigan, C. O., & Grow, J. B. (1980). Cricothyroidotomy revisited again. *Ear, Nose, Throat Journal, 59*, 283–295.

Brown, A. C. D., & Sataloff, R. T. (1981). Special anesthetic techniques in head and neck surgery. *Otolaryngologic Clinics of North America, 14*, 587–590.

De Souza, C. E. & Ogale, S. B. (1995). Tracheostomy. In *Textbook of the ear, nose and throat* (pp. 162–167). Madras, India: Orient Longman.

Fanconi, S., & Duc, G. (1987). Intratracheal suctioning in sick, preterm infants: Prevention of intracranial hypertension and cerebral hypoperfusion by muscle paralysis. *Pediatrics, 79*, 538–541.

Fitton, C. M. (1994). Nursing management of the child with a tracheostomy. *Pediatric Clinics of North America, 41*, 513–523.

Hancock, P. J., & Peterson, G. (1992). Finger intubation of the trachea in newborns. *Pediatrics, 89*, 325–327.

Johnson, J. T. (1985). Antibiotics in tracheostomy. In E. N. Myers, S. E. Stool, & J. T. Johnson (Eds.), *Tracheotomy* (pp. 171–176). New York: Churchill Livingstone.

Johnson, J. T., Rood, S. R., Stool, S. E., Myers, E. N. & Thearle, P. B. (1985). *Tracheotomy self instructional package.* American Academy of Otolaryngology—Head and Neck Surgery Foundation, Inc.

Mallory, G. B., Reilly, J. S., Motoyama, E. K., Mutich, R., Kenna, M. & Stool, S. E. (1985). Tidal flow measurement in the decision to decannulate the pediatric patient. *Annals of Otology, Rhinology and Laryngology, 94*, 454–457.

Mancuso, R. F. (1996). Stridor in neonates. *Pediatric Clinics of North America, 43*, 1339–1356.

McDonald, T. B., & Berkowitz, R. A. (1993). Airway management and sedation for pediatric transport. *Pediatric Clinics of North America, 40*, 381–406.

Myers, E. N., Stool, S. E., & Johnson, J. T. (1985). Technique of tracheotomy. In E. N. Myers, E. N. Stool, & J. T. Johnson (Eds.), *Tracheotomy* (pp. 113–124). New York: Churchill Livingstone.

Pilmer, S. L. (1994). Prolonged mechanical ventilation in children. *Pediatric Clinics of North America, 41*, 473–512.

Rogers, J. H. (1980). Decannulation by external exploration of the tracheotomy in children. *Journal of Laryngology and Otology, 94*, 454–457.

Rogers, J. H. (1988). Tracheostomy and decannulation. In J. N. G. Evans (Ed.), *Scott Brown's Pediatric Otolaryngology* (pp. 471–486). London: Butterworths.

Shribman, A. J., Smith, G., & Achola, K. J. (1987). Cardiovascular and catecholamine responses to laryngoscopy with or without tracheal intubation. *British Journal of Anesthesia, 59*, 295–297.

Tym, G. M. (1988). Home tracheostomy care. In J. N. G. Evans (Ed.), *Scott Brown's Pediatric otolaryngology* (pp. 487–494). London: Butterworths.

Weymuller, E. A., & Cummings, C. W. (1982). Cricothyroidotomy: The impact of antecedent endotracheal intubation. *Annals of Otology, Rhinology and Laryngology, 91*, 437–440.

9

Infections of the Fascial Spaces of the Head and Neck and Cervical Adenopathy in Children

Robert F. Yellon, M.D.

Potent broad spectrum antimicrobial agents have certainly decreased the incidence of deep head and neck space infections, although these potentially life-threatening infections still continue to occur. Familiarity with the important anatomic, etiologic, bacteriologic, and clinical factors, as well as selection of the best diagnostic and therapeutic modalities required for care of infections of the fascial spaces of the head and neck in children, is essential to prevent complications. Knowledge of the differential diagnosis and work-up for cervical adenopathy is also important since cervical adenopathy is so common in childhood, and accurate diagnosis is critical in certain cases, such as those with unusual etiologic organisms or possible malignancy.

ETIOLOGY OF HEAD AND NECK SPACE INFECTIONS

Infection originating in the nose, paranasal sinuses, or nasopharynx can drain via lymphatics to the retropharyngeal lymph nodes, and thus lead to retropharyngeal space infection. Iatrogenic or spontaneous trauma to the pharynx may provide a portal of entry for infection of the retropharyngeal or lateral pharyngeal spaces. Visceral and pretracheal space infections may arise from infection or trauma of the tonsils, laryngotracheal complex, hypopharynx, and esophagus. Infection of the vertebral bodies may cause prevertebral (retropharyngeal) space infections.

Adenotonsillitis is a source of lateral pharyngeal space infection. Infection of the petrous apex of the temporal bone may extend into the lateral pharyngeal space. When infection in the mastoid tip erodes through the cortex to lie between the mastoid tip and mandible, Bezold's abscess occurs, which may also extend into the lateral pharyngeal space. Tonsillitis is the precursor of peritonsillar space infection, which may extend to the lateral pharyngeal space. Lateral pharyngeal space infection may also follow local anesthetic infiltration for tonsillectomy and superior alveolar nerve block.

Mandibular, submandibular, masticator, parotid, lateral pharyngeal, and buccal space infections may arise from dental and gingival infections. Buccal space infections may also occur secondary to infection of the parotid gland or overlying skin, or from adenitis of nodes overlying the adjacent masseter muscle. Bloodborne *Haemophilus influenzae* may also cause buccal space infection in young children. When canine tooth root abscess erodes through the anterior cortex of the maxilla, canine space infection occurs. Sialoadenitis or suppuration of lymph nodes may lead to infections of the parotid space and space of the submandibular gland.

Neck masses such as cystic hygromas and branchial remnants may become infected and lead to infection in adjacent deep neck spaces. The structures of the carotid sheath may become infected via extension from infected adjacent deep neck spaces, suppurative adenitis, intravenous drug abuse, central venous catheter placement, and hypercoagulable states.

BACTERIOLOGY OF INFECTIONS OF HEAD AND NECK SPACES

In our series of 117 children (*N* = 78 cultures) with head and neck space infections seen at Children's Hospital of Pittsburgh during 1986 to 1992 (Table 9–1), the gram-positive aerobic pathogens beta-hemolytic *Streptococci* (18%) and *Staphylococcus aureus* (18%) were most prevalent. *Bacteroides melaninogenicus* (16.7%) and *Veillonella* species (14%) were the predominant anaerobic pathogens (Unkanont et al., 1993). A gram-negative pathogen, *Haemophilus parainfluenzae*, was found in 14% of cultures. In all, gram-negative pathogens were present in 17.9% of cultures. Twenty-two percent of aerobic pathogens produced beta-lactamase. Polymicrobial infections were common, and many of the anaerobes also produced beta-lactamase (Asmar, 1990; Brook, 1987).

ANTIMICROBIAL THERAPY FOR HEAD AND NECK SPACE INFECTIONS

After appropriate cultures are obtained, intravenous antibiotics are indicated for deep head and neck space infection. Oral antibiotics may be adequate for selected patients, such as adolescents, following incision and drainage of peritonsillar abscesses with relief of trismus and good oral intake. Since beta-lactamase producing bacteria are common, penicillin is no longer recommended and agents that inhibit beta-lactamase are more desirable. Clindamycin will provide good coverage for gram-positive organisms and anaerobes. It is not recommended if gram-negative organisms are suspected, in which case clindamycin plus a second or third generation cephalosporin is preferred. Gram-negative aerobic pathogens were found in 17.9% of cultures from 78 in our series of children with head and neck space infections (Table 9–1) (Ungkanont et al., 1993). Ampicillin-sulbactam is also recommended as it has excellent *in vitro* activity against gram-positive, gram-negative, and anaerobic organisms (Reinhardt et al., 1986;

Table 9–1. Bacteriology of head and neck space infections in 78 infants and children at Children's Hospital in Pittsburgh; January 1986 through June 1992.

Organism	No. of Cases (%)
Beta-hemolytic *Streptococcus*	14 (18)
Staphylococcus aureus	14 (18)
Bacteroides melaninogenicus	13 (16.7)
Veillonella species	11 (14)
Haemophilus parainfluenzae	11 (14)
Bacteroides intermedius	6 (7.7)
Micrococcus species	6 (7.7)
Peptostreptococcus species	4 (5)
Fusobacterium species	4 (5)
Candida albicans	4 (5)
Staphylococcus coagulase negative	2 (2.6)
Beta *Streptococcus* group C	2 (2.6)
Hemophilus haemolytica	2 (2.6)
Hemophilus influenzae (nontypable)	2 (2.6)
Bacteroides bivius	2 (2.6)
Eikenella corrodens	2 (2.6)
Escherichia coli	1 (1.3)
Alpha-hemolytic *Streptococcus*[b]	34 (44)
Neisseria species[b]	17 (22)
Diphtheroid species[b]	9 (11.5)
Other[a]	16 (20.5)
No growth	7 (9)

[a]Other organisms consisted of 16 species considered to be normal oropharyngeal flora (one isolate of each species).
[b]Normal oropharyngeal flora.

Retsema et al., 1986; Syriopoulou et al., 1986). The optimum duration for antimicrobial therapy has not been studied, but a total of 10–14 days is recommended. Based on clinical experience, at least 5 days of intravenous antimicrobial agents is recommended to treat any serious deep neck space infection. For oral therapy, amoxicillin-clavulanate, cefuroxime-axetil, or cefprozil are good choices. The combination of erythromycin and sulfisoxazole or clindamycin are appropriate for children with penicillin or cephalosporin allergy.

DIAGNOSTIC STUDIES

Laboratory investigations for children with possible deep neck space infections may include complete blood count with differential, prothrombin time, partial thromboplastin time, electrolytes, and possibly urine specific gravity. Throat, blood, sputum, or wound cultures may be indicated.

Anteroposterior and lateral soft tissue radiographs of the neck and pharynx may be required. It is important that the lateral film be taken with the child's neck in extension and during inspiration, or there may be spurious thickening of the retropharyngeal and retrotracheal spaces, especially in young children. For a properly taken film, if the retropharyngeal space measures more than 7 mm and the retrotracheal space more than 13 mm, an infection in this space is likely (Haug, Wible, & Lieberman, 1991). With retropharyngeal abscess, there is usually loss of the normal curvature and straightening of the cervical spine. Gas in the soft tissues confirms the presence of an abscess. Panorex films are useful to identify mandibular bone erosion or dental infection. A chest radiograph will rule out concomitant pneumonia or mediastinal involvement.

If the presence of an abscess versus cellulitis/adenopathy is still equivocal, further imaging techniques may be indicated. With selected infections such as the cooperative adolescent with a possible peritonsillar abscess, needle aspiration (NA) will be diagnostic if frank pus is obtained, thus obviating the need for imaging studies. When required, axial and coronal CT should be performed with 4–5 mm sections from the cranial base to the upper mediastinum (Weber, Baker, & Montgomery, 1992), which delineates both osseous and soft tissue structures. With intravenous contrast an abscess will appear as a "rim enhancing lesion," with a low-density center. A gas-fluid level or bubbles also confirm the diagnosis of abscess in the absence of trauma. Vascular structures and lymph node anatomy will also be delineated with intravenous contrast.

One hundred seventeen head and neck space infections treated at the Children's Hospital of Pittsburgh were reviewed (Ungkanont et al., 1993). From these cases, a series of 16 CT scans were available from children who had also undergone either open surgical exploration or NA. In this review, the sensitivity of CT for detection of head and neck space abscesses when reviewed by a neuroradiologist in a blinded fashion was 91% with a specificity of 60%. For detection of abscess, the positive predictive value of CT was 83% (Table 9–2). The two false negative cases underwent NA only, without open exploration, and thus it is possible that abscesses that may have been present were not detected.

MRI has also been recommended to distinguish head and neck abscesses from cellulitis/adenopathy. MRI can provide images in multiple planes including axial, coronal, and sagittal. T-1 weighted sequences will delineate major anatomic structures, while the inflammatory tissue has low to intermediate signal intensity. On T-2 weighted images, inflammatory tissue and abscess cavities will generate high-intensity signals. The walls of true abscesses will show "rim enhancement" with gadolinium-DTPA contrast. Sagittal sections using MRI may be particularly valuable for evaluation of retropharyngeal and lateral pharyngeal spaces, although CT and MRI are otherwise equivalent (Weber et al., 1992).

Ultrasonography (US) may also help to differentiate between cellulitis/adenopathy versus abscess dur-

Table 9–2. Sensitivity and specificity of CT scans in distinguishing cellulitis vs. abscesses in head and neck space infections in 16 infants and children at Children's Hospital of Pittsburgh; January 1986 through June 1992.

CT Scan	*Abscess Found at Surgery*	
	YES	NO
Positive	10	2
Negative	1	3

Sensitivity = 10/11 = 91%

Specificity = 3/5 = 60%

Positive Predictive Value = 10/11 = 83%

Negative Predictive Value = 3/4 = 75%

ing head and neck space infections. In one study (Glasier et al., 1992), US vs. CT was compared for the diagnosis of retropharyngeal adenopathy/cellulitis versus abscess in children. All 10 patients had CT scans showing abscesses. US showed only 3 patients with abscesses. For these 3 patients, intraoperative US guided surgical drainage. Two additional children with CTs positive for abscess, but US showing only adenopathy, underwent US guided NA of the retropharyngeal mass, and no pus was obtained. US correctly identified retropharyngeal adenitis/cellulitis in 7 children, whose infections all resolved with antimicrobial agents alone (Ben-Ami, Yousefzadeh, & Aramburo, 1990). In 12 children (Kraus, Han, Babcock, & Oestreich, 1986), US differentiated abscess from adenopathy/cellulitis. Intraoral US has also been used to identify peritonsillar abscess in a series of 12 patients (Haeggstrom, Gustafsson, Engquist, & Engstrom, 1993).

It would appear that, if CT or MRI are not available or are equivocal with regard to the presence of an abscess versus cellulitis/adenopathy, US is indicated to aid in the diagnosis. US also appears to be useful for intraoperative localization of abscess cavities (Glasier et al., 1992; Lewis et al., 1989).

AIRWAY MANAGEMENT FOR HEAD AND NECK SPACE INFECTIONS

A priority for children with head and neck space infections is establishing a stable airway, which may be accomplished when necessary via endotracheal intubation or tracheostomy. When trismus or soft tissue edema precludes endotracheal intubation, tracheostomy is indicated. Securing a tenuous airway should be strongly considered before the child depletes all of his or her respiratory reserve or progresses to complete obstruction, which will precipitate a more risky emergency intubation or tracheostomy. Cricothyroidotomy may be required for severe, acute airway obstruction. Initial intubation with an endotracheal tube or rigid bronchoscope prior to tracheostomy is recommended. However, unsuccessful attempts at intubation may also precipitate acute airway obstruction and thus tracheostomy under local anesthesia has rarely been performed. In selected cases, a nasopharyngeal or oral airway may be useful as a temporizing measure prior to definitive establishment of a secure airway.

SUPERFICIAL FASCIA OF HEAD AND NECK

Comprised of the subcutaneous tissue and fat, the superficial fascia of the head and neck covers the superficial muscles of the head and neck.

DEEP FASCIA OF NECK

Superficial Layer of Deep Cervical Fascia (DCF)

The superficial layer of the deep cervical fascia of the neck is a deeper structure that is distinct from the superficial fascia. The superficial or anterior layer of the DCF arises from the vertebral spinous process and ligamentum nuchae. It then encircles the trapezius, sternocleidomastoid, and omohyoid muscles, and then continues anterior to the strap muscles. It attaches superiorly to the hyoid bone and then splits to attach to both surfaces of the sternum, thus creating the suprasternal space (of Burns).

Middle Layer of Deep Cervical Fascia

The middle, pretracheal, or visceral layer of the DCF is continuous with the superficial layer of the DCF at the lateral borders of the strap muscles. It then forms the pretracheal fascia as it passes posterior to the strap muscles and anterior to the trachea and thyroid gland. Next, it becomes the visceral fascia as it envelops the pharynx and esophagus. The buccopharyngeal fascia is continuous with the middle layer of the DCF. At its superior extent, the middle cervical fascia fuses with the hyoid bone and thyroid cartilage. Inferiorly, it continues deep to the sternum into the superior mediastinum.

Posterior Layer of Deep Cervical Fascia

The posterior or prevertebral layer of the DCF also arises from the vertebral spinous processes and ligamentum nuchae. It then passes deep to the trapezius muscles and overlies the scalenes, levator scapulae, longus colli, brachial plexus, and phrenic nerve. This layer also covers the vertebral column and extends down to the clavicles. The portion that covers the vertebral bodies and longus colli muscles is described by some anatomists (Grodinsky & Holyoke, 1938; Hollinshead, 1982) as two distinct layers with a posterior prevertebral fascia and an anterior alar fascia. However, contemporary head and neck anatomists describe only a single layer of prevertebral fascia without any alar fascia (Drs. Eugene N. Myers and Jonas T. Johnson, personal communication, 1995).

FASCIA OF UPPER NECK, FACE, AND HEAD

Superficial Layer of Deep Cervical Fascia

Superior to the hyoid bone, the superficial layer of the deep DCF extends from the hyoid bone to the mandible and zygomatic arch. This fascia lies under the platysma muscle. It splits to cover both surfaces of the mandible as well as submandibular and parotid glands to form their capsules. The mylohyoid, anterior belly of digastric, lateral aspect of masseter, and medial aspect of the internal pterygoid muscles are also covered by this fascia.

Buccopharyngeal Fascia

The buccopharyngeal fascia covers the pharynx and is continuous with the visceral fascia (middle layer of DCF) covering the esophagus inferiorly. Laterally, it covers the buccinator muscle, and attaches to the pterygomandibular raphe.

SPACES OF NECK, FACE, AND HEAD INCLUDING: ANATOMY, CLINICAL PRESENTATION OF INFECTIONS, AND OPEN SURGICAL PROCEDURES FOR TREATMENT OF INFECTIONS

Peritonsillar Space

The peritonsillar (paratonsillar) space is the most common site of head and neck space infections. This space lies between the capsule of the palatine tonsil and the constrictor muscles. It is anteriorly and posteriorly limited by the tonsillar pillars. Superiorly, it can extend to the level of the hard palate or torus tubarius and inferiorly to the pyriform fossa. Sixty-three percent of 61 children with peritonsillar infection in the Children's Hospital of Pittsburgh series had trismus (Ungkanont et al., 1993), which results from extension of the infection to the lateral pharyngeal space and internal pterygoid muscle.

The presentation of peritonsillar space infections (Quinsy) includes pain, fever, dysphagia, cervical adenopathy, and fetor oris. On clinical exam, the hallmark is swelling of the tissues lateral and superior to the tonsil, with medial and anterior tonsillar displacement. The uvula may be pushed to the side opposite the infection. Hypertrophic, inflamed tonsils are usually present. Abscesses usually (but not always) form at the superior pole of the tonsil.

Some peritonsillar abscesses may be clinically obvious, while for others the clinical distinction between abscess and cellulitis is more difficult. A 12- to 24-hour trial of appropriate intravenous antimicrobials is reasonable in selected patients with no evidence of abscess or complications. If there is suspicion of extension of peritonsillar infection to adjacent deep neck spaces, then CT scan is indicated. If there is no improvement

following a trial of intravenous antimicrobials, NA may be attempted in selected patients in order to identify an abscess. Intraoral US correctly identified 12 out of 12 peritonsillar abscesses in ten adults and two children, and was useful to localize abscesses for NA (Haeggstrom et al., 1993).

Incision and drainage (I&D) via an anterior pillar incision followed by blunt dissection into the abscess cavity with a hemostat has been the standard treatment for peritonsillar abscess. Interval tonsillectomy may then be performed in 4 to 12 weeks if appropriate indications are met (see below) (Paparella, Shumrick, Meyerhoff, & Seid, 1980). Some surgeons advocate immediate tonsillectomy ("Quinsy tonsillectomy," "tonsillectomy *a chaud*") to provide complete drainage and to avoid a second hospitalization for interval tonsillectomy (Beeden & Evans, 1970; Grahne, 1958; McCurdy, 1977; Richardson & Birck, 1981; Templer, Holinger, Wood, Tra, & DeBlanc, 1977). In adults and children, the incidence of bleeding following Quinsy tonsillectomy ranged from 0–7% with an overall incidence of 1% for 1027 patients combined from the above studies. In a study of 55 children who had Quinsy tonsillectomies, no patient had postoperative or delayed bleeding (Richardson & Birck, 1981). No difference in bleeding between Quinsy and interval tonsillectomy was seen in a military population (McCurdy, 1977).

In a study of 41 patients (age not specified), 90% were successfully managed with NA of peritonsillar abscesses at the point of maximum bulging or, if the first aspiration was unsuccessful, 1 cm lower (Herzon, 1984). In a series of 74 patients (adults and children) with peritonsillar infections, NA of the superior, middle, and inferior peritonsillar areas was performed, and pus was aspirated in 70%. Additional aspirations were required for seven (10%) patients on the following day (Schechter, Sly, Roper, & Jackson, 1982).

In 29 children, the incidence of recurrent peritonsillar abscess and recurrent tonsillitis following peritonsillar abscess were each 7% (Holt & Tinsley, 1981). Recurrence of peritonsillar abscess for all ages ranges from 6–36%, with an average of 17% for 526 patients combined from six studies (Beeden & Evans, 1970; Herbild & Bonding, 1981; Holt & Tinsley, 1981; McCurdy, 1977; Nielsen & Greisen, 1981; Templer, 1977). Recurrent tonsillitis prior to or following peritonsillar abscess occurs in 7–50% of patients with an average of 28% for 345 patients combined from four studies (Beeden & Evans, 1970; Holt & Tinsley, 1981; Herbild & Bonding, 1981; Nielsen & Greisen, 1981).

For peritonsillar abscesses, Quinsy tonsillectomy, I&D with or without interval tonsillectomy, and NA have all been shown to be safe and effective. In patients with significant airway obstruction or associated complications, or if I&D have failed, Quinsy tonsillectomy is indicated. In patients with a prior history of recurrent peritonsillar abscess or recurrent tonsillitis warranting tonsillectomy, Quinsy tonsillectomy should be considered to avoid a second period of hospitalization and morbidity. I&D with interval tonsillectomy would also be appropriate for such patients.

NA of peritonsillar abscesses is a minimally invasive treatment which is safe and effective for older, cooperative children without complications. For children with a bleeding diathesis or whose general condition precludes a general anesthetic, NA is the treatment of choice.

Retropharyngeal (Prevertebral, Danger) Space

The cranial base is the superior limit of the retropharyngeal space; inferiorly it continues as the retrovisceral space into the mediastinum to the level of the carina. As described by Grodinsky and Holyoke (1938) and Hollinshead (1982), the posterior layer of the DCF is comprised of two distinct layers with an anterior alar fascia and a posterior prevertebral fascia. Between these two layers is the "danger space," which extends from the cranial base to the diaphragm (Grodinsky & Holyoke, 1938). In the view of these authors, the prevertebral space lies posterior to the prevertebral fascia and anterior to the vertebral bodies.

Contemporary anatomists report that the terms "retropharyngeal," "danger," and "prevertebral" spaces all refer to a single space. In their view, this space lies between a single layer of prevertebral fascia and the buccopharyngeal fascia of the posterior pharyngeal wall. The alar layer is considered to not exist (Drs. Eugene N. Myers and Jonas T. Johnson, personal communication, 1995).

According to the Grodinsky and Holyoke (1938) and Hollinshead (1982) view, infections in the "prevertebral" space (between the vertebral bodies and the prevertebral layer of the DCF) bulge in the midline, are bilateral, and are best approached by the open surgical approach to deep neck infections, as described below, rather than by the transoral approach. This approach avoids the possibility of a persistent draining fistula in the pharynx with the potential for aspiration. Such infections require prolonged antimicrobial therapy for osteomyelitis or tuberculosis of the vertebral bodies (Battista, Baredes, Krieger, & Feldman, 1993).

Children with retropharyngeal infection usually present with irritability, fever, dysphagia, muffled speech or cry, noisy breathing, stiff neck, and adenopathy. Stridor and drooling may be present in more severe cases. In the Children's Hospital of Pittsburgh series of 27 children with retropharyngeal infections, 9 (33%) had torticollis (Ungkanont et al., 1993). Since the buccopharyngeal fascia is adherent to the prevertebral fascia in the midline, infections in the retropharyngeal space are unilateral. If the patient has acute airway obstruction, examination should be performed in the operating room as the child will probably require I&D or an artificial airway. Alternatively, the child might have

supraglottitis if fever, stridor, and drooling are of sudden onset. A localized area of unilateral posterior pharyngeal swelling is usually an enlarged retropharyngeal lymph node. Unilateral swelling that extends from the nasopharynx to the retroesophageal area is usually either cellulitis or an abscess.

A transoral I&D is recommended for abscesses of the retropharyngeal space. Oral intubation may be safely done by introducing the tube on the side opposite the abscess. The Trendelenburg position is employed to avoid aspiration of purulent material. The mouth gag for tonsillectomy is used. Prior to I&D, an NA should be obtained for Gram's stain, culture, and antimicrobial sensitivity studies and to prevent tracheal aspiration of pus at the time of the I&D. A small vertical mucosal incision is made in the lateral aspect of the posterior pharynx between the junction of the lateral one third and medial two thirds of the distance between the midline of the pharynx and the medial aspect of the retromolar trigone. The deep tissues are then bluntly opened to drain the abscess and avoid possible injury to vascular structures. Placement of a drain is not advised as it may be aspirated. If the infection has extended to involve the lateral pharyngeal space, drainage should be performed through an external neck incision, as described below in the section on the open surgical approach to deep neck space infections. In selected cases, both transoral and external neck approaches are performed. If there is early recurrence of the abscess or no improvement following a transoral procedure, then an external approach is used.

Mandibular Space

This space is formed as the two leaflets of the superficial layer of the DCF split at the inferior border of the mandible. The lateral leaflet attaches laterally to the inferior border of the mandible, while the medial leaflet continues medially to the level of the mylohyoid. It is anteriorly limited by the attachment of the anterior belly of the digastric, and posteriorly limited by the attachment of the medial pterygoid to the mandible.

Most commonly, mandibular space infections occur when a suppurative dental process erodes through the lingual cortex of the mandible to create an abscess between the mandible and the inner leaflet of fascia. This painful intraoral swelling lies more anterior than that seen during infection of the more posterior medial portion of the masticator space. No external facial swelling is present unless the submandibular space is also involved. Mandibular space abscesses are drained by intraoral incision along the body of the mandible.

Masticator Space

The masticator space contains many structures including fat, loose connective tissue, the ramus of the mandible, the temporalis muscle, mandibular nerve, and internal maxillary artery. It is created by the splitting of the superficial layer of the DCF around the masseter and internal pterygoid muscles. This space extends anteriorly as the fascia covers the buccal fat pad and then ends as the fascia attaches to the maxilla and buccinator fascia. It ends at the back along the posterior border of the mandible. In its superior portion, the medial aspect of the masticator space is limited by the origin of the temporalis muscle from the skull, and laterally by the temporalis fascia. It extends medially to include the pterygopalatine fossa. Masticator space infection may occur medial or lateral to the mandible. The superior portion is referred to as the temporal space with compartments medial and lateral to the temporalis muscle.

Infections of the masticator space usually arise from dental pathology. Osteomyelitis or subperiosteal abscess of the mandible may occur. Pain usually occurs along the ascending ramus of the mandible. Trismus, sore throat, dysphagia, and pain on moving the tongue are commonly found. Swelling is observed in the retromolar trigone if the medial compartment is involved, which mimics peritonsillar abscess. Swelling of the floor of mouth and lateral pharyngeal wall may also be seen. With lateral compartment infection, swelling will be externally seen overlying the masseter.

For drainage of the lateral portion of the masticator space, an incision is made below and parallel to the body of the mandible. The facial vein, and possibly the facial artery, are then identified and ligated. They are then elevated with the platysma and the capsule of the gland to protect the marginal mandibular nerve. The masseter tendon is detached from the mandible, thus draining the lateral portion of the masticator space. Iodoform packing is placed. The medial portion of this space is approached by incision medial to the ascending ramus of the mandible in the retromolar trigone.

The temporal space may be approached via preauricular or hairline incisions through the temporalis fascia in order to reach abscesses lateral to the temporalis muscle or through the temporalis muscle to reach medially located abscesses. Iodoform packing is placed.

Buccal Space

Lateral to the buccinator muscle lies the buccopharyngeal fascia, which comprises the medial wall of the buccal space. The lateral aspect is formed by the skin of the cheek. Inferiorly, the buccal space is limited by the lower border of the mandible. The pterygomandibular raphe forms the posterior limit. The buccal fat pad, Stenson's duct, and facial artery lie within the buccal space (Topazian & Goldberg, 1981).

Infections in the buccal space present with swelling of the cheek. Trismus from inflammation of the masseter muscle is often present. Intraoral swelling

is usually minimal. Buccal space infections may occasionally be associated with the maxillary sinus, orbit, preseptal orbital tissues, or cavernous sinus.

Buccal space abscesses are usually in a subcutaneous location and are drained by skin or intraoral incision with blunt dissection parallel to the facial nerve branches.

Canine Space

The canine space is a potential space that lies anterior to the canine fossa of the maxilla. Dental infection usually precedes canine space infection. Swelling, which may be mistaken for dacryocystitis, is present adjacent to the nose, and spontaneous drainage may occur just inferior to the medial canthus of the eye. When the infection extends inferiorly, swelling is present in the labial sulcus.

Canine space infections may be approached by incision in the labial sulcus through the periosteum. Dissection continues superiorly to drain the abscess. Treatment of the associated dental infection is required (Topazian & Goldberg, 1981).

Parotid Space

The superficial layer of the DCF splits to cover the medial and lateral surfaces of the parotid gland to form the parotid space. This space contains the periparotid lymph nodes, the facial nerve, and may contain the auriculotemporal nerve, external carotid and superficial temporal arteries, and retromandibular vein. Pain, redness, and edema over the parotid are the usual findings with parotid space infection. Even when abscess is present, the thick fascia covering the gland prevents palpation of fluctuation.

Parotid space abscesses are drained via parotidectomy-type incision. The parotid fascia is detached from the tragus and sternocleidomastoid muscle to drain superficial abscesses. If necessary, the facial nerve is identified to allow drainage of abscesses that lie in the deep aspect of the parotid space. Intraparotid abscesses may be drained by gentle blunt dissection parallel to the branches of the nerve.

OPEN SURGICAL APPROACH TO DEEP NECK SPACE INFECTIONS

Although first described in 1929, Mosher's (1929) open surgical approach to deep pus in the neck is still useful today, with modification, for drainage of visceral, submandibular, and lateral pharyngeal space infections; infections of the carotid sheath; and selected infections of the retropharyngeal space. The majority of retropharyngeal abscesses may be transorally drained as described above. Mosher's T-shaped incision has been modified in that the horizontal limb is lower in relation to the body of the mandible and the vertical limb is omitted. After incising skin and platysma, dissection proceeds anterior to the sternocleidomastoid and postero-inferior to the submandibular gland. It is not unusual for the fascial layers to be extremely thickened. The facial artery should be identified and avoided or ligated during elevation of the gland. If the abscess is in the space of the submandibular gland, the capsule of the gland is incised along its lower border for drainage, or the gland may be excised. The carotid sheath contents are identified opposite the tip of the greater horn of the hyoid bone and may require I&D if there is infection in that space. Next, finger dissection superiorly along the carotid sheath allows drainage of the lateral pharyngeal space up to the cranial base. The visceral space may then be drained by blunt dissection medial to the carotid sheath in an inferior direction. Iodoform packing is placed for several days and the wounds are loosely closed. Packing should be left in place but advanced for at least 4 or 5 days. Early removal of the packing may result in reaccumulation of the abscess.

Head and neck space abscesses in any location that are obviously pointing may be managed by incision of skin and subcutaneous tissue with evacuation of pus. Digital exploration of any abscess cavity is important to drain any areas of loculation. Packing is then placed.

Lateral Pharyngeal Space

The lateral pharyngeal (parapharyngeal) space is shaped like an inverted pyramid and extends from the cranial base to the hyoid bone. It lies lateral to the buccopharyngeal fascia, and medial to the pterygoid muscles and fascia on the medial surface of the parotid. Anterosuperiorly, it extends to the pterygomandibular raphe, and posteriorly to the posterior surface of the carotid sheath. The styloid process and attached fascia of the tensor veli palatini muscle divide the lateral pharyngeal space into a prestyloid compartment containing the internal maxillary artery, maxillary nerve, and tail of parotid gland, and a poststyloid compartment which contains the carotid artery, internal jugular vein, cervical sympathetic chain, and cranial nerves IX–XII.

Pain, fever, and stiff neck are the usual presentation of lateral pharyngeal space infection. Trismus is caused by inflammation of the internal pterygoid muscle. Perimandibular edema may be present. Lateral pharyngeal wall swelling is noted which is frequently posterior to the tonsil. The tonsil is usually displaced in a medial and anterior direction. CT, MRI, or US may help to determine whether abscess or cellulitis is present. Complications such as airway obstruction or neuropathies may be present. When necessary, lateral pha-

ryngeal space infections are drained by the open surgical approach described above.

Carotid Sheath

The carotid sheath receives contributions from all three layers of the DCF. It contains the carotid artery, internal jugular vein, and vagus nerve. Neck stiffness, swelling, and torticollis are the frequent findings with carotid sheath infection. If thrombosis of the internal jugular vein occurs, spiking ("picket fence") fevers are common as septic emboli seed the pulmonary circulation. An open surgical approach to this deep neck space infection is required as described above.

Visceral Space

Within the visceral space are found the thyroid gland, trachea, and esophagus. The visceral space is divided into pretracheal and retrovisceral spaces, which are superiorly in continuity. Above the level where the inferior thyroid artery enters the thyroid gland, there is only one visceral compartment, defined anteriorly by the middle layer of the DCF, laterally by the carotid sheath, and the posterior layer of the DCF. Inferior to the level where the inferior thyroid artery enters the thyroid gland, dense connective tissue attaches the lateral aspect of the esophagus to the prevertebral layer, thus creating a pretracheal space anteriorly and a retrovisceral space posteriorly. The pretracheal portion extends superiorly to the attachment of the strap muscles to the thyroid cartilage and hyoid bone and inferiorly to the anterior mediastinum. Superiorly, the retrovisceral portion is continuous with the retropharyngeal space. Inferiorly, it extends to the carina and is a common pathway for the spread of deep neck infection into the mediastinum.

Neck swelling, pain, and dysphagia may occur with visceral space infection. Hoarseness due to glottic edema may progress to airway obstruction. Visceral perforation can lead to mediastinal and neck emphysema or pneumothorax. An open surgical approach is required as described above.

Submandibular Space Infections and Ludwig's Angina

The submandibular space is superiorly limited by the mucosa of the floor of the mouth and the tongue and the superficial layer of DCF as it runs from the hyoid bone to the mandible. In the interpretation of Hollinshead (1982), the sublingual space is the portion of the submandibular space that lies superior to the mylohyoid muscle which contains the sublingual glands, the lingual and hypoglossal nerves, and a portion of the submandibular gland and duct. Contemporary authorities divide the submandibular space into a supramylohyoid portion that is equivalent to the sublingual space, and an inframylohyoid portion that contains the structures lateral to the digastric muscle and medial to the mandible as well as the submental space, between the anterior bellies of the digastric muscles (Drs. Eugene N. Myers and Jonas T. Johnson, personal communication, 1995). The supramylohyoid and inframylohyoid portions of the submandibular space are in continuity posterior to the mylohyoid muscle which allows for easy spread of infection from one portion to the other.

When infection of the supramylohyoid portion occurs, there is induration and edema of the floor of mouth and tongue. When the inframylohyoid portion is involved, induration and edema lie inferior and medial to the mandible.

Bilateral involvement of the submandibular spaces may cause massive edema of the tongue and floor of mouth with posterior displacement of the tongue which, combined with trismus from involvement of the internal pterygoid muscles and possibly glottic edema, cause severe airway obstruction. The tissues are extremely indurated. This constellation of findings is called Ludwig's angina which, by definition, is a bilateral process. Cellulitis is sufficient to make a diagnosis of Ludwig's angina, and an abscess need not be present. In Ludwig's angina, release of tension in the edematous tissues is the basic surgical principle (Tschiassny, 1947). It is important to surgically explore for abscesses and drain them if present. Even if imaging studies do not show an abscess, open surgical intervention is indicated in all but the rare mild, early case of Ludwig's angina. Early establishment of a secure airway is advised. A horizontal incision is made approximately 1 cm above the hyoid bone, which may be extended to explore the space of the submandibular gland, if needed. The superficial layer of the DCF is incised in the midline from the mandibular symphysis to the hyoid bone. The digastric, mylohyoid, and a portion of the tongue are divided in the sagittal plane to decompress the floor of the mouth. Blunt dissection between the layers of muscles laterally will drain any possible abscesses. Iodoform packing is placed and the wounds left open. If an abscess is pointing within the oral cavity, it may be drained transorally.

Space of Submandibular Gland

As the superficial layer of the DCF splits to form a capsule around the submandibular gland and lymph nodes, the space of the submandibular gland is formed.

This space lies within the inframylohyoid portion of the submandibular space. On its posteromedial surface, the fascia is transversed by the submandibular duct, which allows spread of infection above the mylohyoid muscle. If necessary, this space is drained by the open approach described above.

SURGICAL VS. NONSURGICAL THERAPY FOR HEAD AND NECK SPACE INFECTIONS

Controversy exists concerning the need for, and timing of, surgical intervention in head and neck space infections in children. Some clinicians are advocating treating even documented abscess with an intravenous course of antimicrobial agents without surgical drainage. One author (Broughton, 1992) reported resolution of seven small, early, CT-documented retropharyngeal and parapharyngeal abscesses in children with intravenous antibiotics as the only treatment. In 65 children with retropharyngeal abscesses (Thompson, Cohen, & Reddix, 1988), 73% were treated with I&D, while 27% were treated with intravenous antimicrobials. In another series of 17 children with retropharyngeal abscesses (Morrison & Pashley, 1988), 82% were treated with I&D, and 18% with antimicrobials alone. All had a favorable outcome.

Antimicrobials are highly effective in treating most patients with uncomplicated cellulitis or adenopathy; however, when patients have a compromised airway or fail to rapidly improve on antimicrobial therapy, I&D are indicated, despite the lack of evidence from imaging that an abscess is present. Continued medical treatment of children despite lack of improvement over a reasonable period (24–72 hours) puts the child at risk for catastrophic complications. In patients with documented abscesses, surgical drainage is indicated. When the imaging studies are negative or equivocal for abscess, a trial of medical management is appropriate. Repeat of imaging studies during antimicrobial treatment can be helpful when a child is not rapidly improving and may be positive for abscess. The most effective method to determine causative organisms and to direct antimicrobial therapy is to obtain a culture during NA or I&D, which would be indicated when an unusual organism is suspected, as in the immunocompromised patient. NA in the awake infant or young child is not recommended and can be dangerous, but it is an option for selected older children. One or two NAs in conjunction with intravenous antimicrobials were successful in 56% of 18 neck abscesses in 17 children (Brodsky et al., 1992). Unilocular and small abscesses had a higher response rate to NA than multilocular and large abscesses that often required I&D.

For abscesses associated with complications and for those that fail NA, I&D is necessary. For uncomplicated head and neck space abscesses, the choice of intravenous antimicrobials alone vs. NA or I&D plus intravenous antibiotics is left to the judgment of the clinician, although I&D is strongly recommended.

COMPLICATIONS OF HEAD AND NECK SPACE INFECTIONS

Complications such as airway obstruction during a head and neck space infection are potentially fatal and require an open surgical approach. An intrathoracic complication during a head and neck space infection requires consultation with a chest surgeon. Bleeding from the pharynx or ear may be a harbinger of arterial erosion and massive hemorrhage. Arteriography may help to identify the bleeding vessel if there is sufficient time for this examination. Obtaining access to the great vessels for ligation and control of hemorrhage is critical in this situation. Thrombosis of the internal jugular vein is characterized by spiking fevers ("picket-fence fevers"), chills, and facial and orbital swelling, with evidence of septic emboli in the pulmonary, and occasionally the systemic circulation. The diagnosis of internal jugular vein thrombosis may be made on the basis of the typical clinical picture plus findings consistent with thrombosis using CT with contrast (Merhar, Colley, Clark, & Herwig, 1981), US (Bach, Roediger, & Rinder, 1988), or MRI with flow sensitive pulse sequences. Arteriography and venography are unnecessarily invasive and risky for most cases of internal jugular vein thrombosis as CT and MRI are reliable and safer (Dr. Hugh Curtin, personal communication, 1995). Internal jugular vein thrombosis may require systemic anticoagulation, ligation, or possible excision of the vein if emboli continue (Bach et al., 1988). An abscess may rupture into the airway and possibly cause asphyxiation, pneumonia, lung abscess, or empyema. Inflammatory torticollis with possible cervical vertebral subluxation requiring cervical traction and fusion has been reported to occur during head and neck space infections (Breden, Kamp, & Maceri, 1990). Neuropathies may be associated with lateral pharyngeal space infections (Langenbrunner & Dajani, 1971; Varghese, Hengerer, Putnam, & Colgan, 1982). It is the responsibility of the surgeon to prevent or minimize complications by making a rapid diagnosis and by delivering effective and timely medical and surgical interventions.

CERVICAL ADENOPATHY

Possible etiologies of cervical adenopathy in children include congenital, infectious, inflammatory, iatrogenic, and neoplastic causes. The stem cells for the T-lymphocytes arise in the thymus, whereas B-lymphocytes are produced in the fetal liver and bone marrow.

The primary lymphoid cells then migrate into the secondary lymphoid tissues including lymph nodes, tonsils, adenoids, spleen, and Peyer patches in the gut. There are 300 lymph nodes in the head and neck region that are grouped into specific regions with specific drainage patterns. These drainage patterns are described in the section on the etiology of head and neck space infections above.

In response to an antigenic or infectious stimulus, T- and B-lymphocytes are activated to produce germinal centers and numerous antibody-producing plasma cells. The lymph nodes significantly increase in size and are seen clinically as lymphadenopathy.

Congenital etiologies of lymphadenopathy are rare. Congenital agammaglobulinemia is a disorder with X-linked recessive inheritance with absence of production of gamma globulin. Recurrent bacterial infections are treated with antimicrobials and gamma globulin injections. Primary immunodeficiencies involving the phagocytic system are associated with lymphadenopathy (Adamkiewicz & Quie, 1992). Chronic granulomatous disease is due to an inability of phagocytes to generate free radicals for bacterial killing. The diagnosis is made by a positive finding on the nitroblue tetrazolium test. Chediak-Higashi syndrome, a disorder of the lysosomal membrane of neutrophils, is inherited in autosomal recessive manner, and is associated with recurrent bacterial infections. Metabolic storage disorders such as Gaucher or Neimann-Pick diseases may also present with generalized adenopathy.

INFECTIOUS ETIOLOGIES OF CERVICAL ADENOPATHY

Among the inflammatory etiologies of cervical adenopathy, viral infections account for the vast majority of cases. Adenovirus, rhinovirus, and enterovirus can all cause pharyngitis and cervical lymphadenopathy. These infections usually resolve within 10 days. Measles, rubella, varicella, zoster, mumps, and herpes simplex also may cause cervical lymphadenopathy. Mumps is typically associated with parotitis and rubella with postauricular lymphadenopathy. Human immunodeficiency virus causes the acquired immunodeficiency syndrome (AIDS) in which generalized lymphadenopathy may be prominent. EBV infection may lead to infectious mononucleosis, which clinically presents as fever, weakness, hepatosplenomegaly, and generalized lymphadenopathy. Tonsillitis with bacterial superinfection or tonsillar hypertrophy may occur. The diagnosis is made by the typical clinical picture, the finding of atypical lymphocytes on the peripheral blood smear and a positive monospot test. Ampicillin and amoxicillin usually will cause a rash. If treatment with antibiotics does not result in improvement, corticosteroids are indicated. If airway obstruction persists, endotracheal intubation, adenotonsillectomy, or even tracheostomy may be required (Stevenson, Webster, & Stewart, 1992).

Bacterial cervical lymphadenitis in children is also very common. Peak ages for these infections are 1–5 years. Submandibular and upper jugular lymph nodes are most frequently affected. The most prevalent organisms are *Staphylococcus aureus* and Group A streptococci (Barton & Feigin, 1974; Wright & Reid, 1987). Anaerobes are also possible (Brooks, 1980). When cervical lymphadenitis occurs in neonates, *S. aureus* and Group B streptococci predominate (Baker, 1982); however, gram-negative organisms are not uncommon.

Empiric therapy for routine cases of bacterial cervical adenitis would include 10 days of a second generation cephalosporin, amoxicillin-clavulanate, or one of the newer broad spectrum macrolides. Intravenous antimicrobial therapy is indicated when cervical lymphadenopathy is associated with severe pain, dysphagia, cellulitis, or systemic toxicity. In selected, older cooperative children, NA may help to obtain material for culture to direct more specific antimicrobial therapy. If an abscess is suspected, or if clinical improvement does not occur rapidly on intravenous antimicrobials, CT scan, MRI, or US may be helpful to differentiate lymphadenopathy/cellulitis vs. abscess. If abscess is documented on an imaging study, I&D are strongly recommended (see Surgical vs. Nonsurgical Therapy for Head and Neck Space Infections, above).

Mycobacteria can also cause cervical adenitis called scrofula. The offending pathogens may be *Mycobacterium tuberculosis* or atypical mycobacteria. Cervical adenopathy caused by atypical mycobacteria often shows redness and swelling without pain. Draining sinus formation is common.

Diagnosis of infection by *Mycobacterium tuberculosis* may be made by skin testing with purified protein derivative (PPD). Needle aspiration may show acid-fast bacteria. Histopathology of mycobacterial cervical adenitis shows granulomas with caseating necrosis. Chest radiography may disclose pulmonary manifestations. Other manifestations of systemic mycobacterial disease should be sought. Testing for AIDS is recommended. Long-term multidrug chemotherapy and infection control measures are required (Jawahar et al., 1990).

Nontuberculous or atypical mycobacteria generally produce mild disease in otherwise healthy children. The adenopathy and draining sinuses usually resolve over 9-12 months. Surgical excision of affected lymph nodes and sinuses is usually rapidly diagnostic and curative for infections with *M. avium intracellulare* or *M. scrofulaceum*. Curettage or needle aspiration are acceptable for lesions in critical locations where excision may be dangerous (Alessi & Dudley, 1988; Kennedy, 1992). Local recurrence of disease is possible in some cases (Joshi et al., 1989; Sigalet, Lees, & Fanning, 1992). Disseminated or severe atypical mycobacterial infec-

tion should raise suspicion of AIDS. Disseminated atypical mycobacterial infections and those caused by *M. kansasii* require antimicrobial therapy.

Cat scratch disease is another common bacterial cause of cervical lymphadenopathy in children. The offending pathogen, *Bartonella henselae* (formerly called *Rochalimaea henselae*) has been isolated from cats and fleas, and contact with an infected domestic cat is the most common cause of infection (Margileth & Hayden, 1993; Zangwill et al., 1993). The majority of children develop an inoculation papule following exposure. Although adenopathy may be extensive, most patients are otherwise asymptomatic. Enlarged lymph nodes may initially be tender, but then tenderness resolves. Suppuration of nodes may occur. Some patients may develop systemic signs including fever, malaise, and anorexia. Parinaud's oculoglandular syndrome occurs in 6% of patients and consists of conjunctival involvement and preauricular adenopathy. Severe manifestations such as encephalopathy or neuroretinitis are possible but not common.

Diagnosis is usually made on the basis of the typical history and clinical findings. If malignancy is suspected, lymph node biopsy is indicated. The definitive diagnosis may be made by identification of small, pleomorphic bacilli in excised lymph node sections using the Warthin-Starry stain. Serologic and skin tests are available in some centers (Zangwill et al., 1993).

Manifestations of cat scratch disease usually regress spontaneously after 2 to 6 months, although prolonged lymphadenopathy is possible. Antibiotic therapy may be helpful and may include trimethoprim/sulfamethoxazole, rifampin, ciprofloxacin, or aminoglycosides (Jackson, Perkins, & Wenger, 1993).

Other possible bacterial etiologies of cervical lymphadenopathy in children include *Yersinia pestis, Francisella tularensis,* and *Brucella. Yersinia pestis* causes bubonic plague. Rodents, fleas, cats, dogs, and squirrels transmit the plague bacillus to humans. The diagnosis is usually made by identification of Gram stain and culture of these gram-negative organisms from suppurating nodes called buboes. Streptomycin is effective for antimicrobial therapy. Contacts may need prophylaxis (Brubaker, 1991; Butler, 1989).

Francisella tularensis, a gram-negative coccobacillus, is the causative agent of tularemia. Exposure to rabbits, ticks, and contaminated water are the usual modes of transmission (Rohrback, Westerman, & Istre, 1991). The presentation may include fever, nausea, vomiting, tonsillitis, and painful ulcer at the site of inoculation, and cervical lymphadenopathy, which may suppurate.

Presumptive diagnosis is made from history of exposure to animals or biting insects in conjunction with the physical findings. Definitive diagnosis is made from special cultures from blood, gastric washings or draining wounds, or from a serum agglutination test (Sato et al., 1990). Streptomycin, gentamicin, and fluoroquinolones are acceptable for treatment (Scheel et al., 1993).

Several species of the gram-negative bacillus *Brucella* cause brucellosis in children. Contact with infected cattle or swine, including dairy product ingestion without pasteurization, are the usual modes of transmission. Fever, malaise, depression, and cervical adenopathy are common. Blood cultures and serologic tests are available for diagnosis. Doxycycline plus aminoglycoside or trimethoprim/sulfamethoxazole plus rifampin are usually effective (Al-Eissa et al., 1990; Montejo et al., 1993).

Cervicofacial actinomycosis ("lumpy jaw") is caused by the gram-positive organism *Actinomyces israelii*. Infections usually follow oral trauma, and mixed infections with other organisms are common. Material obtained from lesions shows the characteristic "sulfur granules." Treatment with penicillin is effective (Friduss & Maceri, 1990; Hong, Mezghebe, Gaiten, & Lofton, 1993).

Mycoplasma pneumoniae, which is a common cause of bronchopneumonia, pharyngitis, and bronchitis in school-age children, may cause a prolonged period of cough that is associated with cervical adenopathy. Serum cold agglutinins usually help to make the diagnosis. Macrolides and tetracyclines are effective for treatment (Fernald, Collier, & Clyde, 1975).

Congenital syphilis and the secondary stage of acquired syphilis caused by the spirochete *Treponema pallidum*, can present with fever, malaise, sore throat, rash, weight loss, and generalized lymphadenopathy. Peg-shaped (Hutchinson) teeth and saddle nose deformity may be present in congenital syphilis. The Venereal Disease Research Laboratory (VDRL) test is a serologic test that is useful as a screen but is nonspecific. The fluorescent treponemal antibody absorption (FTA-ABS) test is more specific; however, positive serologic tests in the child may result from transmission of maternal antibodies. Dark field microscopy of scrapings from lesions may show mobile spirochetes. Penicillin is effective for treatment (Zenker & Berman, 1991).

Fungal cervical adenopathy usually affects children with either a primary immunodeficiency or immunodeficiency acquired by iatrogenic immunosuppression or AIDS. Types of fungal organisms that can cause cervical adenopathy include *Candida, Aspergillus, Histoplasma,* and *Cryptococcus*. Systemic antifungal therapy with agents such as amphotericin-B, itraconazole, ketoconazole, or fluconazole is required (Como & Dismukes, 1994; Leggiadro, Barrett, & Hughes, 1992; Walmsley et al., 1993; Wheat, 1992).

Parasitic infection resulting in cervical adenopathy in children is usually caused by *Toxoplasma gondii*. Infection with this protozoan is usually acquired by ingestion of tissue cysts in undercooked meat or from oocytes in cat feces. Acquired toxoplasmosis in immunocompetent children usually causes asymptomatic cervical lymphadenopathy with or without malaise. The nodes do not suppurate. Most patients sponta-

neously recover without treatment. More severe manifestations occasionally occur in immunocompetent hosts but usually occur in the immunosuppressed population. Manifestations may include fever, stiff neck, myalgia, arthralgia, rash, hepatitis, pneumonia, myocarditis, meningitis, and chorioretinitis. Congenital infection with *T. gondii* may cause prematurity, jaundice, microcephaly, seizures, and eye problems.

For diagnosis, *T. gondii* organisms may be isolated from blood or tissue. Serologic tests are also useful. Pyrimethamine plus sulfadiazine are used as combination therapy (McCabe, Brooks, Dorfman, & Remington, 1987).

INFLAMMATORY/IDIOPATHIC TYPES OF CERVICAL ADENOPATHY

Kawasaki's disease (mucocutaneous lymph node syndrome) is a usually self-limited, but potentially fatal, idiopathic vasculitis, usually occurring before the age of 5. Clinical manifestations include fever, conjunctivitis, oral changes, edema and desquamation of hands and feet, rash, cervical adenopathy, and coronary vasculitis. Thrombocytosis is common. Antibiotics are ineffective. Coronary artery aneurysm, thrombosis, and infarction are possible and echocardiography is indicated. The diagnosis is mainly clinical. Intravenous gamma globulin and salicylates are used for treatment (Gersony, 1991).

Sinus histiocytosis with massive lymphadenopathy (Rosai-Dorfman disease) is an idiopathic disorder with massive enlargement of nontender cervical nodes. Typical findings on histologic examination of excised nodes include dilated sinuses, increased plasma cells, and sinusoidal histiocytes. Most cases are self-limited, but severe cases may require operative intervention, radiation, or chemotherapy (Komp, 1990).

Kikuchi-Fujimoto disease is a rare type of cervical adenopathy usually occurring in Asians that spontaneously resolves. Excised lymph nodes usually show necrosis in the paracortical or cortical areas (Garcia, Girdhar-Gopal, & Dorfman, 1993).

Sarcoidosis may also cause cervical adenopathy. There may be associated enlargement of the parotid gland and perihilar adenopathy on chest radiography (Kendig, 1974). Patients with histiocytosis-X (DiNardo & Watmore, 1989), systemic lupus erythematosus, and rheumatoid arthritis also may present with cervical adenopathy.

IATROGENIC CAUSES OF CERVICAL ADENOPATHY

Iatrogenic cervical adenopathy is frequently due to drugs including phenytoin, isoniazid, pyrimethamine, allopurinol, and phenylbutazone (Treyve & Duckert, 1981). In the transplant population, the immunosuppressive drugs FK 506 and cyclosporine are known to cause cervical adenopathy as part of the posttransplant lymphoproliferative disease (Armitage et al., 1993). Serum sickness following drug administration is also associated with lymphadenopathy. Other iatrogenic causes of cervical lymphadenopathy include vaccination with *Bacillus Calmette-Guerin* (BCG) (Oguz et al., 1992), as well as DPT vaccination (Omokolev & Castello, 1981).

NEOPLASTIC/MALIGNANT CERVICAL LYMPHADENOPATHY

Malignant cervical lymph nodes are usually firm and nontender, enlarge rapidly, and may be matted and fixed to the skin and surrounding structures. There is no response to antimicrobials. A review of pediatric head and neck malignancies disclosed that 60% of malignancies were lymphoma, 15% rhabdomyosarcoma, 10% thyroid malignancy, 5% neuroblastoma, and 5% nasopharyngeal carcinoma (Cunningham, Myers, & Bluestone, 1987).

DIAGNOSTIC APPROACH TO CERVICAL LYMPHADENOPATHY

Normal cervical lymph nodes are 1 cm or less in diameter. Acute, localized, unilateral cervical lymphadenopathy is usually due to infection by gram-positive bacteria. In contrast, acute viral and systemic infections usually cause bilateral cervical or generalized lymphadenopathy. A careful history including questions to determine duration of the mass, changes in size, constitutional symptoms, exposure to animals or insects, ingestion of unusual foods, or history of infections in the mother or family should be performed. In the differential diagnosis of pediatric neck masses, congenital etiologies should also be considered. Congenital neck masses would include thyroglossal duct cysts and epidermoid cysts in the midline, and branchial cleft remnants in the lateral neck. A pit or draining sinus along the anterior border of the sternocleidomastoid muscle suggests branchial cleft remnant. A careful physical exam may disclose associated findings such as an infected scalp lesion or systemic manifestations such as hepatomegaly. Nodes that are firm and nontender, enlarge rapidly, and are matted and fixed to the skin and surrounding structures suggest malignancy. If the affected nodes have failed to decrease in size following a 10-14 day course of antimicrobials that would cover staphylococci and streptococci, further evaluation may be needed.

Complete blood count with differential may help the evaluation point toward bacterial vs. viral infection,

or possibly toward noninfectious etiologies. Serologic tests for EBV, toxoplasmosis, cat scratch disease, syphilis, tularemia, brucellosis, histoplasmosis, AIDS, and anti-streptolysin-0 should be considered. Mycobacterial skin tests and chest radiography may be indicated.

Imaging studies including CT, MRI, and US may help to define anatomy and clarify whether the mass is cystic or solid, whether an abscess is present, or whether malignant necrosis is present within nodes (see Diagnostic Studies, above). Imaging studies will be useful to diagnose hemangiomas and lymphangiomas.

I&D are strongly recommended for abscesses (see Surgical vs. Nonsurgical Therapy for Head and Neck Space Infections, above). NA may be effective for small, unilocular abscesses (Brodsky, 1992). Diagnostic fine-needle aspiration may be useful in selected, cooperative, older children, but may be dangerous in uncooperative children. Incisional or, if possible, excisional biopsy should be considered if the history and physical exam are suspicious for malignancy, or if the child is ill and a diagnosis has not been reached by other means. Indications for incisional or excisional biopsy may include large, hard fixed nodes, fever, weight loss, night sweats, low neck adenopathy, continued increase in size of nodes despite antimicrobials, and failure of nodes to decrease in size after 6 to 8 weeks (Knight, Mulune, & Vassy, 1982). In a series of biopsies of pediatric neck masses, the incidence of malignancy was approximately 15% (Knight et al., 1982; Moussatos & Baffes, 1963).

REFERENCES

Adamkiewicz, T., & Quie, P. G. (1992). When to evaluate a child with recurrent infections for immunodeficiency. *Report—Pediatric Infectious Disease, 2,* 26.

Al-Eissa, Y. A., Kambal, A. M., Al-Nasser, M. N., Sulaiman, A., Al-Mabib, S. A., Ibrahim, M., Al-Fawaz, I. M., Fahad, A., & Al-Zamil F.A. (1990). Childhood brucellosis: A study of 102 cases. *Pediatric Infectious Disease Journal, 9,* 74.

Alessi, D. P., & Dudley, J. P. (1988). Atypical mycobacteria-induced cervical adenitis: Treatment by needle aspiration. *Archives of Otolaryngology—Head and Neck Surgery, 114,* 664.

Armitage, J. M., Fricker, F. J., Kurland, G., Michaels, M., Morita, S., Hardesty, R., Starzl, T. E., Yousem, S. A., Jaffe, R., & Griffith, B. P. (1993). Pediatric lung transplantation: The years 1985 to 1992 and the clinical trial of FK 506. *Journal of Thoracic and Cardiovascular Surgery, 105,* 337.

Asmar, G. I. (1990). Bacteriology of retropharyngeal abscess in children. *Pediatric Infectious Disease Journal, 9*(8), 595–597.

Bach, M. C., Roediger, J. H., & Rinder, H. M. (1988). Septic anaerobic jugular phlebitis with pulmonary embolism: Problems in management. *Reviews of Infectious Diseases, 10*(2), 424–427.

Baker, C. J. (1982). Group B streptococcal cellulitis-adenitis in infants. *American Journal of Diseases of Children, 136,* 631.

Barton, L. L., & Feigin, R. D. (1974). Childhood cervical lymphadenitis: A reappraisal. *Journal of Pediatrics, 84,* 846.

Battista, R. A., Baredes, S., Krieger, A., & Feldman, R. (1993). Prevertebral space infections associated with cervical osteomyelitis. *Otolaryngology—Head and Neck Surgery, 108*(2), 160–166.

Beeden, A. G., & Evans, J. N. G. (1970). Quinsy tonsillectomy—A further report. *Journal of Laryngology and Otology, 84,* 443–448.

Ben-Ami, T., Yousefzadeh, D. K., & Aramburo, M. J. (1990). Pre-suppurative phase of retropharyngeal infection: Contribution of ultrasonography in the diagnosis and treatment. *Pediatric Radiology, 21,* 23–26.

Bredenkamp, J. K., & Maceri, D. R. (1990). Inflammatory torticollis in children. *Archives of Otolaryngology—Head and Neck Surgery, 116,* 310–313.

Brodsky, L., Belles, W., Brody, A., Squire, R., Stanievich, J., & Volk, M. (1992). Needle aspiration of neck abscesses in children. *Clinical Pediatrics, 31*(2), 71–76.

Brook, I. (1980). Aerobic and anaerobic bacteriology of cervical adenitis in children. *Clinical Pediatrics, 19,* 693–696.

Brook, I. (1987). Microbiology of abscesses of the head and neck in children. *Annals of Otology, Rhinology, and Laryngology, 96,* 429–433.

Broughton, R. A. Nonsurgical management of deep neck infections in children. *Pediatric Infectious Disease Journal, 11*(1),14–18.

Brubaker, R. R. (1991). Factors promoting acute and chronic diseases caused by Yersinia. *Clinical Microbiology Reviews, 4,* 309.

Butler, T. (1989).The black death past and present. Plague in the 1980s. *Transactions of the Royal Society of Tropical Medicine and Hygiene, 83,* 458.

Como, K. A., & Dismukes, W. E. (1994). Oral azole drugs as systemic antifungal therapy. *New England Journal of Medicine, 330,* 263.

Cunningham, M. J., Myers, E. N., & Bluestone, C. D. (1987). Malignant tumors of the head and neck in children. A twenty-year review. *International Journal of Pediatric Otorhinolaryngology, 13,* 279.

DiNardo, L. J., & Wetmore, R. F. (1989). Head and neck manifestations of histiocytosis-X in children. *Laryngoscope, 99,* 721.

Fernald, G. W., Collier, A. M., & Clyde, W. A., Jr. (1975). Respiratory infections due to *Mycoplasma pneumoniae* in infants and children. *Pediatrics, 55,* 327.

Friduss, M. E., & Maceri, D. R. (1990). Cervicofacial actinomycosis in children. *Henry Ford Hospital Medical Journal, 38,* 28.

Garcia, C. E., Girdhar-Gopal, H. V., & Dorfman, D. M. (1993). Kikuchi-Fujimoto disease of the neck: Update. *Annals of Otology, Rhinology, and Laryngology, 102,* 11.

Gersony, W. M. (1991). Diagnosis and management of Kawasaki disease. *JAMA, 265,* 2699.

Glasier, C. M., Stark, J. E., Jacobs, R. F., Mancias, P., Leithiser, R. E., Seibert, R. W., & Seibert, J. J. (1992). CT and ultrasound imaging of retropharyngeal abscesses in children. *American Journal of Neuroradiology, 13,* 1191–1195.

Grahne, B. (1958). Abscess tonsillectomy. *Archives of Otolaryngology, 68,* 332–336.

Grodinsky, M., & Holyoke, E. (1938). The faciae and fascial spaces of the head, neck and adjacent region. *American Journal of Anatomy 63,* 367.

Haeggstrom, A., Gustafsson, O., Engquist, S., & Engstrom, C.-F. (1993). Intraoral ultrasonography in the diagnosis of peritonsillar abscess. *Otolaryngology and Head and Neck Surgery, 108*(3), 243–247.

Haug, R. H., Wible, R. T., & Lieberman, J. (1992). Measurement standards for the prevertebral region in the lateral soft tissue radiograph of the neck. *Journal of Oral and Maxillofacial Surgery, 49,* 1149–1151.

Herbild, O., & Bonding, P. (1981). Peritonsillar abscess: Recurrence rate and treatment. *Archives of Otolaryngology—Head and Neck Surgery, 107,* 540–542.

Herzon, F. S. (1984). Permucosal needle drainage of peritonsillar abscesses. *Archives of Otolaryngology—Head and Neck Surgery, 110,* 104–105.

Hollinshead, W. (Ed.). (1982). *Anatomy for surgeons* (Vol. I), (3rd ed., pp. 269–289). Philadelphia: Harper and Row.

Holt, G. R., & Tinsley, P. P. (1981). Peritonsillar abscesses in children. *Laryngoscope, 91,* 1226–1230.

Hong, I. S., Mezghebe, H. M., Gaiter, T. E., & Lofton, J. (1993). Actinomycosis of the neck: Diagnosis by fine-needle aspiration biopsy. *JAMA, 85,* 145.

Jackson, L. A., Perkins, B. A., & Wenger, J. D. (1993). Cat scratch disease in the United States: An analysis of three national databases. *American Journal of Public Health, 83,* 1707.

Jawahar, M. S., Sivasubramanian, S., Vijayan, V. K., Ramakrishnan, C. V., Paramasivan, C. N., Selvakamar, V., Paul, S., Tripathy, S. P., & Prabhakar, R. (1990). Short course chemotherapy for tuberculous lymphadenitis in children. *British Medical Journal, 301,* 359.

Joshi, W., Davidson, P. M., Jones, P. G., Campbell, P. E., & Roberton, D. M. (1989). Non-tuberculous mycobacterial lymphadenitis in children. *European Journal of Pediatrics, 148,* 751.

Kendig, E. L. (1974). The clinical picture of sarcoidosis in children. *Pediatrics, 54,* 289.

Kennedy, T. L. (1992). Curettage of nontuberculous mycobacterial cervical lymphadenitis. *Archives of Otolaryngology—Head and Neck Surgery, 118,* 759.

Knight, P. J., Mulune, A. F., & Vassy, L. E. (1982). When is lymph node biopsy indicated in children with enlarged peripheral nodes? *Pediatrics, 69,* 391.

Komp, D. M. (1990). The treatment of sinus histiocytosis with massive lymphadenopathy (Rosai-Dorfman disease). *Seminars in Diagnostic Pathology, 7,* 83.

Kraus, R., Han, B. K., Babcock, D. S., & Oestreich, A. E. (1986). Sonography of neck masses in children. *American Journal of Radiology, 146,* 609–613.

Langenbrunner, D. J., & Dajani, S. (1971). Pharyngomaxillary space abscess with carotid artery erosion. *Archives of Otolaryngology—Head and Neck Surgery, 94,* 447–457.

Leggiadro, R. J., Barrett, F. F., & Hughes, W. T. (1992). Extrapulmonary cryptococcosis in immunocompromised infants and children. *Pediatric Infectious Disease Journal, 11,* 43.

Lewis, G. J. S., Leithiser, R. E., Glasier, C. M., Iqbal, V., Stephenson, C. A., & Seibert, J. A. (1989). Ultrasonography of pediatric neck masses. *Ultrasound Quarterly, 7*(4), 315–335.

Margileth, A. M., & Hayden, G. F. (1993). Cat scratch disease from feline affection to human infection. *New England Journal of Medicine, 329,* 53.

McCabe, R. E., Brooks, R. G., Dorfman, R. F., & Remington, J. S. (1987). Clinical spectrum in 107 cases of toxoplasmic lymphadenopathy. *Reviews of Infectious Diseases, 9,* 754.

McCurdy, J. A. (1977). Peritonsillar abscess: A comparison of treatment by immediate tonsillectomy and interval tonsillectomy. *Archives of Otolaryngology, 103,* 414–415.

Merhar, G. L., Colley, D. P., Clark, R. A., & Herwig, S. R. (1981). Computed tomographic demonstration of cervical abscess and jugular vein thrombosis. *Archives of Otolaryngology—Head and Neck Surgery, 107,* 313–315.

Montejo, J. M., Alberola, I., Glez-Zarate, P., Alvarez, A., Alonso, J., Canovas, A., & Aguirre, C. (1993). Open, randomized therapeutic trial of six antimicrobial regimens in the treatment of human brucellosis. *Clinical Infectious Diseases, 16,* 671.

Morrison, J. E. & Pashley, N. R. T. (1988). Retropharyngeal abscesses in children: A 10-year review. *Pediatric Emergency Care, 4,* 9–11.

Mosher, H. (1929).The submaxillary fossa approach to deep pus in the neck. *Transactions of the American Academy of Ophthalmology and Otolaryngology, 34,* 19–36.

Moussatos, G. H., & Baffes, T. G. (1963). Cervical masses in infants and children. *Pediatrics, 32,* 251.

Nielsen, V. M., & Greisen, O. (1981). Peritonsillar abscess. I. Cases treated by incision and drainage: A follow-up investigation. *Journal of Laryngology and Otology, 95,* 801–807.

Oguz, F., Mujgan, S., Alper, G., Alev, F., & Neyzi, O. (1992). Treatment of *Bacillus Calmette-Guerin* associated lymphadenitis. *Pediatric Infectious Disease Journal, 11,* 887.

Omokoku, B., & Castells, S. (1981). Post-DPT inoculation cervical lymphadenitis in children. *New York State Journal of Medicine, 81,* 1667.

Paparella, M. M., Shumrick, D. A., Meyerhoff, W. L., & Seid, A. B. (Eds.). (1980). *Otolaryngology* (Vol. 3, 2nd ed., pp. 2272–2273). Philadelphia: W. B. Saunders.

Reinhardt, J. F., Johnston, L., Ruane, P., Johnson, C. C., Ingram-Drake, L., MacDonald, K., Ward, K. W., Mathisen, G., George, W. L., Finegold, S. M., & Mulligan, M. E. (1986). A randomized, double-blind comparison of sulbactam/ampicillin and clindamycin for the treatment of aerobic and aerobic-anaerobic infections. *Reviews of Infectious Diseases, 8* (Suppl. 5), S569–S575.

Retsema, J. A., English, A. R., Girard, A., Lynch, J. E., Anderson, M., Brennan, L., Cimochowski, C., Faiella, J., Norcia, W., & Sawyer, P. (1986). Sulbactam/ampicillin in vitro spectrum, potency, and activity in models of acute infection. *Reviews of Infectious Diseases, 8* (Suppl. 5), S528–S534.

Richardson, K. A., & Birck, H. (1981). Peritonsillar abscess in the pediatric population. *Otolaryngology—Head and Neck Surgery, 89,* 907–909.

Rohrback, B. W., Westerman, E., & Istre, G. R. (1991). Epidemiology and clinical characteristics of tularemia in Oklahoma, 1979 to 1985. *Southern Medical Journal, 84,* 1091.

Sato, T., Fujita, H., Ohara, Y., & Homma, M. (1990). Microagglutination test for early and specific serodiagnosis of tularemia. *Journal of Clinical Microbiology, 28,* 2372.

Schechter, G. L., Sly, D. E., Roper, A. L., & Jackson, R. T. (1982). Changing face of treatment of peritonsillar abscess. *Laryngoscope, 92,* 657–759.

Scheel, O., Hoel, T., Sanvik, T., & Berdol, B. P. (1993). Susceptibility pattern of Scandinavian *Francisella tularensis* isolates with regard to oral and parenteral antimicrobial agents. *APMIS, 101,* 33.

Sigalet, D., Lees, G., & Fanning, A. (1992). Atypical tuberculosis in the pediatric patient: Implications for the pediatric surgeon. *Journal of Pediatric Surgery, 27,* 1381.

Stevenson, D. S., Webster, G., & Stewart, I. A. (1992). Acute tonsillectomy in the management of infectious mononucleosis. *Journal of Laryngology and Otology, 106,* 989.

Syriopoulou, V., Bitsi, M., Theodoridis, C., Saroglou, I., Krikos, X., & Tzanetou, K. (1986). Clinical efficiency of sulbactam/ampicillin in pediatric infections caused by ampicillin-resistant or penicillin-resistant organisms. *Reviews of Infectious Diseases, 8* (Suppl. 5), S630–S633.

Templer, J. W., Holinger, L. D., Wood, R. P., Tra, N. T., & DeBlanc, G. B. (1977). Immediate tonsillectomy for the treatment of peritonsillar abscess. *American Journal of Surgery, 134,* 596–598.

Thompson, J. W., Cohen, S. R., & Reddix, P. (1988). Retropharyngeal abscess in children: A retrospective and historical analysis. *Laryngoscope, 98,* 589–592.

Topazian, R., & Goldberg, M. (Eds.). (1981). *Management of infections of the oral and maxillofacial regions* (pp. 196–199). Philadelphia: W. B. Saunders.

Treyve, E., & Duckert, L. G. (1981). Phenytoin-induced lymphadenopathy appearing as a nasopharyngeal malignant neoplasm. *Archives of Otolaryngology, 107,* 392.

Tschiassny, K. (1947). Ludwig's angina—A surgical approach based on anatomical and pathological criteria. *Annals of Otology, Rhinology and Laryngology, 56,* 937–945.

Ungkanont, K., Yellon, R. F., Weissman, J. L., Casselbrant, M. L., Gonzalez-Valdepena, H., & Bluestone, C. D. (1993). Deep neck infections in infants and children: The Pittsburgh experience. Unpublished manuscript.

Varghese, S., Hengerer, A. S., Putnam, T., & Colgan, M. T. (1982). Neck abscess causing Horner's syndrome. *New York State Journal of Medicine, 82*(13),1855–1856.

Walmsley, S., Devi, S., King, S., Schneider, R., Richardson, S., & Ford-Jaras, L. (1993). Invasive *Aspergillus* infections in a pediatric hospital: A ten-year review. *Pediatric Infectious Disease Journal, 12,* 673.

Weber, A. L., Baker, A. S., & Montgomery, W. W. (1992). Inflammatory lesions of the neck, including fascial spaces—Evaluation by computed tomography and magnetic resonance imaging. *Israel Journal of Medical Science, 28,* 241–249.

Wheat, L. J. (1992). Histoplasmosis in Indianapolis. *Clinical Infectious Diseases, 14* (Suppl. 1), S91.

Wright, J. E., & Reid, I. S. (1987). Acute cervical lymphadenitis in children. *Australian Paediatric Journal, 23,* 193.

Zangwill, K. M., Jamilton, D. H., Perkins, B. A., Regnery, R. L., Plikaytis, B. D., Hadler, J. L., Carter, M. L., & Wenger, J. D. (1993). Cat scratch disease in Connecticut: Epidemiology, risk factors, and evaluation of a new diagnostic test. *New England Journal of Medicine, 329*(1), 8–13.

Zenker, P. N., & Berman, S. M. (1991). Congenital syphilis: Trends and recommendations for evaluation and management. *Pediatric Infectious Disease Journal, 1,* 105.

10

Neoplastic Disease of the Head and Neck in Children: Incidence and Assessment

Phillip K. Pellitteri, D.O.

Head and neck malignant disease represents approximately 5–6% of all cancers occurring in the pediatric population. The two most common head and neck malignant neoplasms in children are lymphoma and rhabdomyosarcoma (Jaffe & Jaffe, 1973). The age at which children develop malignant disease in the head and neck varies with the type of tumor. Sarcomas, neuroblastomas, and malignant teratomas may appear in the newborn, while lymphomas generally present after the age of 2 and continue through childhood. Malignancies of the thyroid gland, nasopharynx, and salivary glands present later in childhood, affecting older children and adolescents. Forty percent of pediatric malignancies occur in children less than 5 years of age.

The two most common sites of presentation for head and neck cancers in children are the neck (70%) and the nasopharynx and oropharynx (16%) (Cunningham, Myers, & Bluestone, 1987). The usual presenting sign is the appearance of a mass, either in the neck or the pharynx. Most head and neck masses in children are inflammatory, and it may be difficult to distinguish between neoplastic disease and infection. Often, the neoplastic mass is asymptomatic and not otherwise associated with regional or systemic inflammatory symptoms. However, this is not always the case; lymphoma may be associated with tender lymphadenopathy and systemic illness may be manifested by fever and weight loss. It is imperative that the examiner conduct a comprehensive methodological work-up consisting of a complete history, comprehensive head and

neck examination, and appropriate supportive laboratory studies. Only after the comprehensive assessment is completed should attempts at diagnostic biopsy be considered, as these procedures often require sedation or general anesthesia in order to safely be performed in a child.

The history should include the setting in which discovery of the mass was made, as well as the date of onset and duration. Changes in the size and consistency of the mass, together with rate of growth, should be elicited. Associated regional and systemic symptoms should be sought, including epistaxis; nasal obstruction; dysesthesia; abnormalities of vision, speech, or swallowing; airway obstruction; weight loss; and fever.

A thorough head and neck examination includes otoscopy, rhinoscopy, and examination of the oral cavity, nasopharynx, laryngopharynx (either indirectly or directly), and the neck. Older children and adolescents are usually examined without difficulty, including indirect mirror examination; however, the younger child may not allow the performance of such methods. The examiner should not be deterred, and fiberoptic examination of these important areas must be performed. In rare instances, the young or uncooperative child may require sedation or general anesthesia in order to secure an adequate examination. A thorough cranial nerve evaluation is mandatory to assess the extent of disease and skull base involvement. Cranial nerve palsy may represent the heralding event in both malignant and benign disease, such as schwannoma/neurofibroma and nasopharyngeal carcinoma. In suspected cases of lymphoma, all lymphatic stations should be assessed, and there should be a thorough examination for hepatic and/or splenic enlargement as well.

The presence of additional lymphatic enlargement and/or hepatosplenomegaly with or without additional signs (i.e., Horner's syndrome and head and neck venous engorgement) make rapid diagnosis necessary. In more seemingly innocuous cases of lymphatic enlargement, the experience of the examiner, the response to antimicrobial therapy, and the results of adjunctive laboratory studies determine the timing as to when to perform diagnostic biopsy. In many instances, the size, consistency, growth rate, and location of the mass will prompt the performance of a diagnostic procedure early in the course of evaluation as suspicion for a neoplastic process is high. Large, rapidly growing, multiple masses in the posterolateral neck in a child with no identifiable source of infection is usually an indication of a malignant process and, as such, demands more urgent diagnosis. The more usual scenario involves lymphadenopathy, which may have evolved around an episode of remote upper respiratory tract infection, that has persisted, and may have slowly enlarged. Biopsy in this setting should be considered for enlarged lymph nodes still present or increasing in size 3 to 4 weeks following a 2-week course of antibiotics.

The presence of a mass, together with symptoms of nasal or pharyngeal obstruction or cranial nerve palsy, demands urgent diagnosis. Patients with this presentation are candidates for immediate aspiration or surgical biopsy to obtain suitable amounts of tissue.

Adjunctive laboratory and imaging studies may serve to support the clinical impression or determine the extent of a neoplastic process. In situations where lymphoma is suspected, a complete blood count with peripheral smear, chemistry for hepatic and renal function, and a chest x-ray should be obtained. If a neoplastic process other than lymphoma is suspected, as with the presence of upper airway obstruction/dysfunction or cranial nerve abnormality, a CT or MRI scan is usually indicated to assess the area of concentration and extent of disease.

The diagnostic procedure chosen greatly depends on the age of the child, the site of involvement, and the experience of the consulting cytopathologist. Fine needle aspiration (NA) is a minimally invasive and valuable procedure for many neoplastic processes affecting the neck and superficially accessible areas of the head and face. Its accuracy is directly dependent on the experience of the cytopathologist reading the aspirate—especially in cases of lymphoma and salivary and thyroid gland malignancy. The ability to perform flow cytometric studies on material aspirated from lymph nodes suspected of harboring lymphoma has enhanced the diagnostic capability of this procedure. In many cases of lymphoma, however, open surgical biopsy is required to accurately characterize and type the disease so that appropriate management may be instituted.

In patients suspected of salivary or thyroid gland malignancy, fine NA may not be diagnostic, even though ample tissue is obtained for cytologic review. In these instances, excisional biopsy from the remaining glandular tissue, as in parotidectomy or thyroidectomy, is diagnostic and therapeutic. In younger children, fine NA may require sedation and, in some cases, general anesthesia to be safely and efficiently performed. Masses that present in regions inaccessible by fine NA generally require endoscopic evaluation and biopsy to secure a diagnosis. These procedures are performed under general anesthesia and include endoscopic nasal/paranasal sinus procedures (including transnasal nasopharyngeal biopsy) and transoral endoscopic pharyngeal and laryngeal procedures. It is important to mention that, in many instances, these upper aerodigestive tract masses may pose a threat to the airway; therefore precautions for securing an airway and assessing the extent of the lesion by way of imaging prior to biopsy should be performed. This includes an assessment as to whether or not the mass represents a vascular neoplasm (i.e., angiofibroma, cavernous or plexiform hemangioma) or anomaly so that catastrophic hemorrhage is avoided.

Once the histologic diagnosis is secure, the disease process, if malignant or advancing on essential structures, is staged and recommendations for management are made. Staging for lymphomatous disease is generally made on the basis of imaging studies to assess extent of regional and distant lymphatic stations and hepatosplenic involvement, together with bone marrow assessment. For malignant lesions other than lymphoma, or histologically benign processes that encroach on important adjacent head, neck, and central nervous system structures, imaging forms the basis for evaluation of extent of disease in the absence of coexisting systemic symptoms.

Following histologic classification and staging, the child is presented to a multidisciplinary head and neck tumor conference for therapeutic recommendations and planning. This board is comprised of individuals from a variety of disciplines, including otolaryngology/head and neck surgery, radiation oncology, medical oncology, pathology, radiology, oromaxillofacial surgery, and appropriate healthcare support personnel from speech pathology, nutrition, and rehabilitative and social services. Children diagnosed with lymphoma are generally referred directly to the pediatric oncology service as these patients generally do not require extirpative surgery and reconstruction as part of the accepted therapeutic regimen. The staging of nonlymphatic pediatric head and neck malignancies is somewhat different from that which is used for adult carcinoma. In several instances the histologic type of malignancy has greater prognostic significance and may represent the determinative factor in treatment planning. Management schemes must also take into consideration the effect of therapy, whether surgical, radiotherapeutic, or chemotherapeutic, on normal growth in the head and neck. In general, most pediatric head and neck malignancies require multimodality therapy, but these therapeutic measures may occur in stages separated by long periods of time so as not to produce severe treatment-induced growth morbidity. In similar fashion, extensive extirpative surgery is usually reserved for tumors unresponsive to chemotherapy and is seldom required in the treatment of these childhood neoplasms. The following chapters offer a discussion on specific tumors of the head and neck in children, and their evaluation and management.

References

Cunningham, M. J., Meyers, E. S., & Bluestone, C. D. (1987). Malignant tumors of the head and neck in children: A twenty-year review. *International Journal of Pediatric Otorhinolaryngology, 13,* 279–285.

Jaffe, B. F., & Jaffe, N. (1973). Diagnosis and treatment: Head and neck tumors in children. *Pediatrics, 51,* 731–737.

11

Neoplasms of Lymphatic and Hematopoietic Origin

Phillip K. Pellitteri, D.O.

LYMPHOMA

Lymphoma is the most common pediatric malignancy of the head and neck and the second most common solid malignancy in children. It is subdivided into Hodgkin's and non-Hodgkin's lymphoma, with the former predominantly occurring in adolescence and the latter most commonly occurring in early childhood. Hodgkin's disease is considered a lymphoreticular malignancy and is thought to originate in a solitary node or dominant nodal group, usually cervical, and subsequently spread via contiguous lymphatics. Non-Hodgkin's lymphoma tends to be widespread at diagnosis,

with cervical adenopathy representing a part of the disease spectrum. The Ann Arbor staging system is now shared by both Hodgkin's and non-Hodgkin's lymphoma for staging purposes (Carbone et al., 1971) (Table 11–1).

Hodgkin's Lymphoma

Hodgkin's disease occurs at an incidence of 5.8 cases per million and follows a bimodal distribution. The first peak occurs in adolescents and young adults with a 3:1 male predominance and carries with it a good prognosis; this is followed by a second peak in individuals

Table 11–1. Ann Arbor staging system for Hodgkin's and non-Hodgkin's lymphoma.

Stage	Clinical Description
I	Single lymph node region or extralymphatic site (IE).
II	Two or more lymphatic regions or extralymphatic sites (IIE) on the same side of the diaphragm.
III	Nodal regions or extralymphatic sites (IIIE) on both sides of the diaphragm; spleen may be involved (S).
IV	Disseminated disease.

Subclasses for each stage:	A.	Absence of systemic symptoms
	B.	Presence of fever, night sweats, weight loss greater than 10%.

age 40 or older and is associated with a poorer prognosis (MacMahon, 1966). It is characterized by the presence of Reed-Sternberg cells, which are large, multinucleated cells with eosinophilic cytoplasm and perinucleolar areas, as well as mononucleolar variants of these cells (Figure 11–1). It commonly involves cervical, supraclavicular, and mediastinal nodal groups. Four histologic subtypes of Hodgkin's disease exist: lymphocyte predominant, nodular sclerosing, mixed cellularity, and lymphocyte depletion. Nodular sclerosing occurs in greater frequency in teenage children and young adults, and is associated with a more favorable prognosis. It is characterized by the presence of a thickened nodal capsule, which may divide the tumor into discrete nodules or lobules, and the lacunar cell, a variant of the Reed-Sternberg cell.

Mixed cellularity and lymphocyte predominant subtypes follow next in order of frequency and demonstrate a clear male predominance (approximately 5.5:1 and 4:1, respectively); whereas nodular sclerosing displays a reduced ratio of about 2:1 (Poppema & Lennert, 1980). Lymphocyte-depleted Hodgkin's disease is the least frequently encountered subtype (4–5%) and is differentiated from its predominant cousin by the relative proportions of neoplastic, Reed-Sternberg cells, and normal lymphocytes. As the percentage of normal lymphocytes decreases and the Reed-Sternberg cells increase, the prognosis worsens.

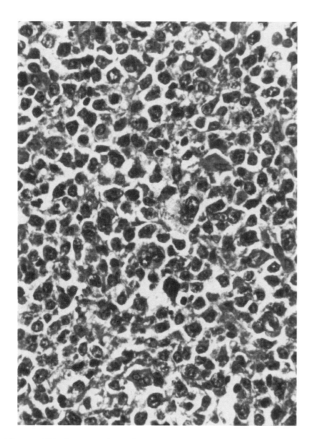

Figure 11–1. Hodgkin's lymphoma demonstrating large multinucleated Reed-Sternberg Cells. (Courtesy A. Garbes, M.D.)

Eighty to 90% of patients with Hodgkin's lymphoma present with painless cervical adenopathy. Lymphatic spread associated with supraclavicular adenopathy on the right may herald mediastinal disease; spread on the left may be associated with abdominal disease (Figure 11–2).

Patients may demonstrate systemic symptoms, in addition to adenopathy, consisting of fever, night sweats, and weight loss. The fever produced is characteristic, occurring in a relapsing fashion with elevations in the late afternoon and evening and is referred to as Pel-Epstein fever.

Laboratory examinations that need to be performed include a complete blood count with peripheral smear, liver chemistry, erythrocyte sedimentation rate, and serum copper level. These latter two examinations are useful in following the course of disease after therapy (Hrgovcic & Tessmer, 1968). A bone marrow test may not be useful in patients without systemic dissemination of disease and is carried out in those patients exhibiting systemic symptoms (Rosenberg, 1971).

Controversy exists as to whether staging laparotomy with splenectomy should be carried out on patients with Hodgkin's disease. Significant morbidity may attend up to 50% of children undergoing splenectomy (Chilcote, Baehner, & Hammond, 1976), and laparotomy changes the staging in approximately 20% of patients following the procedure. Thus, the benefit of determining the presence of disease below the diaphragm must be weighed against the potential morbidity or failure to upstage associated with performing this procedure. CT has advanced sufficiently in its ability to resolve discrete pathologic processes in the abdomen and pelvis so as to supplant the need for staging laparotomy and splenectomy in most situations.

Staging of Hodgkin's disease follows the Ann Arbor staging system seen in Table 11–1. Stages I–IV are subdivided into A or B with A representing patients without symptoms and B patients exhibiting fever, night sweats, or weight loss. The majority of children present with Stage I or II disease (approximately 70%), with Stage IV disease presenting in less than 10% of children at the time of diagnosis.

Treatment of Hodgkin's disease is very much dependent on stage at presentation. Stage I-A and II-A disease is usually well controlled with localized administration of 3500-4000 cGy of ionizing radiation alone. This may be directed toward the involved nodal groups or extended to address adjacent groups of nodes not clinically involved. Prognosis for early (I-A, II-A) disease treated with appropriate radiotherapy is excellent with a 10-year survival rate of 95% and relapse-free survival rate of 85–90% (Hellman & Mauch, 1982). Relapses may be effectively treated with chemotherapy. Advancing stage disease (I, II-B, III-A) usually requires the use of both irradiation and chemotherapy consisting of MOPP (nitrogen mustard, vincristine, procarbazine, and prednisone) or ABVD (Adriamycin, Bleomycin, vin-

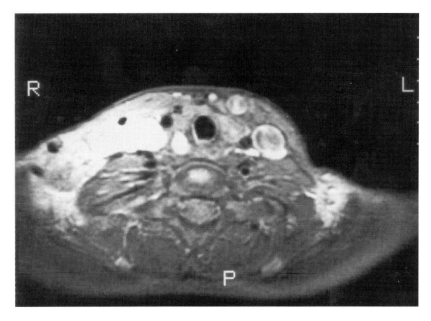

Figure 11–2. Axial MRI demonstrating Hodgkin's lymphoma involving supraclavicular lymph nodes extending to involve superior mediastinum.

blastine, dacarbazine) (De Vita & Simon, 1980). MOPP has also been shown to be effective in treating patients with early stage disease who have relapsed following radiation (Santoro, BonFante, & Bonnadonna, 1982). Late stage disease (III-B, IV) is usually treated using chemotherapy alone. High remission rates over 5 years may be seen in patients with advanced stage disease, although relapse rates are also significant in these patients. Children with the lymphocyte-depletion subtype and Stage III and IV disease have a poor prognosis (35%) despite combined therapy, whereas early stage disease exhibiting the lymphocyte-predominant histology demonstrates an excellent (> 90%) overall survival rate.

Morbidity and long-term sequelae of therapy for Hodgkin's disease are significant. These include infertility, immunosuppression, depression, and the development of a second malignancy. Patients treated with combined radiation and chemotherapy have an increased risk of developing a second malignancy compared to patients treated with either modality alone. Most commonly, leukemia represents the acquired malignancy and may occur in about 5% of patients on average of 5 to 7 years following treatment (Coleman et al., 1977). The development of leukemia appears to be related to an alkylating agent used in MOPP. Trials with ABVD and radiotherapy have not demonstrated development of leukemia in patients receiving this therapy (Valagussa et al., 1982).

Non-Hodgkin's Lymphoma

Non-Hodgkin's lymphoma is a rapidly progressive disease that often presents with widespread systemic and bone marrow involvement. Approximately 15% of patients with lymphoma will demonstrate head and neck disease at the time of presentation. Non-Hodgkin's lymphoma occurring in children is distinctly different from that encountered in adults in that the nodular and well-differentiated patterns are rarely found in childhood (Crist et al., 1981).

Non-Hodgkin's lymphoma may be practically divided into three distinct histologic types: (1) lymphoblastic (35% of patients), (2) undifferentiated small cell (Burkitt's and non-Burkitt's type) (40–50% of patients), and (3) large cell immunoblastic (15–20% of patients).

Malignant lymphomas of the lymphoblastic type morphologically resemble acute lymphoblastic leukemia. They are characterized histologically by diffuse uniform cells with minimal cytoplasm and rare nuclei. These lymphomas exhibit a paracortical pattern in affected lymph nodes with some sparing of nonneoplastic germinal centers.

The undifferentiated type (small noncleaved cell) consists of both Burkitt's lymphoma and non-Burkitt's type. Burkitt's type exhibits a diffuse homogeneous pattern of primitive cells with multiple nuclei. Frequently a starry-sky pattern of phagocytic histiocytes is present (Figure 11–3). There is a high mitotic index present, and a B-cell origin is suggested by monoclonal surface immunoglobulins of the IgM class. There is great nuclear pleomorphism associated with the non-Burkitt's type, and this entity is more rare than the Burkitt's type.

Diffuse large cell immunoblastic lymphomas are the least common histologic type encountered in children and are similar to their counterparts found in adults. Previously termed "histiocytic lymphomas," the majority exhibit lymphoid elements rather than true histiocytes.

Aside from the presence of a tumor mass, symptoms associated with advancement on adjacent vital

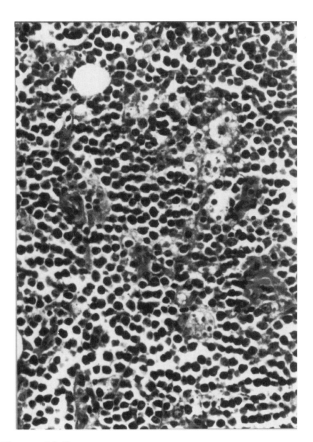

Figure 11–3. Burkitt's lymphoma demonstrating a typical "starry sky" pattern. (Courtesy A. Garbes, M.D.)

kin's disease. Treatment, however, should be instituted without delay and elaborate staging procedures postponed or conducted during the institution of therapy. Usually, patients are categorized into localized and non-localized disease for purposes of deciding on therapy at the initial staging (Anderson et al., 1983).

The treatment of lymphoma rarely involves surgery as a primary modality aside from surgical biopsy. Surgical resection in the head and neck is performed for relief of compressive symptoms (i.e., tracheal) or, in the instance of Burkitt's lymphoma, where the prognosis is directly dependent upon the volume of tumor present at initiation of treatment (Magrath & Lee, 1980). For rapid temporary relief of mediastinal compressive symptoms (i.e., tracheal, superior vena cava), a single administration of 500 cGy of external irradiation is usually adequate.

Chemotherapy using a four-drug combination, COMP (cyclophosphamide, vincristine, methotrexate, prednisone) or a 10-drug combination, LSA_2-L_2 (Table 11–2) remains the mainstay of therapy for lymphoma. COMP has demonstrated greater activity against non-lymphoblastic subtypes and has shown less toxicity. LSA_2-L_2 has been shown to produce improved treatment results against lymphoblastic lymphoma subtype in nonlocalized disease. Overall, neither treatment is superior for localized disease with both combinations demonstrating 84% disease-free survival over 2 years (Anderson et al., 1983). Two-year relapse-free survival rates for lymphoblastic and nonlymphoblastic lymphoma utilizing these treatment regimens are 76% and 57%, respectively, according to a Children's Cancer Study Group investigation (Anderson et al., 1983).

Burkitt's lymphoma is treated with intensive chemotherapy following surgical debulking, if feasible. The initial response to chemotherapy is quite important prognostically as those who fail to respond to initial treatment die within several months. High doses of cyclophosphamide, either alone or in combination with the other agents in COMP, are required and represent effective regimens.

Aside from the toxicity of chemotherapy, side effects related to massive tumor lysis may be encountered with treatment of systemic widespread disease. Hyperuricemia is common and can affect renal function,

structures may occur. Tracheal compression or superior vena cava syndrome can frequently occur in head and neck and mediastinal disease. Neoplastic involvement of Waldeyer's ring may present with eustachian tube obstruction and middle ear effusion, nasal obstruction, and, rarely, airway obstruction secondary to faucial tonsil and lingual tonsil involvement. Burkitt's lymphoma occurring in American children differs from the typical African variety in that neck masses are more common; however, tumor mass will nevertheless infrequently present in the jaw or parotid area.

Diagnosis is based on biopsy of the cervical/facial mass, usually in the form of open surgical biopsy to obtain sufficient tissue to subtype histology, or endoscopic biopsy of Waldeyer's ring tissue. The disease is rapidly progressive and may be widespread at the time of diagnosis, thus treatment should be embarked on without the delay that may result from elaborate staging procedures. Laboratory evaluations that are important for treatment include complete blood cell count with peripheral smear, liver, renal, and urine chemistries, and determination of serum uric acid, calcium, and phosphorus. Performance of a bone marrow examination is mandatory, and examination of cerebrospinal fluid (CSF) may be necessary if central nervous system (CNS) involvement is suspected.

The staging system utilized for non-Hodgkin's lymphoma is now essentially the same as that for Hodg-

Table 11–2. Multiple drug chemotherapy regimens for non-Hodgkin's lymphoma.

COMP	LSA_2-L_2	
Cyclophosphamide	Cyclophosphamide	Cytarabine
Oncovin	Vincristine	Thioguanine
Methotrexate	Methotrexate	Asparaginase
Prednisone	Daunomycin	Carmustine
	Prednisone	Hydroxyurea

necessitating dialysis. Renal function should be monitored and allopurinol administered to promote uric acid excretion. In addition, adequate hydration and prevention of hyperkalemia, hyperphosphatemia, and hypocalcemia must be undertaken to avoid electrolyte-associated morbidity.

HISTIOCYTOSIS-X

Histiocytosis-X represents a spectrum of syndromes characterized by histiocytic proliferation due to an unknown etiology. Three groups comprise this spectrum of disease, including, in progressive order of malignancy: (1) eosinophilic granuloma, (2) Han-Schuller-Christian disease, and (3) Letterer-Siwe disease. All components of this triad histologically represent a continuum and involve infiltration of Langerhans histiocytes into tissues and bone (Favara, 1981). Multinucleated giant cells are frequently seen, especially in solitary lesions; eosinophils and lymphocytes are also characteristic. Although the clinical picture may vary depending on the severity of the disease, the presentation usually involves a soft tissue mass with a typical well-circumscribed lytic lesion affecting the underlying bone. The head and neck is the sight of involvement for approximately 15% of all patients with histiocytosis-X, but may occur in 80% of patients if other associated findings are present (McCaffrey & McDonald, 1979). Other findings may include seborrheic skin lesions, "floating" multiple teeth, lymphadenopathy, otorrhea, diabetes insipidus, anemia, hepatomegaly, and pulmonary abnormalities.

Eosinophilic granuloma is a benign process most commonly characterized by lytic lesions of skull, mandible, spine, and long bones. Lesions are usually solitary, but may be multiple. When the calvarium is involved, the process begins in the diploic space and spreads to involve inner and outer tables with the latter more severely affected. This creates the typical beveled edge appearance on radiographs of the skull. There is usually an adjacent soft tissue mass in association with a bony sequestrum. The maxilla and mandible may be involved with the mandibular alveolar surface more frequently encountered. Involvement of the alveolar margin creates the lytic lesion which destabilizes the teeth, resulting in the characteristic mobilization seen on x-ray.

Otologic symptoms may be seen in up to 60% of patients due to involvement of the mastoid and temporal bones, which demonstrate characteristic changes on CT. Systemic involvement generally does not accompany eosinophilic granuloma. Roentgenographic characteristics of Han-Schuller-Christian disease are similar to that of eosinophilic granuloma, but may be limited to the axial skeleton. Although Letterer-Siwe disease represents systemic disease involving liver and bone marrow involvement, no distinct radiographic features are noted. The diagnosis of histiocytosis-X with identification of the affecting component disorder is based on surgical biopsy demonstrating the Langerhans histiocyte, roentgenographic findings, and the degree of systemic involvement.

The treatment of the solitary bone lesion of eosinophilic granuloma is generally curettage, although low-dose radiotherapy may be used. Multifocal lesions and patients with systemic disease are treated with chemotherapy using single or multiple drug regimens, including prednisone, vincristine, vinblastine, methotrexate, and cyclophosphamide.

The prognosis greatly depends on the extent of disease and age at onset. In general, the younger the patient, the poorer the prognosis, with children under age 2 or 3 failing therapy in most circumstances. The number of organ systems involved also influences the prognosis, with demonstrable organ dysfunction in any major system (i.e., liver, lung, bone marrow) representing an ominous prognosis. In a study reporting on 50 patients without organ dysfunction, 66% responded to treatment with a mortality rate of 4%. This is in direct contrast to patients with organ dysfunction, where only 33% responded to treatment and in whom a 66% mortality rate was noted (Lahey, 1975).

On the basis of age at onset and the presence or absence of organ dysfunction, patients with histiocytosis-X may be divided into three prognostic groups (Table 11–3) (Komp, 1981). Overall survival rates are listed relative to these groups.

Table 11–3. Histiocytosis X-prognostic groups with reference to age and organ system dysfunction.

Group	Organ Dysfunction	Age
Good risk	Absent	> 2 years
Intermediate risk	Absent	< 2 years
Poor risk	Present	All ages

Source: Adapted from "A Staging System for Histiocytosis X: A Southwest Oncology Group Study," by D.M. Komp, J. Herson, K. A. Starling, T. J. Vietti, and E. Hvizdala, 1981, *Cancer, 47*, pp. 798–800.

References

Anderson, J. R., Wilson, J. F., Jenkin, D. T., et al. (1983). Children's non-Hodgkin's lymphoma. The results of a randomized therapeutic trial comparing four 4-drug regimen (COMP) with a 10-drug regimen (LSA$_2$-L$_2$). *New England Journal of Medicine, 308*, 559–565.

Carbone, P. P., Kaplan, H. S., Musshoff, K., et al. (1971). Report on the committee on disease staging classification. *Cancer Research, 31*, 1860–1878.

Chilcote, R. R., Baehner, R. L., & Hammond, D. (1976). Septicemia and meningitis in children splenectomized for Hodgkin's disease. *New England Journal of Medicine, 295*, 798–800.

Coleman, C. N., Williams, C. J., Flint, A., et al. (1977). Hematologic neoplasia in patients treated for Hodgkin's disease. *New England Journal of Medicine, 297*, 1249–1252.

Crist, W. M., Kelly, D. R., Ragab, A. S., et al. (1981). Predictive ability of Lukes-Collins classification for immunologic phenotypes of childhood non-Hodgkin's lymphoma: An institutional series and literature review. *Cancer, 48,* 2070–2075.

De Vita, V., & Simon, R. M. (1980). Curability of advanced Hodgkin's disease with chemotherapy. Long-term follow-up of MOPP-treated patients at the National Cancer Institute. *Annals of Internal Medicine, 92,* 587–595.

Favara, B. E. (1981). The pathology of "histiocytosis." *American Journal of Pediatric Hematology/Oncology, 3,* 45–51.

Hellman, S., & Mauch, P. (1982). Role of radiation therapy in the treatment of Hodgkin's disease. *Cancer Treatment Reports, 66,* 915–921.

Hrgovcic, M., & Tessmer, C. F. (1968). Serum copper levels in lymphoma and leukemia. Special reference to Hodgkin's disease. *Cancer, 21,* 743–746.

Komp, D. M., Herson, J., Starling, K. A., et al. (1981). A staging system for histiocytosis X: A Southwest Oncology Group study. *Cancer, 47,* 798–800.

Lahey, M. E. (1975). Histiocytosis X—analysis of prognostic factor. *Journal of Pediatrics, 85,* 184–189.

MacMahon, B. (1966). Epidemiology of Hodgkin's disease. *Cancer Research, 26,* 1189–1195.

Magrath, I., & Lee, Y. J. (1980). Prognostic factors in Burkett's lymphoma: Importance of the tumor burden. *Cancer, 45,* 1507–1515.

McCaffrey, T. V., & McDonald, T. J. (1979). Histiocytosis X of the ear and temporal bone. Review of 22 cases. *Laryngoscope, 89,* 1735–1740.

Poppema, S., & Lennert, K. (1980). Hodgkin's disease in childhood. Histopathologic classification in relation to age and sex. *Cancer, 45,* 1443–1447.

Rosenberg, S. A. (1971). Hodgkin's disease of the bone marrow. *Cancer Research, 31,* 1733–1738.

Santoro, A., Bonfante, V., & Bonnadonna, G. (1982). Salvage chemotherapy with ABVD in MOPP-resistant Hodgkin's disease. *Annals of Internal Medicine, 96,* 139–143.

Valagussa, P., Santoro, A., Bellasi, F., et al. (1982). Absence of treatment-induced second neoplasms after ABVD in Hodgkin's disease. *Blood, 59,* 488–490.

12

Neoplasms of Soft Tissue

Phillip K. Pellitteri, D.O., and
Thomas L. Kennedy, M.D., F.A.C.S.

MALIGNANT LESIONS

Rhabdomyosarcoma

Rhabdomyosarcoma represents over half of the soft tissue sarcomas occurring in children under the age of 15, with the head and neck region being the most common site of involvement (38%) (Table 12–1). The annual incidence approaches 5 per million in white children and 1.5 per million in black children under 15 years of age, with a peak incidence occurring around 5 years of age (Young & Miller, 1975). There is a slight male predominance. This malignant tumor arises from embryonic mesenchyme or mesodermal tissue that is destined to become striated muscle. It may originate in virtually any anatomic location, and it is disseminated at the time of diagnosis in approximately 20% of patients.

The clinical presentation will vary according to the head and neck site involved. The most common primary site in the head and neck region is the orbit, followed by the pharynx and soft tissues of the face and neck (Sutow, 1964). Parameningeal involvement, particularly when the orbit is involved, is frequently encountered. These tumors may arise in any site containing striated muscle or its precursor cells.

Rhabdomyosarcoma may histopathogically be classified into four subtypes: (1) embryonal, (2) botryoid, (3) alveolar, and (4) pleomorphic. These subtypes share certain histologic elements; however, certain features may be uniquely characterized for each group of neoplasms (Gonzales-Cruss & Black-Schaffer, 1979).

Embryonal tumors represent the majority of rhabdomyosarcomas found in the head and neck in childhood. These tumors are composed of densely packed cells, which are similar in size to lymphocytes and contain hyperchromatic oval nuclei. They are arranged in an interlacing syncytial pattern (Figure 12–1) within a myxoidlike background. The botryoid subtype may be considered a variant of the embryonal, which occurs when the tumor arises beneath mucous membrane to form a polypoid growth.

The alveolar subtype exhibits cells that are moderate-sized and are separated by septated fibrous bands with alveolar clusters. Cellular nuclei are blunted and grooved with multinucleation frequently found. There may be evidence of rhabdomyoblastic differentiation with various cell forms, including straplike cells, racket cells, and multinucleated cells lined by peripherally located nuclei termed "spider cells."

Pleomorphic rhabdomyosarcoma demonstrates a distinctly different histologic pattern than the other three

Table 12–1. Frequencies of rhabdomyosarcoma in the pediatric population based on site of involvement

Anatomic Site	Occurrence (%)
Head and neck	38
Genitourinary	21
Extremities	18
Trunk	7
Retro-peritoneum	7

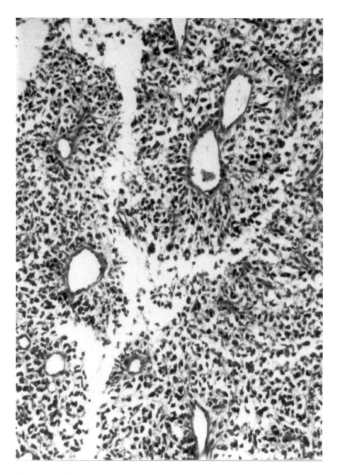

Figure 12–1. Embryonal rhabdomyosarcoma. (Courtesy of A. Garbes, M.D.)

subtypes. The tumor is composed of larger, morphologically bizarre cells, which appear to have characteristic differentiating features of skeletal muscle and, in distinction from the previous groups, appear to arise within mature skeletal muscle. Because these tumors do not arise in embryonic tissue, as do the other three, they are essentially limited to adults.

Alveolar rhabdomyosarcoma occurs predominantly in older children, has the worst prognosis, and is found in approximately 20% of head and neck rhabdomyosarcomas. The disease may be difficult to characterize histologically, with only 20–30% of specimens demonstrating cross-striations or features of striated muscle on biopsy. An adequate specimen from biopsy should be supplied to the pathologist.

The clinical manifestations are dependent on the anatomic site of involvement. Orbital involvement is heralded by a rapidly developing proptosis, which usually facilitates early diagnosis. Soft tissue tumors involving the deep face or neck usually present as a painless, relentlessly enlarging mass (Figure 12–2). Difficulty may be encountered with tumors of the nasopharynx or middle ear as the symptoms will mimic intercurrent upper respiratory infection. Nasal obstruction, otorrhea, and bloody rhinorrhea will ultimately lead to the dis-

covery of a mass in the middle ear or nasopharynx, thus reinforcing the necessity of a careful ear, nose, and throat evaluation in a child with delayed resolution of an upper respiratory tract or middle ear inflammatory process.

Surgical biopsy is required to establish diagnosis and characterize subtype. The staging evaluation is based primarily on extent of disease at the time of treatment initiation following biopsy or resection if localized disease is present. Imaging with CT or MR (particularly for parameningeal involvement) is the most effective means of establishing tumor extent, defining ports of radiation treatment, and assessing treatment response. CT findings may demonstrate a noncalcified enhancing mass in the orbit, deep tissues of the neck or face, or nasopharynx, which may invade and destroy adjacent structures. Direct intracranial extension may be noted and should be evaluated by MRI to assess dural integrity and possible parenchymal brain involvement. A chest x-ray is necessary to eliminate metastasis and should be combined with a chest CT if suspicious. Other measures to assess potential metastasis (i.e., bone marrow aspirate, liver scan or abdominal CT, lumbar puncture, bone scan) should be directed by associated systemic symptoms.

The Intergroup Rhabdomyosarcoma Study Group (IRS) previously advocated a clinical pathologic staging system that is dependent on therapeutic decisions made before categorization (Table 12–2) (Maurer et al., 1988). This clinical pathologic grouping of patients, made after initial surgical efforts are carried out, has prognostic significance. This does not represent an ideal system as most patients undergo biopsy rather than resection because of the improvement in chemotherapeutic regimens. Nevertheless, survival has been shown by most studies using the group classification to decrease as groups progress from stage I to IV. A more reliable pretreatment staging system has been developed by the IRS to classify patients based on presurgical findings and clinical presentation (Maurer & Abdelsalam, 1988b).

Cure is achievable for the majority of patients who present with localized disease. Therapy should be directed through a multidisciplinary approach coordinating surgery, chemotherapy, and radiation therapy to obtain maximum benefit from each modality.

Surgery should be directed at the performance of biopsy and determination of histopathology for tumor classification and, if feasible, total tumor resection with a margin of normal tissue. This is rarely achievable in the head and neck secondary to the proximity of adjacent vital structures and the difficulty in obtaining clear normal tissue margins. Should total resection with margins (I) or gross tumor removal with residual microscopic disease (II) be possible, the prognosis is favorable with a 3-year survival rate approaching 90% (Maurer et al., 1988a). Most children with head and neck disease are unresectable for the aforementioned reasons and fall into clinical group III. Open surgical biopsy is usually

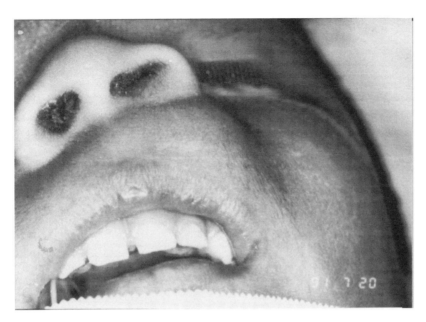

Figure 12–2. Rhabdomyosarcoma involving the maxilla in a young boy.

Table 12–2. Intergroup Rhabdomyosarcoma Study Group (IRS) clinical groups.

Group	Clinical Description
III	Localized disease, completely removed, no regional nodes involved. A. Confined to organ of origin. B. Contiguous involvement with infiltration outside organ or origin.
II	A. Gross removal of disease with microscopic residual; no gross residual, no nodal involvement. B. Regional disease, completely removed; no microscopic residual disease. C. Regional disease grossly removed, microscopic residual disease.
III	Incomplete removal or biopsy with gross residual disease.
IV	Distant metastatic disease present at diagnosis.

Source: Adapted from "The Intergroup Rhabdomyosarcoma Study—I: A Final Report," by H. M. Maurer, M. Beltangady, E. A. Gehan, W. Crist, D. Hammond, D. M. Hays, R. Heyn, W. Lawrence, W. Newton, J. Ortega, et al., 1988, *Cancer, 61,* pp. 209–220.

the only initial surgical procedure performed and is subsequently followed by chemotherapy/radiotherapy. Neck dissection is usually not performed because of the low incidence of lymph node metastasis from the head and neck primary sites.

Radiation therapy is delivered to the primary tumor and any suspicious lymph node groups with the intent of obtaining tumor control. Local relapse-free rates are generally higher when more than 4000 cGy of external beam radiation is administered to patients 6 years of age or older. The dose is determined primarily by the size of the primary tumor (less than or greater than 5.0 cm) and the age of the child (age 6). For tumors more than 5.0 cm, 4500 cGy is administered to children under 6 years of age and 5040 cGy to children 6 years or older. When tumor size is less than 5.0 cm, children

under age 6 receive 4140 cGy and those 6 or older receive 4500 cGy (Maurer & Abdelsalam, 1991). Radiation is generally administered to all patients except clinical group I and alveolar rhabdomyosarcoma. Patients with alveolar lesions in group I receive radiation therapy because of the increased risk of local relapse attributed to this histologic pattern.

All patients with rhabdomyosarcoma receive chemotherapy, as there has been sufficient evidence shown that it significantly improves survival rate (Heyn, 1994). The primary role of chemotherapy is to eradicate microscopic residual tumor. The standard chemotherapeutic agents currently used for rhabdomyosarcoma include: vincristine, actinomycin-D, cyclophosphamide, and doxorubicin—in two, three, or four drug combinations (Maurer et al., 1988a, 1988b). In general, patients in clinical groups

I and II with the embryonal histologic pattern receive less intensive therapy than those in groups III and IV, and patients in groups I and II with the alveolar pattern.

Three-year survival rates in head and neck disease are good with reported rates (IRS) of 85–90% (groups I–II) and 70–75% (group III) (Maurer et al., 1988a). Patients in clinical group IV in general fare poorly with 3-year survival rates of 30%; however, multimodality therapy is being developed using new combinations of chemotherapeutic agents in conjunction with bone marrow transplantation and may offer improved survival.

Survival following relapse is generally poor for rhabdomyosarcoma, with a combined group survival after recurrence of approximately 17% (Maurer et al., 1988a). Aggressive therapy is required following relapse, including surgical resection of tumor. The risk of relapse increases as patients progress in groups from I to IV.

In addition to rhabdomyosarcoma, a number of other soft part malignant lesions may arise in the head and neck in children. These include fibrosarcoma, liposarcoma, synovial cell sarcoma, malignant fibrous histiocytoma, alveolar soft part sarcoma, and hemangiopericytoma. These tumors are most frequently encountered in the trunk and extremities; however, they may occasionally involve the head and neck. The pattern of spread is usually in contiguity with rare distant metastasis from head and neck sites. Local recurrence is a common source of treatment failure. Surgical resection and adjuvant radiotherapy represent the main modalities of treatment for most of these neoplasms.

Fibrosarcoma

Fibrosarcoma is a rare lesion in children, but its clinical representation and general characteristics are essentially the same as those of adults. The tumors are composed of densely packed anaplastic spindle cells arranged in an interwoven herringbone pattern (Figure 12–3). Histologic grade is determined from cellularity, mitotic index, anaplasia, and morphologic differentiation. The tumor may originate from bone or soft tissue, but is usually associated with fibrous soft tissue. Low-grade lesions demonstrate uniform spindle cells arranged in a monotonous herringbone pattern, with high-grade lesions displaying increased pleomorphism, greater cellularity, and increased mitotic activity. Tumor necrosis may be demonstrated in high-grade lesions and has been found to be a reliable indicator of aggressive behavior (Costa et al., 1984).

Fibrosarcoma may occur in any anatomic site in the head and neck but most commonly appears in the neck and paranasal region. Regional lymphatic metastases are rarely seen as the tumor uncommonly metastasizes via a hematogenous route.

The mainstay of therapy remains surgical resection with disease-free margins when feasible. For lesions involving or in close proximity to vital structures (i.e.,

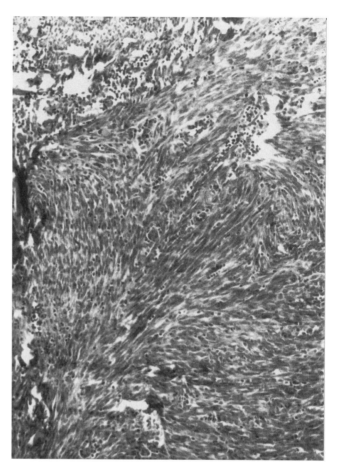

Figure 12–3. Fibrosarcoma demonstrating characteristic spindle cells in an interwoven herringbone pattern. (Courtesy of A. Garbes, M.D.)

orbit, brain, carotid artery), the extensiveness of resection is controversial. For low-grade lesions, surgical resection with clear margins seems sufficient, whereas for high-grade lesions and low-grade lesions with positive margins, or those associated with vital unresected structures, postoperative radiotherapy is recommended (Costa et al., 1984).

Unlike rhabdomyosarcoma, the role of chemotherapy for fibrosarcoma is unclear. It does not currently represent a primary adjuvant modality, but may play a palliative role in metastatic disease. Survival has been most closely associated with tumor grade, size, and the adequacy of surgical margins. Low-grade lesions that are less than 5 cm and can be completely resected offer survival rates ranging from 60% to 90% over 5 years (Farr, 1981; Greager et al., 1985).

Liposarcoma

Liposarcomas represent a group of malignant mesenchymal neoplasms that are more common in adults than in children. Those affecting the head and neck region are even more rare. A review of 17 lesions occurring in children from the files of the Armed Forces Institute of Pathology revealed only one to involve a head and neck region (Schmookler & Enzinger, 1983). Typically, liposarcomas occurring in childhood demonstrate a predominant myxoid characteristic, which conveys a more favorable outlook. The treatment centers around radical excision, with adjunctive postoperative radiation therapy for unresectable disease or positive margins. Survival statistics regarding head and neck disease cannot be quantified because of the paucity of lesions collected. In general, survival rates for the myxoid type vary from 50–70% depending upon anatomic location.

Synovial Cell Sarcoma

Synovial cell sarcoma is a slow-growing tumor arising in or near tendons or tendon sheaths. These tumors occur in the soft tissues of the neck in proximity to musculotendinous structures when the head and neck is the primary region involved. They grossly appear as well-circumscribed solitary lesions, often found in the retropharyngeal area in children. Histologically, these tumors display a characteristic biphasic pattern of epithelioid cells forming clefts that are surrounded by fibrosarcomalike cells.

The treatment is primarily surgical via wide local resection. The local recurrence rate is high, and thus surgical resection should be accompanied by adjunctive radiotherapy for large lesions or those with positive margins. Recurrence usually will manifest within 2 years and should be treated with reexcision and chemotherapy in a manner similar to that of the treatment for rhabdomyosarcoma.

Malignant Fibrous Histiocytoma

Malignant fibrous histiocytoma is an extremely rare tumor of childhood. The origin of the tumor resides in primitive undifferentiated mesenchymal cells showing partial fibroblastic and histiocytic differentiation. A series of 200 cases reviewed by the Armed Forces Institute of Pathology yielded a 3% incidence involving patients under the age of 20 and only 3% with head and neck involvement (Weiss & Enzinger, 1978). The most common symptom at presentation was that of a painless enlarging mass, which may grow in a slow or rapid manner. Three histologic subtypes are described based on growth patterns: (1) storiform, (2) pleomorphic, and (3) fascicular, with the first group being most frequently encountered (Figure 12–4). The risk of metastasis is dependent upon the depth of tumor invasion, with deeper tumors displaying increased rates of metastasis.

Radical resection represents the mainstay of therapy. Radiation therapy and chemotherapy have shown little benefit in treating these neoplasms. Most tumors

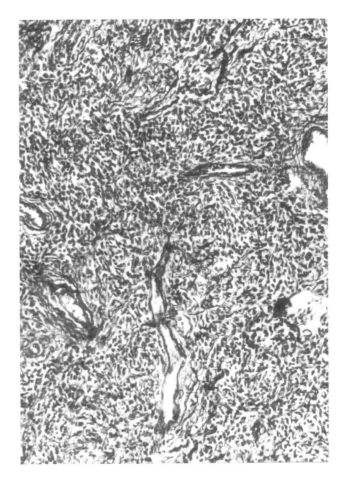

Figure 12–4. Hemangiopericytoma demonstrating thin walled endothelial-lined channels with surrounding densely packed pericytes. (Courtesy A. Garbes, M.D.).

locally recur within 2 years of treatment, but some may occur in delayed fashion. The 2-year survival in the AFIP series was noted to be approximately 40%, a significant number of which patients were alive with disease (Weiss & Enzinger, 1978).

Alveolar Soft Part Sarcoma

Alveolar soft part sarcoma is a tumor of uncertain histologic origin occurring (rarely) in adolescents and young adults. The predominant region involved in the head and neck is the orbit. The tumor is noted to be well circumscribed and quite vascular with a characteristic microscopic appearance of polygonal cells containing cytoplasmic crystalline structures arranged in a pseudoalveolar pattern. Delayed metastasis, 10 years or more following primary therapy, has been noted, making evaluation for primary therapy difficult. Surgery and radiation therapy for unresectable or recurrent disease form the basis for treatment.

Hemangiopericytoma

Hemangiopericytoma is a vascular neoplasm of mesenchymal origin which is found primarily in adults and is rare in children. The cell of origin is thought to be the pericyte of Zimmerman, a mesenchymal cell similar to primitive fibroblasts, which can be found at the periphery of developing capillaries. The tumor cells may be difficult to distinguish from fibroblasts, endothelial cells, and histiocytes, which they resemble. The diagnosis is predominantly based on ultrastructural studies and recognition of a distinct architectural pattern. The tumor differs between adults and children in regard to several aspects but, as in adults, may occur as both benign and malignant neoplasms in children.

Hemangiopericytoma of childhood generally occurs early in life during the 1st year after birth. These tumors are characteristically limited to the subcutis and are multilobulated with distinct intravascular and perivascular satellite nodules outside the main tumor mass (Weiss & Enzinger, 1988). The tumor microscopically consists of densely packed cells located around thin-walled endothelium-lined vascular channels of varying dimensions (see Figure 12–4). There may be areas of spindle cell aggregation, but not the interwoven or fascicular pattern that is seen in fibrosarcoma or synovial sarcoma. Solid areas of tumor may mimic a neural tumor because of a focal palisading nature. Mitotic activity is useful in distinguishing between benign and malignant tumors. Less than three mitotic figures per high-power field usually indicate a benign lesion, whereas more than four mitotic figures per high-power field are indicative of a rapidly growing tumor capable of metastasis. Malignant lesions tend to be more cellular with greater pleomorphism and focal areas of necrosis and hemorrhage. Ultrastructural studies of the tumor cells confirm the cell of origin to be the pericyte of Zimmerman. The cells have pale-staining cytoplasm with large round or oval nuclei and are situated in the peripheral location around thin-walled, endothelial cell-lined, vascular sinusoids and channels. Microscopically, the infantile hemangiopericytoma closely resembles the adult type, except for endovascular proliferation of tumor cells, increased mitotic activity, and focal necrosis, all of which represent features that indicate malignancy in the adult form. Most infantile lesions follow a relatively benign course without recurrence after wide local incision. The vascular nature of this tumor must be taken into consideration when planning excision in a small child or infant.

BENIGN LESIONS

Hemangiomas

As the most common tumor of infancy, hemangiomas occur in a number of different head and neck locations. These lesions are actually separate from the so-called vascular malformations, which are structural anomalies due to an error in vascular morphogenesis. Hemangioma, on the other hand, implies a growth potential characterized by endothelial proliferation that can, and usually does, undergo slow regression. Although malformations are present from birth, hemangiomas may not appear for 3 to 6 weeks and sometimes appear later. They usually go through rapid growth the 1st year and then stabilize before showing any regression. More than 80% are localized to a single site with the eyelids and larynx causing the most functional concern.

These lesions have been classified as capillary and cavernous in the past, based on the vessel size and location in the skin or subcutaneous tissue. It is now felt that a more appropriate description should be based on the depth of involvement of the lesion. Lesions close to the surface would be classified as superficial, those well under the skin would be deep, and mixed hemangiomas would refer to a combination of the two (McGill & Mulliken, 1993). The more common anatomical locations for hemangiomas in the child include the parotid, cheek, nasal, labial and vestibular, eyelids, and airway (Figure 12–5). The most common airway presentation that can be life-threatening involves the laryngeal subglottis. Treatment consideration depends on the location and depth of the hemangioma, the likelihood of regression, and the functional disability. Treatments have included surgical excision (single or staged removal), sclerosing agents, radiotherapy, and laser surgery. Most lesions are cared for with laser surgery or a combination of excision and laser treatments.

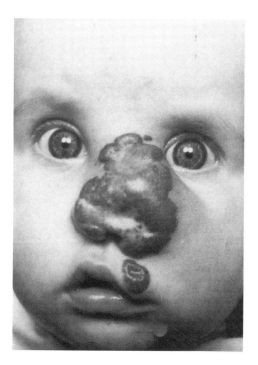

Figure 12–5. Nasal hemangioma.

Juvenile Nasopharyngeal Angiofibroma (JNA)

JNA is a rare benign vascular tumor that originates in the lateral aspect of the nasopharynx in adolescent males. It has been felt to be hormonally dependent by some, showing the presence of dihydrotestosterone receptors. The histogenesis is unknown and the histology includes fibrous tissue stroma and vascular channels. Because of the lack of smooth muscle around the vessels, bleeding is common. The presenting symptoms of epistaxis and nasal blockage are the hallmarks of this disease. The same symptoms are so common in this age group that the diagnosis is usually delayed for months and sometimes years. The initial diagnosis is suspected when a soft rubbery-appearing lesion is seen in the nasal cavity or nasopharynx. A biopsy in the office can sometimes lead to significant embarrassing bleeding and, therefore, is done in the operating room at the time of surgical removal. Diagnostic investigations should include a CT, MRI, and arterial contrast study (Figure 12–6). The arteriogram is held until the day before or the morning of surgery. This enables embolization of the feeding vessels with Gelfoam or plastic discs just prior to the surgery and significantly cuts down on the intraoperative bleeding (Jones, DeSanto, Bremer, & Neal, 1986).

The management of these neoplasms has evolved over the years. Radiotherapy, which was once condemned, is now used for tumors that have extended into the intracranial space. This change in philosophy has resulted from improved techniques in radiotherapy and reported studies showing good long-term results (Briant, Fitzpatrick, & Berman, 1978). Intracranial spread of tumor usually means vascular involvement with the cavernous sinus and internal carotid artery increasing the surgical complications significantly. Most, however, would still limit radiotherapy's use to those lesions that have intracranial extension because of the potential side effects of radiation in the pediatric age group. In general, the treatment of JNA has dramatically improved because of the cooperative efforts of the neuroradiologist, radiotherapist, and the head and neck surgeon.

Lipoma

Lipomas are uncommon lesions in the pediatric population. These growths are benign and require treatment only when the diagnosis is uncertain or a major cosmetic deformity results. They may be found in the facial area, especially around the parotid gland, neck, oral area and oropharynx, and rarely in the larynx and tracheobronchial area. These lesions are much more common in the adult and should be considered a reportable case in the child.

Cystic Hygroma

Hygroma cysticum coli, or cystic hygroma, is a complex lymphatic malformation, which is part of a larger spectrum that includes lymphangiomas. This idea was brought about by a unified concept described by Bill and Sumner (1965) that considered lymphangiomas and cystic hygromas as variations of a single entity. A common classification for these lesions set forth by Lauding and Farber (1965) includes three types: lymphangioma simplex, cavernous lymphangioma, and cystic lymphangioma or cystic hygroma. These three groups are sometimes found together in the same lesion. The majority of the lymphangiomas occur in the head and neck, with more than 90% reported in the cervical region. These malformations are felt to be an arrest in the development of the connecting lymphatics to the venous system. The reported incidence for lymphangiomas is low and even less for cystic hygromas. Actual percentages are not available, but one study found 21 cases of cervical hygromas in 2519 patients with neck masses in Atlanta hospitals in the years 1954–1963 (Skandalakis & Gray, 1972). The male-to-female ratio appears to be equal in most reported series. The cervical region is the most common site for cystic hygroma (Figure 12–8) and the lips, cheek, tongue, and parotid are frequent locations for the cavernous lymphangioma (Figure 12–9). Most lesions are seen in early childhood with 65–75% diagnosed at birth.

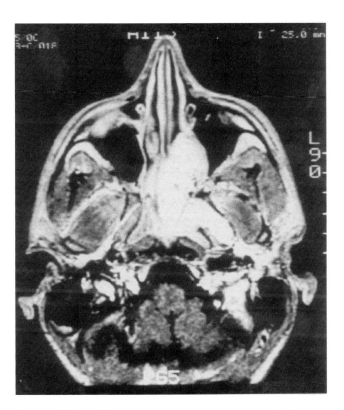

Figure 12–6. MRI of a juvenile nasopharyngeal angiofibroma.

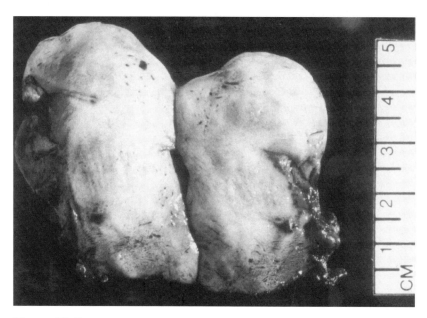

Figure 12–7. Gross pathology from Figure 12–8.

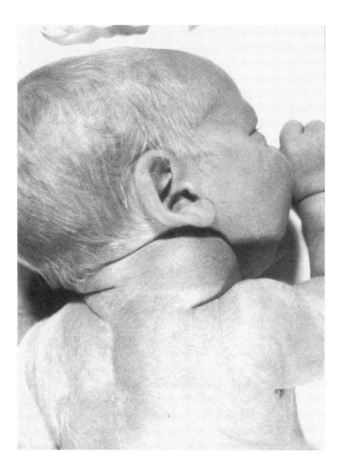

Figure 12–8. Cystic hygroma.

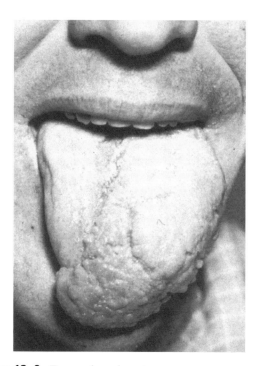

Figure 12–9. Tongue lymphangioma.

The presenting sign is a mass with second and third symptoms causing obstruction to the airway and difficulty in swallowing. Inflammation and infection in the cysts, bleeding into the cystic spaces, difficulty with speech, and compression of other vital structures are all possible symptoms and complications. Diagnosis rarely presents a problem, especially for the large hygromas. The most common incorrect diagnosis in the neck is a lipoma. Treatment is surgical removal if a major function is interfered with or the resulting cosmetic defect is felt to be significant. Management is a challenge and should not be carried out by the occasional operator in the neck.

References

Bill, A. H. Jr., & Sumner D. S. (1965). A unified concept of lymphangioma and cystic hygroma. *Surgery, Gynecology and Obstetrics, 120,* 79–86.

Briant, T. D. R., Fitzpatrick, P. J., & Berman, J. (1978). Nasopharyngeal angiofibroma: A 20 year study. *Laryngoscope, 88,* 1247–1251.

Costa, J., Wesley, R. A., Glatesein, E., et al. (1984). The grading of soft tissue sarcomas: Results of a clinicohistopathologic correlation in a series of 163 cases. *Cancer, 53,* 530–541.

Farr, H. W. (1991). Soft tissue sarcoma of the head and neck. *Seminars in Oncology, 8,* 185–189.

Gonzales-Cruss, F., & Black-Schaffer, S. (1979). Rhabdomyosarcoma of infancy and childhood, problems of morphologic classification. *American Journal of Surgical Pathology, 3,* 157–161.

Greager, J. A., Patel, M. K., Brieve, H. A., et al. (1985). Soft tissue sarcoma of the adult head and neck. *Cancer, 56,* 820–824.

Heyn, R. (1994). The role of combined chemotherapy in the treatment of rhabdomyosarcoma in children. *Cancer, 34,* 2128–2131.

Jones, G. C., DeSanto, L. W., Bremer, J. W., & Neal, H. B. III. (1986) Juvenile angiofibromas: Behavior and treatment of extensive and residual tumors. *Archives of Otolaryngology—Head and Neck Surgery, 112,* 1191–1193.

Lauding, B. H., & Farber, S. (1956). *Tumors of the cardiovascular system. Atlas of tumor pathology.* Washington, DC: Armed Forces Institute of Pathology.

Maurer, H. M., et al. (1988). Intergroup rhabdomyosarcoma study (IRS)—II: A final report. *Proceedings of the American Society of Clinical Oncology, 7,* 255–262.

Maurer, H. M. & Abdelsalam, H. R. (1991). Rhabdomyosarcoma. In D. S. Fernraut & T. J. Vietti (Eds.), *Clinical pediatric oncology* (4th ed., pp. 491–515). St. Louis: C.V. Mosby.

Maurer, H. M., Abdelsalam, H. R., et al. (1991). The intergroup rhabdomyosarcoma study—I: A final report. *Cancer, 61,* 209–215.

McGill, T. J. I., & Mulliken, J. B. (1993). Vascular anomalies of the head and neck. In C.W. Cummings, J. M. Fredrickson, L. A. Harker, C. J. Krause, & D. E. Schuller (Eds.), *Otolaryngology head and neck surgery* (2nd ed., pp. 333–346). St. Louis: Mosby Year Book Inc.

Schmookler, B. M., & Enzinger, F. M. (1983). Liposarcomas occurring in children. *Cancer, 52:*567–573.

Skandalakis, J. E., & Gray, S. W. (1972). *Embryology for surgeons* (pp. 695–714). Philadelphia: W. B. Saunders.

Sutow, W. W. (1964). Cancer of the head and neck in children. *JAMA, 190,* 414–420.

Weiss, S. W., & Enzinger, F. M. (1978). Malignant fibrous histiocytoma in children. *Cancer, 41,* 2250–2258.

Weiss, S. W., & Enzinger, F. M. (1988). Hemangiopericytoma. In S. W. Weiss & F. M. Enzinger (Eds), *Soft tissue tumors* (2nd ed., pp. 596–613). St. Louis: C. V. Mosby.

Young, J. L., Jr, & Miller, R. W. (1975). Incidence of malignant tumors in U.S. in children. *Journal of Pediatrics, 86,* 254–258.

13

Neoplasms of Neural Origin

Thomas L. Kennedy, M.D., F.A.C.S.

MALIGNANT NEURAL LESIONS

Neuroblastoma

Neuroblastomas are aggressive malignant tumors in young children with a peak age range from 1 to 5 years of age. An undifferentiated sympathetic nervous system precursor cell of the neural crest is the cell of origin (Batsakis, 1974a). Although the adrenal gland is the most common site, these tumors present in the cervical neck regions in 2–4% of cases and metastasize to the head and neck with a slightly higher frequency (Batsakis, 1974a). These neoplasms arise in the cervical sympathetics when they present as primary head and neck lesions. They may spread locally, invading surrounding structures and extend into the neural foramina of the spine. Horner's syndrome and upper cranial nerve deficits are commonly manifested. When the tumor is metastatic to the neck, these neural changes can be absent until the metastatic focus becomes quite large. The primary tumors may also have a tendency to spread to regional lymphatics.

The work-up for neuroblastomas includes an intravenous pyelography (IVP); CT scans of the abdomen, chest, neck, and brain; and, sometimes, a metastatic evaluation. Because these lesions secrete catecholamines, a 24-hour urine collection for vanillylmandelic acid is obtained. Treatment depends on the site of the primary lesion and the evidence of metastatic disease. A localized lesion in the neck should be surgically removed. More advanced lesions may require a combination of surgery, radiation, and chemotherapy. The prognosis for these neoplasms is influenced by many factors, including the stage of the disease, age of the pa-

tient, primary site of involvement, and the histological grade of the tumor. Infants fare better than older children and primary lesions of the head and neck have a better outcome. The improved results in the head and neck are probably related to the earlier presentation of the patient. Prognosis is predicated by the stage of the malignancy; the survival ranges from 5 to 85% for 2 years with the early tumors responding better (Cotton et al., 1987). The only exception to this is stage IV-S disease, which occasionally shows spontaneous resolution in children under 1 year of age. In general, however, the outlook for children over 1 year of age with neuroblastomas is poor.

Neurofibromatosis

Von Recklinghausen's disease, or neurofibromatosis, is considered under the heading of malignant lesions because of its progressive nature, associated mortality, and its sarcomatous potential. This genetic hamartomatous disorder is a result of an autosomal dominant trait with variable penetrance (Greinwald, Derkay, & Schechter, 1996). The incidence is one case in 3,300 to 4,000 births, and there are thought to be spontaneous mutations in those patients with a negative family history (Greinwald et al., 1996).

A neurofibroma is usually the initial finding, followed by an examination revealing café-au-lait spots. Almost half the patients show some findings at birth with two thirds manifesting signs by their first year. The neural tumors consist of pedunculated skin appendages and subcutaneous nodules. The disease is associated with other abnormalities and tumors such as gliomas, acoustic neurofibromas, meningiomas, hemangiomas, spina bifida, and syndactyly. Williams and Pollack (1966) reported a neuropolyendocrine syndrome of mucosal neuromas, pheochromocytoma, and medullary thyroid carcinoma. The disease runs a slow course and the tumors continue to increase in size, occasionally leading to disfigurement and significant disabilities. Although small, there is a malignant potential for these lesions to change to neurogenic sarcomas with an incidence of 5.5–16% of patients. When needed, surgery is the only treatment and is rarely considered curative (Batsakis, 1974b).

BENIGN NEURAL LESIONS

Schwannoma

A schwannoma or neurilemmoma has a cell of origin, the Schwann cell, which is the same parent cell of the neurofibroma, even though these two tumors are pathologically and clinically different lesions. The schwannoma is solitary, encapsulated, and attached or surrounding a nerve. It has rarely shown malignant potential and is not associated with von Recklinghausen's disease. The tumor may show cystic degeneration in places with hemorrhagic necrosis. They tend to be centrifugally distributed and can present with symptoms of pain and tenderness. They have a characteristic pathological slide appearance with Antoni type A and B cells and a palisading pattern of its nuclei around a mass of cytoplasm (Verocay body). In the head and neck region, these tumors are seen in the neck affecting the vagus nerve and sympathetic chain. Their location near the base of skull in the parapharyngeal space is common and the primary diagnosis for a retrostyloid compartment tumor. Their location within the larynx, as shown in Figure 13–1, is extremely rare. Treatment is surgical excision with unlikely recurrence (Figure 13–2).

Neurofibroma

Neurofibroma can present in three different ways: as a solitary neurofibroma, as multiple neurofibromas (von Recklinghausen's disease), and as an uncommon presentation of multiple neurofibromas without the association of von Recklinghausen's (Batsakis, 1974b). As mentioned in the discussion on schwannomas, the Schwann cell is also the cell of origin of neurofibromas and the histology manifests a spindle cell pattern in a mass without a true capsule (Figure 13–3). The nerve fibers pass through and can be involved in the makeup of the lesion. These lesions tend to be compact and primarily centripetal in location. Their association with neurofibromatosis and possible malignant transformation has already been discussed. When these lesions are solitary their surgical removal is readily performed and curative with minimal disability except for the nerve involved.

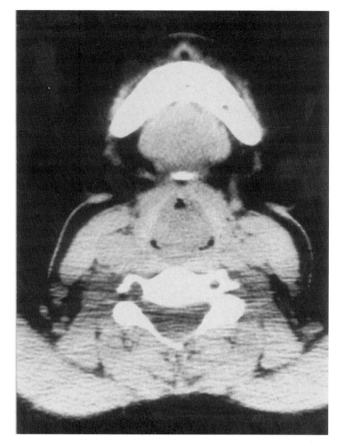

Figure 13–1. CT of a laryngeal schwannoma causing airway obstruction.

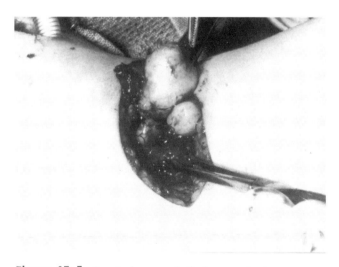

Figure 13–2. Surgical removal of a laryngeal schwannoma.

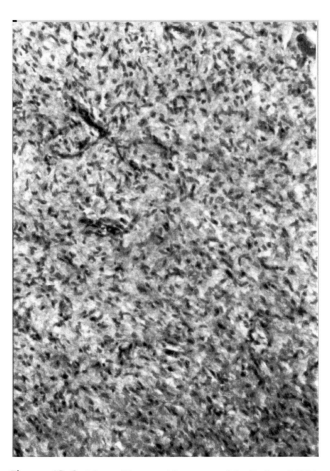

Figure 13–3. Neurofibroma. (Courtesy of A. Garbes, M.D.)

References

Batsakis, J. G. (1974a). Other neuroectodermal tumors and related lesions of the head and neck. In J. G. Batsakis (Ed.), *Tumors of the head and neck: Clinical and pathological considerations* (pp. 250–263). Baltimore: Williams & Wilkins.

Batsakis, J. G. (1974b). Tumors of the peripheral nervous system. In J. G. Batsakis (Ed.), *Tumors of the head and neck: Clinical and pathological considerations* (pp. 231–249). Baltimore: Williams & Wilkins Company.

Cotton, R. T., Ballard, E.J ., Going, J. A., Myer, C. M., III, Towbin, R. B., & Wong, K. Y. (1987). Tumors of the head and neck in children. In S. E. Thawley, W. R. Panje, J. G. Batsakis, & R. D. Lindberg (Eds.), *Comprehensive management of head and neck tumors* (Vol. 2, pp. 1770–1825). Philadelphia: W. B. Saunders.

Greinwald, J., Derkay, C. S., & Schechter, G. L. (1996). Management of massive head and neck neurofibromas in children. *American Journal of Otolaryngology, 17(2)*, 136–142.

Williams, E. D. & Pollack, D. J. (1966). Multiple mucosal neuromata with endocrine tumor: A syndrome allied to Von Recklinghausen's disease. *Journal of Pathology and Bacteriology, 91*, 71–74.

14

Neoplasms of Epithelial Origin

**Thomas L. Kennedy, M.D., F.A.C.S.,
Phillip K. Pellitteri, D.O.,
and Brad Millman, M.D.**

MALIGNANT NEOPLASMS

Squamous Cell Carcinoma

The diagnosis of squamous carcinoma outside of the nasopharynx is sporadically made in children and is quite rare. Potential anatomic sites of involvement include the larynx, paranasal sinuses, oral cavity, and skin of the face and neck. An association between this development and exposure to immunosuppressive agents has been demonstrated (Clark, Rosen, & Lapierriere, 1982). Squamous carcinoma has been reported to develop in severe burn scars and in patients with preexisting xeroderma pigmentosum, a condition that makes the patients susceptible to the carcinogenic effects of ultraviolet radiation from sunlight (Novick et al., 1977; Sutow & Montague, 1967). With the increased use of smokeless tobacco products by older children and adolescents has come an increase in the development of oral carcinoma in these children, as well as an increase in the risk for developing the disease as adults.

The incidence of squamous carcinoma of the larynx occurring in a child has been comprehensively reviewed (Ohlms, McGill, & Nealy, 1994) in the literature and offers perspectives for treatment. In general, squamous carcinoma of the head and neck in children is treated similarly as it is in adults. Surgery and radiotherapy represent the major modalities used for treatment. The larynx, as an organ vital to both respiration and phonation, represents a challenge in treatment when dealing with squamous carcinoma in children. Organ preservation protocols consisting of chemothera-

py and radiotherapy, used concurrently or in sequence, should be considered, even in the presence of advanced local regional disease. Concurrent chemoradiotherapy using cisplatin and 5-FU and 6600 cGy of external beam radiation has been shown to be effective in preserving laryngeal function, although long-term survival data cannot be assessed secondary to an insufficient follow-up. Children with squamous carcinoma of the head and neck should be evaluated by a multidisciplinary tumor board so that multimodality treatment may be better coordinated.

Nasopharyngeal Carcinoma

Nasopharyngeal carcinoma (NPC) accounts for approximately one third of the nasopharyngeal neoplasms occurring during childhood. Even so, it is rare, with an incidence reported from major institutional reviews of less than one case per year (Cunningham, Myers, & Bluestone, 1987; Fernandez, 1976). An increased incidence has been noted among black adolescents.

The cells of origin from NPC are the epithelial cells within the respiratory epithelium of the nasopharynx. The tumors are composed of small, uniform, undifferentiated cells that fail to show squamous characteristics. A wide spectrum of cell patterns may be seen, including typical squamous carcinoma, transitional cell, spindle cell, clear cell, and pleomorphic cell patterns. Three types of NPC have been classified by the World Health Organization: (1) keratinizing squamous carcinoma; (2) nonkeratinizing carcinoma, and (3) undifferentiated carcinoma, which is sometimes referred to as lymphoepithelioma in older literature (Weiland, 1985). The majority of NPC occurring in children and adolescents is of the undifferentiated type, making the distinction of NPC from non-Hodgkin's lymphoma and rhabdomyosarcoma sometimes difficult.

A strong serologic correlation between NPC types II and III and EBV has been established, suggesting that the virus may act as a tumor promoter following infection. Antibody titers to the virus (anti-EBV) tend to parallel the tumor burden and show a decrease when therapy reduces the volume of tumor. Recurrence of disease has been heralded by a rise in antibody titer, and thus it is a useful indicator of disease activity (Naegele, Champion, & Murphy, 1982). The keratinizing type of NPC has not been shown to have an association with elevated EBV titers.

Most commonly, NPC presents with cervical lymphadenopathy, which may be unilateral or bilateral, and represents metastatic tumor involvement. There may be concurrent nasal obstruction and epistaxis and, infrequently, cervical pain that radiates to the ear and skull. Unilateral secretory otitis representing tumor obstruction at the eustachian tube orifice is a common physical finding. Deep pain and the presence of cranial nerve palsies, usually cranial nerves V and VI, are ominous findings, indicating skull base involvement by tumor. In essence, any symptom in the head and neck may be attributed to NPC, and this process must be ruled out when symptoms and clinical findings cannot be reconciled by identifying an inflammatory or other benign source. Most children with NPC are treated for an inflammatory disorder for a variable period of time prior to diagnosis. Delay in diagnosis following presentation has been reported to be an average of 18 weeks (Pager & McClatchey, 1981). The most common anatomic sites of nasopharyngeal wall involvement are, in decreasing order, lateral wall, posterosuperior wall, posterior wall, and anterior wall (Batsakis, Solomon, & Rice, 1981).

The diagnosis is secured by direct nasopharyngeal examination and biopsy, which is usually performed under sedation or general anesthesia. MRI is usually the imaging method of choice because of improved soft tissue resolution and an indication of intracranial involvement, dural or parenchymal. Intracranial extension as indicated by clinical symptoms or imaging should prompt the performance of CSF examination. The presence of metastatic disease in bone, lung, and liver should be ruled out by appropriate imaging, such as chest x-ray, CT scan, and bone scan.

The extensiveness of NPC involvement at diagnosis is best characterized by the TNM (primary tumor [T], nodal metastasis [N], distant metastasis [M]) staging system. In general, however, this system has limited prognostic and therapeutic usefulness because most children present with advanced disease at diagnosis—Stage III or IV. Radiation represents the mainstay of therapy for NPC, for both adults and children. In particular, undifferentiated, or type III, NPC is a very radiosensitive tumor and, as such, has demonstrated excellent response rates to irradiation. Radiation primarily addresses local regional disease and does not resolve the problem of distant metastasis. Chemotherapy has not been demonstrated to improve survival in randomized trials (Kim et al., 1989; Pao et al., 1989). Recent efforts at developing a chemoradiotherapy protocol for primary therapy by the South West Oncology Group (SWOG) have yielded promising findings in terms of response and survival (Shuller, personal communication, 1996). These results may herald the recommendation that patients with NPC be treated in a combined fashion in an effort to improve survival.

The development and subsequent refinement in cranial base surgery has offered another modality with which to treat patients with recurrent, local, or local regional disease and, in many situations, represents an effective form of adjuvant therapy. Children with NPC have an overall 5-year survival rate of approximately 40%. Favorable prognostic characteristics include histologic types II and III and tumors confined to the nasopharynx without CNS extension or cervical metastasis.

Thyroid Carcinoma

Carcinoma of the thyroid occurs rarely during childhood, constituting 0.5% to 3% of all childhood malignancies (Millman & Pellitteri, 1995). It is more common in females and mainly occurs in children 10 years of age or older. The peak incidence of childhood thyroid cancer occurred in the mid-1950s and has markedly decreased since then. The annual incidence currently is less than one case per million children under age 14, and approximately three cases per million adolescents between ages 15 and 21. Although thyroid cancer is thought to be a disease of adulthood, approximately 10% of all thyroid malignancies occur in patients under the age of 21. Thyroid cancer is usually found in older children and adolescents, but has been reported to occur in neonates (DeKeyser & Van Herle, 1985). A female predominance exists, but not to the same degree as found in adults. The ratio in children is approximately 2:1 compared with a 3:1 or 4:1 female predominance in adults.

Several causative factors for the development of thyroid carcinoma in children have been proposed, including radiation exposure, genetics, dysfunctional iodine metabolism, and other endocrinopathies. Ionizing radiation to the head and neck was commonly used for many benign childhood ailments prior to 1960 in the United States of America. Accordingly, thousands of children received low-dose radiation to the head and neck, most commonly for tonsillar and nasopharyngeal lymphoid hyperplasia and neonatal thymic enlargement. The association between radiation exposure and thyroid carcinoma was confirmed by a number of animal and human studies, and a high percentage of children with thyroid carcinoma were found to have prior radiation exposure (Buckwalter, Thomas, & Freeman, 1975; DeKeyser & Van Herle, 1985). Winship and Rosvall (1970), in a landmark 20-year study, obtained a history of prior radiation exposure in 80% of patients in whom an attempt was made to elicit this information in a history. The average dose was 512 cGy, and the average interval from irradiation to diagnosis of thyroid carcinoma was 8.5 years. Ionizing radiation-induced carcinoma is usually represented by papillary or follicular cancers. Although head and neck irradiation for benign disease has declined and is no longer used, radiation exposure to the lower neck and mediastinum still occurs as a consequence of the treatment for Hodgkin's disease and other malignancies of the head and neck in children. Following treatment of these nonthyroid cancers, long-term survivors are at risk for development of thyroid malignancy up to 10 to 15 years following irradiation.

Genetic influences have been postulated in the development of thyroid cancer. Both Pendred's and Gardner's syndromes have been associated with thyroid carcinoma. Medullary thyroid carcinoma is associated with the multiple endocrine neoplasia syndrome type II, although it may occur in both a sporadic and familial form as well.

Carcinoma of the thyroid is generally divided into four groups: papillary, follicular, medullary, and undifferentiated or anaplastic. Although the pathologic types found in children are the same as in adults, the relative frequencies differ, with a greater proportion of differentiated tumors occurring in children. Greater than 70% of thyroid malignancies in children are of the papillary type with 15–20% being follicular and approximately 3% each being medullary and anaplastic. In about 5% of cases, the tumor cannot be typically classified (Figure 14–1).

Children with thyroid cancer most commonly present with a lateral cervical mass, with or without a thyroid nodule. Cervical lymphatic metastasis is common and is found in up to 90% of children at time of diagnosis, compared to 20–30% of adults. The absence of a palpable thyroid mass does not eliminate the possibility of thyroid cancer, as has been noted in children presenting with cervical metastases and no palpable thyroid nodules (Millman & Pellitteri, 1995; Zohar, Strauss, & Lamian, 1986). Distant metastases, commonly to the lungs, are present in 10–20% of the patients at diagnosis. Bony metastases, not uncommon in adults, are rarely found in children with thyroid cancer.

The differential diagnosis of a solitary thyroid nodule includes congenital anomalies, cysts, thyroid inflammatory disease, colloid nodules, adenomatoid nodules, Hashimoto's thyroiditis, and benign and malignant neoplasms. Nuclear scintigraphy was once utilized as a determinative study in conjunction with thyroid suppression to decide on surgical resection of

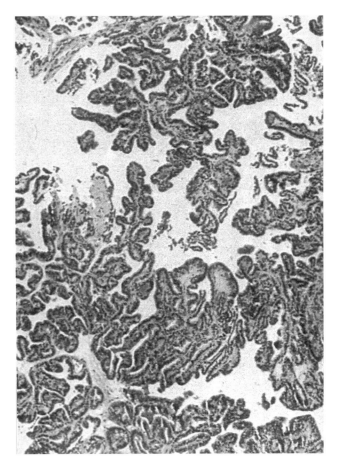

Figure 14–1. Papillary carcinoma of the thyroid.

thyroid disease. It is now used as an adjunctive or correlative study or in patients with dysthyroid metabolic abnormalities. The majority of children with thyroid malignancy are euthyroid and demonstrate a hypofunctioning nodule on scintigraphy using radioiodine. However, approximately 85% of benign nodules will also demonstrate a "cold" appearance on scan; thus the utility of a determinative test for surgical resection is low. With the advent and refinement of fine needle aspiration (FNA) biopsy, all other adjunctive studies have become subordinate. Most studies indicate an approximate 90% specificity and sensitivity in detecting the presence of neoplastic disease within a thyroid nodule using FNA biopsy (Millman & Pellitteri, 1995). The diagnostic accuracy is directly dependent on the expertise and experience of the interpreting cytopathologist. Difficulty with FNA occurs in determining whether a follicular neoplasm represents a carcinoma or an adenoma, as a pathologist will often require an intact complete surgical specimen to define capsular, lymphatic, and/or vascular invasion by a carcinoma. Other limitations include insufficient sample size and a lesion less than 5 mm in diameter. Ultrasound-guided FNA for thyroid nodules is a useful adjunct for obtaining a sufficient sample in smaller lesions or in patients in whom position or body habitus presents a problem in performing biopsy.

The incidence of malignancy in a solitary thyroid nodule increased in the 1950s to a high of approximately 70% and has decreased since then. Most studies now quote an incidence in the 20–30% range. A recent review of 71 children over 20 years noted an incidence of malignancy in a solitary thyroid nodule of 36% (Millman & Pellitteri, 1995). Surgery is the mainstay of treatment for thyroid cancer, with total thyroidectomy being the most frequently recommended procedure. This posture is somewhat controversial with regard to papillary carcinoma isolated to one lobe of the thyroid gland. In this setting subtotal thyroidectomy has been advocated (J. Shah, personal communication, 1995; Withers & Rosenfeld, 1979). In general, however, total thyroidectomy is advocated for all histologically proven thyroid carcinoma (Figure 14–2). Total thyroidectomy not only extirpates clinical disease but also surgically samples and removes any remaining occult carcinoma in the opposite lobe. This appears to be especially relevant for children where the incidence of occult bilateral disease is greater than for adults and where life expectancy is an additional 50–60 years. Total thyroidectomy also promotes increased efficiency for radio-iodine scanning and subsequent ablation by minimizing the amount of residual normal thyroid tissue.

Regional cervical disease should be addressed by modified or selective lymphadenectomy with preservation of structures such as the spinal accessory nerve, internal jugular vein, and the sternocleidomastoid muscle, where feasible (Figure 14–3). For patients with medullary carcinoma, total thyroidectomy should be attended by meticulous central compartment nodal dissection, including the paratracheal region and superior mediastinum. The potential for recurrence following long periods of quiescence, as may occur with thyroid malignancy, together with the attendant catastrophic sequelae, such as laryngotracheal invasion and carotid artery involvement, make this surgical approach even more important in children (Figure 14–4). Surgical extirpation of cancer and remaining normal thyroid tissue should be followed by postoperative uptake scanning (radio-iodine, I^{123}) with subsequent radio-ablation if there is evidence of residual or persistent disease. Therapy with postoperative radio-iodine has been shown to be safe and effective when carefully administered. Surgical removal of all thyroid tissue, normal and neoplastic, not only extirpates disease but offers an advantage for radio-iodine scanning in that a more accurate determination of potential residual or recurrent disease is provided. If radio-ablation is required, I^{131} is used for treatment purposes, and the patient is sequestered through radio-isolation protocol for several days. A baseline serum thyroglobulin is subsequently measured, and replacement/suppression therapy with thyroid hormone is initiated. Six months following the first treatment, the child is again thyroid deprived to elevate thyroid-stimulating hormone and subsequently undergoes total body scintigraphy to assess the possible presence of recurrent disease. Long-term thyroid hormone replacement is mandatory, with regular serum thyroglobulin determinations and scintigraphy as indicated constituting long-term follow-up evaluation for differentiated thyroid carcinoma. Serum calcitonin measurements are advocated at regular intervals for patients with medullary carcinoma. Although most

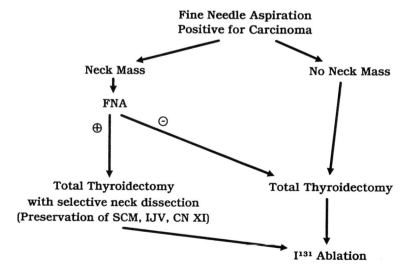

Figure 14–2. Algorithm for management of thyroid malignancy in children.

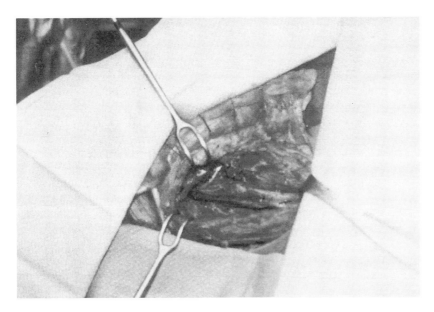

Figure 14–3. Selective neck dissection for metastatic thyroid carcinoma preserving internal jugular vein, spinal accessory nerve (CN XI), and sternocleidomastoid muscle in an 8-year-old girl.

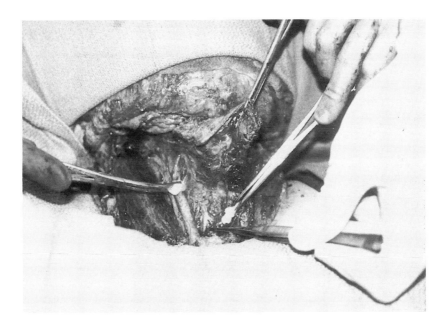

Figure 14–4. Bilateral neck dissection for extensive recurrent regional metastatic thyroid carcinoma in a teenage girl. Note recurrent laryngeal nerve medial to common carotid artery.

children present with more extensive disease, the overall prognosis for differentiated thyroid cancer is excellent. In most long-term series, survival rates exceeding 90% at 15–20 years following therapy are demonstrated, despite the presence of regional or distant disease at diagnosis (Goepfert, Dichtel, & Samaan, 1984; Gorlin & Sallan, 1990; Zohar et al., 1986). Medullary thyroid carcinomas are much more life-threatening, with a reported survival rate of 50% at 5 years (Goepfert et al., 1984). This is primarily due to the fact that medullary thyroid carcinoma is not radiosensitive, and thus radio-iodine therapy is not useful.

BENIGN NEOPLASMS

Benign Thyroid Neoplasms

The majority of thyroid nodules (60–70%) occurring in children are benign, with a smaller percentage comprised of benign neoplasms and adenomatoid goiter. Follicular adenoma and rare Hürthle cell neoplasms constitute the population of benign thyroid neoplasms that occur in children. Follicular neoplasms are difficult to histologically characterize as to the presence of malignant or benign disease by FNA. The tumors generally require excision for accurate histologic determination as the examination must include the entire capsule of the nodule to determine the extent of tumor involvement. Invasion of the capsule by tumor, whether in the presence of vascular/lymphatic invasion or not, generally constitutes malignancy and the diagnosis of follicular carcinoma (Figure 14–5). If no capsular invasion is apparent, the diagnosis is generally held to be follicular adenoma. The diagnosis often is not made until the final permanent pathologic evaluation has been completed following resection. In a setting of lobectomy or subtotal resection, final pathologic determination of malignancy mandates completion thyroidectomy. For this reason, two surgical approaches have been advocated. In the presence of a fine-needle aspirate suggestive of follicular neoplasm, total or near total thyroidectomy is initially carried out, thereby avoiding a second procedure in the event the pathology is malignant. Unfortunately, frozen section analysis of the nodule at the time of surgery rarely yields a sufficient sampling to eliminate the possibility of malignancy. The second approach is to surgically resect the nodule via partial thyroidectomy and await permanent histologic analysis—if benign, the procedure is sufficient; if malignant, completion thyroidectomy is performed. The risk of malignancy in a follicular neoplasm is approximately 25–30%, so consideration should be given to a more conservative procedure depending upon the surgeon's preference and experience in dealing with these neoplasms in children. Long-term suppressive therapy with thyroid hormone is usually recommended for both benign and malignant disease.

Hürthle cell neoplasms are rare in children and represent a variant of follicular neoplasm. They are composed of large, frequently polygonal, eosinophilic cells with an abundance of fine granular cytoplasm. Hürthle cells may be associated with nonneoplastic thyroid processes such as thyroiditis, Graves' disease, goiter, and nodular lesions of the thyroid. There is considerable controversy as to whether benign and malignant Hürthle cell neoplasm may be reliably differentiated on the basis of cellular histologic findings. In the final analysis, the diagnosis and prognosis of a Hürthle cell neoplasm, on which therapy should be based, depends on the clinical findings in the patient and the histopathologic findings at resection. Similar to follicular neoplasms, evidence of gross breach of the thyroid capsule, lymph node involvement, or capsular/vascular invasion on microscopic evaluation implies malignancy.

Treatment of malignant Hürthle cell neoplasms is primarily surgical and requires total thyroidectomy. Regional metastatic disease should be addressed by neck dissection. One of the distinguishing features of this neoplasm, as compared to follicular carcinoma, has been its apparent inability to concentrate I^{131}; thus adjunctive radio-iodine therapy has not played a significant role in treating these tumors.

MALIGNANT SALIVARY GLAND LESIONS

The malignant salivary gland tumors that are found in the pediatric population are no less variable in their histological and biological behavior than those seen in adults. The vast majority of these lesions in children are of parotid origin with submandibular and minor salivary tumors occurring much less frequently. Fifty percent of parotid lesions are vascular or lymphatic in nature with solid neoplastic growths making up the other half. Before reviewing the more common pe-

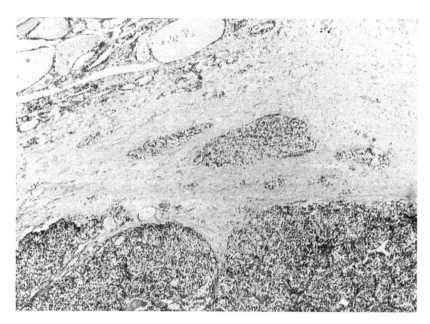

Figure 14–5. Follicular thyroid carcinoma demonstrating tumor invading thyroid capsule.

diatric malignant lesions, some comparisons with the adult counterpart need to be made. In a review at the Armed Forces Institute of Pathology of 10,000 salivary tumors, only 54 malignancies related to children were found (Foote & Frazell, 1953). Although there are less total numbers of malignant tumors in the younger age group, this group is more likely to have a cancerous lesion when they present with a solid tumor in the parotid. Fifty percent of these solid tumors in the pediatric age group will be malignant. This is in contrast to the adult population, where 20% of solid lesions are malignant. The same association continues in the submandibular and minor salivary gland tumors, where the larger the gland, the more likely it will be malignant in the child. The reverse holds in adult tumors. Mucoepidermoid is the most common malignancy in both the adult and child (Shikhani & Johns, 1988). The second most common malignant tumor in adults is adenoid cystic; whereas acinic or acinous cell ranks second in large pediatric series (Shikhani & Johns, 1988). Adenoid cystic carcinoma is a rare malignancy in the child; and because of the need for a more aggressive treatment plan, it becomes a challenge for physician, family, and patient.

Mucoepidermoid Carcinoma

Mucoepidermoid carcinoma has many faces, and it is a common malignant lesion in both the adult and pediatric age groups. It tends to have a wide range of malignant potential, which is in part related to its cell mix. The name mucoepidermoid was first coined by Stewart in 1945, thereby emphasizing the two main cell types of mixed epidermoid and mucous-secreting cells (Stewart,

Foote, & Becker, 1945). At least six different cell differentiations have been described in the histogenesis of mucoepidermoid carcinoma. The maternal cell is the cell of origin of all the other cell types, leading to the formation of the intermediate, epidermoid, and the mucous cell lines. Foote and Frazell (1953) used these three cell lines to classify mucoepidermoid lesions into low-grade (mostly mucinous), intermediate-grade (mostly mucinous and epidermoid), and high-grade (mostly epidermoid). Others have tried to classify these tumors based on invasive characteristics, such as deeply invasive, and whether there was evidence for neural invasion. Although most pathologists follow the cell type classification, the best answer lies in a combination of cell predominance and the tumor's invasive nature (Figure 14–6).

The signs and symptoms related to mucoepidermoid tumors are similar to other salivary gland lesions, with the major complaint being that of a mass. This could be a mass in the parotid or in the palate, which are the two most common locations. Pain usually, but not always, indicates a high-grade malignant lesion. Facial paralysis is a poor prognostic sign and can indicate perineural spread of tumor. Lymph node metastasis has been reported in 10 to 66% and can occur in tumors that have been classified as low-grade (Batsakis, 1974). A history of rapid growth, fixation to surrounding structures, and/or skin changes over the lesion are usually reserved for advanced high-grade malignancies. Generally, even the high-grade tumors in the pediatric population are brought to medical attention when they are at the early mass stage and it is unusual to see a child present with a fixed mass or facial paralysis.

Management of mucoepidermoid carcinoma is the same in the adult and pediatric age groups. Surgery is

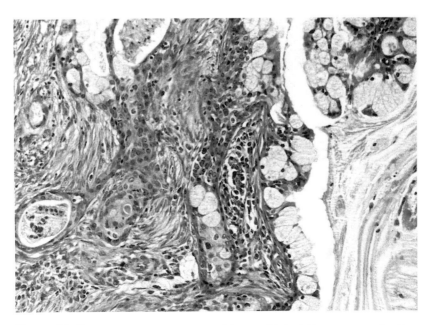

Figure 14–6. Mucoepidermoid carcinoma of the parotid gland. Note mucous and epidermoid components. (Courtesy of A. Garbes, M.D.)

the primary treatment modality. In the case of a parotid lesion, it usually consists of a total parotidectomy. Some studies have shown a higher recurrence rate in both enucleation and superficial parotidectomy, 48.3% and 30.7%, respectively, when compared to total parotidectomy, irrespective of whether the tumor was a deep lobe or superficial lesion (Shikhani & Johns, 1988). Radiation therapy is postoperatively recommended in high-grade tumors and those showing perineural invasion. However, more rigid criteria for recommending irradiation in the pediatric age group are followed because of the long-term effects of ionizing radiation in this group. Chemotherapy may play a role in patients with such problems as distant metastasis and base of skull extension. The overall success rate varies with the grade of the lesion, approaching 90% for 5 years in all patients (Batsakis, 1974).

Acinic Cell Carcinoma

Acinous cell, or as more commonly referred to, acinic cell, is the second most common malignant tumor of salivary origin in the pediatric population. In a 1988 review of malignant salivary lesions in children by Shikhani and Johns, 30 of 246 malignancies were found to represent acinic cell tumors (Shikhani & Johns, 1988). This tumor's behavior is similar in children and adults, with a biological course that is difficult to predict. These lesions are located almost exclusively in the parotid gland because of the cell of origin, the serous cell of the gland acini (Figure 14–7). Characteristics of this lesion include its reported bilateral parotid involvement, female dominance, slow growth, benign appearing cells with infrequent mitosis, superficial lobe location, and

usual lack of any definable capsule around the lesion. Grossly, these lesions are solid, but can be cystic to the point of confusion with more malignant tumors such as a mucoepidermoid carcinoma. Pain and facial paralysis are late in the course of the disease and carry an extremely bad prognosis. As with other salivary lesions, the first presenting complaint is a mass in the parotid gland.

Treatment for these growths is surgical removal and most surgeons favor a total or near total parotidectomy with preservation of the uninvolved facial nerve. Cervical metastasis is uncommon, but, if present at the time of surgery, necessitates a neck dissection. Radiation therapy is used cautiously in children and usually reserved for patients with aggressive lesions that present with nodal disease or facial paralysis. Survival figures for acinic cell lesions, as well as other malignant salivary lesions in children, are hard to determine because of the small numbers and the lack of acceptable follow-up. The survival in adults ranges from close to 90% in 5 years to 50% after 25 years (Eneroth, Hamberger, & Jakobsson, 1966). If the same figures can be applied to children, then we should assume that this tumor represents a serious tumor for the pediatric population.

Adenoid Cystic Carcinoma

Although adenoid cystic carcinoma is the second most common malignant tumor in the adult population, it ranks fourth in patients under 20 years of age. Because of the small number of case reports, it is difficult to understand the biological behavior of this tumor in the pediatric age. Long-term follow-ups are just not available and we must assume that this tumor behaves

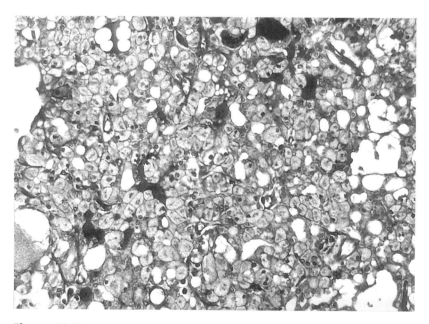

Figure 14–7. Acinic cell carcinoma—parotid gland. (Courtesy of A. Garbes, M.D.)

as it does in the adult. This malignant epithelial tumor is more common in the minor salivary tissue, but has been reported as the most common malignant lesion of the submandibular gland in large groups. Although rare as a primary parotid lesion, Figure 14–8 represents an adenoid cystic lesion of the parotid and parapharyngeal space on a CT scan of a 9-year-old African-American girl. The cell of origin of adenoid cystic carcinoma is felt to be located at the canaliculi and the intercalated ducts of the peripheral duct system (Batsakis, 1974). Microscopically, the pattern may be dominated by a solid epithelial cell component, indicating a high-grade lesion, or a basaloid cell (cribriform) pattern, suggesting a lower grade malignancy (Figure 14–9). The more aggressive tumors are also manifested by rapid growth, pain, and facial nerve weakness. Perineural invasion is a common finding with this neoplasm and can be present with or without a preoperative facial paralysis.

Surgical removal followed by adjunctive radiotherapy is the treatment no matter what the age. Most feel that this tumor is radiosensitive but not radiocurable. A controversy does remain on a radical vs. a more conservative approach to surgery for this tumor. Recurrence rate does not appear to have changed with either type of surgical treatment, as long as spillage of tumor does not occur and the gross disease has been removed with acceptable margins. Perineural spread is probably the single most important factor for recurrence at the primary site. As the tumor recurs, the chances for distant metastases to such areas as the lung and spine increase. Although a high percentage are alive in 5 years, the long-term survival over 20 years is only 13% (Blanck, Eneroth, Jakobsson, & Jakobsson, 1967).

BENIGN SALIVARY GLAND LESIONS

Childhood head and neck neoplasms are rare lesions, with 8% consisting of salivary gland tumors (Rush, Chambers, & Rovitch, 1963). Only tumors of the nasopharynx, skin, and thyroid rank higher in the pediatric age group. In a review published by Shikhani and Johns in 1988, the total number of benign lesions, including 18 from Johns Hopkins, was 247 (Shikhani & Johns, 1988). This included an extensive review of the world literature, but did not include such lesions as hemangiomas and lymphangiomas. Solid salivary neoplasms make up 50% of the major salivary lesions, with vascular and lymphatic lesions comprising the rest. The more common benign major salivary gland lesions will be discussed in more detail.

Hemangioma

Vascular neoplasms are the most common growths found in the parotid gland in children. In a report by Schuller and McCabe (1977), 111 pediatric patients out of 428 were found to have hemangiomas. These lesions are usually noted at birth or shortly after birth and rarely present a difficult diagnosis. Frequently, there is an associated smaller skin telangiectasia or capillary lesion signifying a larger underlying lesion (Figure 14–10). These tumors are soft, compressible, and turn blue with increased blood flow when the child cries or gets upset. There is debate concerning the true neoplastic nature of these lesions, as well as lymphangiomas. Most, however, feel these lesions are distinct from vascular malformations and represent neoplastic growth. Treatment is considered only in cases that are life-threatening or severely disfiguring; and this is, in part, due to the fact that spontaneous regression is not uncommon.

Lymphangiomas

Although lymphangiomas are rare lesions, they rank second in nonsolid neoplasms of the parotid gland. These lesions are considered malformations resulting from a congenital arrest of development in the

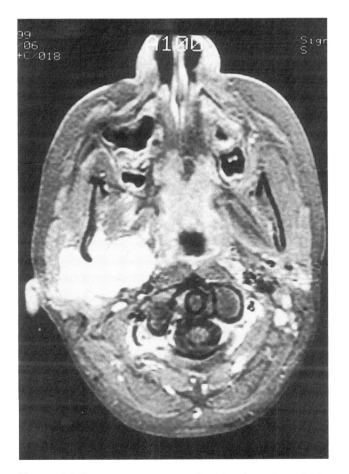

Figure 14–8. CT scan showing an adenoid cystic carcinoma in the parotid and parapharyngeal space of a child.

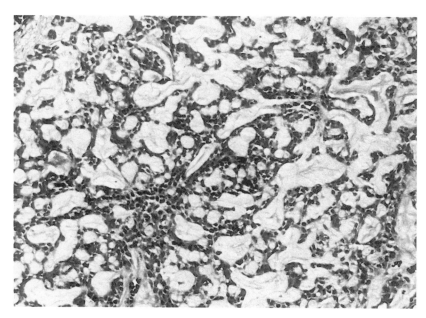

Figure 14–9. Adenoid cystic carcinoma. Note characteristic cribriform cellular pattern. (Courtesy of A. Garbes, M.D.)

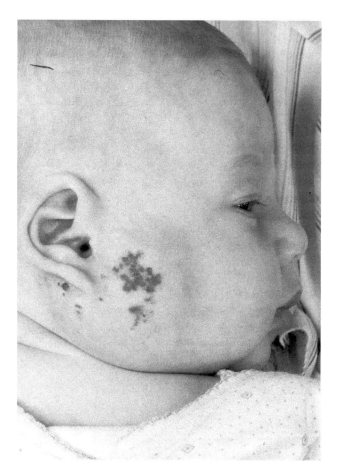

Figure 14–10. Parotid hemangioma in an infant.

drainage channels of the lymphatics. When this occurs at birth it can be associated with a much larger lesion in the neck called a cystic hygroma. Details on the theories

of development of these lesions can be found in more detailed accounts of lymphangiomas (Kennedy, 1989). Isolated lymphangiomas of the parotid may be noticed weeks to several months after birth, but can also spontaneously show up at age 6 or older. The latter presentation is usually associated with a prior infection, such as a cold or upper respiratory tract infection. Either the inflammation or a congenital partial lymphatic obstruction leads to the development of the mass. Observation is the best treatment for these cases, as a large percentage will resolve with time.

The most prominent finding at presentation is a mass. These lesions fluctuate with lymphatic stimulation and, therefore, may increase with infectious or inflammatory processes within the head and neck. Cystic or lymphangiomatous lesions occasionally become infected, and recurrent infections are one of the indications for surgery. Airway embarrassment and a severe cosmetic deformity are the two other reasons to carry out surgery. If surgical removal is required, it should be reserved for surgeons experienced in this type of exercise due to the complex architecture of the lymphatic structures throughout the parotid parenchyma.

Benign Mixed Tumor

Pleomorphic adenoma is the most common solid tumor of salivary origin in the pediatric population. Although this is also true in the adult, the child has a greater chance of having a malignant lesion, as the second most common solid lesion in the younger age group is mucoepidermoid carcinoma. As of 1988, the total number of reported benign salivary gland neoplasms in children was 247, with 214 representing benign mixed tumors (Shikhani & Johns, 1988). In the same study of 246 malignant lesions, 219 were of salivary gland tissue, 122 of which were mucoepidermoid neoplasms. These numbers also indicate the rare occurrence of salivary gland tumors in children, with a reported incidence of < 5% of salivary gland lesions in all age groups (Castro, Huvos, Strong, & Foot, 1972; Jaques, Krolls, & Chambers, 1976). Sex predilection favors females, and the age of onset ranges from 8 to 20 years with few reports of a child under the age of 8 (Figure 14–11).

These tumors are composed of epithelial and myoepithelial cells, both derived from the intercalated duct reserve cell. The histological appearance contains these two cell components in a loose myxoid stroma (Figure 14–12). The usual presenting symptom is a nonpainful mass. Differential diagnosis includes such things as an enlarged inflammatory lymph node and a type 1 branchial cleft anomaly. Treatment is surgical excision in all cases. Fine-needle biopsy is helpful prior to excision and can be carried out in this age group with about a 94% accuracy. Recurrences in children are hard to determine due to the small number of cases reported and little follow-up data.

Other Solid Salivary Neoplasms

The remaining benign salivary lesions are extremely rare and need only be mentioned. Warthin's tumor,

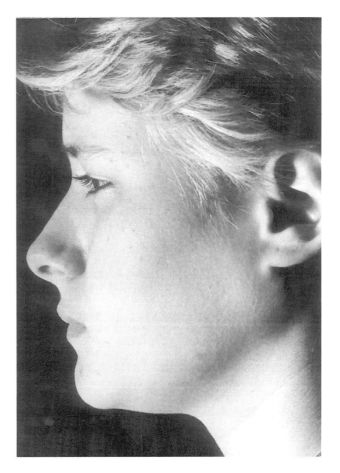

Figure 14–11. Benign mixed tumor of the parotid gland in a young girl.

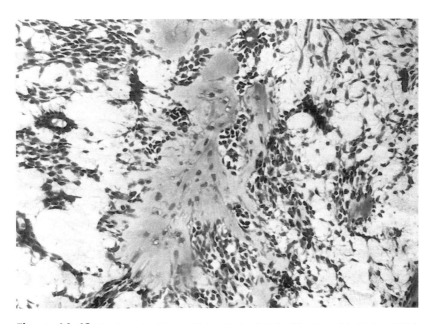

Figure 14–12. Benign mixed tumor. Note mixed cellularity. (Courtesy of A. Garbes, M.D.)

oncocytoma, and neural tumors occur much less frequently than benign mixed tumors and some of the malignant lesions. They behave as in the adult and require surgical removal for treatment.

References

Batsakis, J. G., Solomon, A. R., & Rice, D. H. (1981). The pathology of head and neck tumors: Carcinoma of the nasopharynx, Part II. *Head and Neck Surgery, 3,* 511–517.

Batsakis, J. G. (1974). Tumors of the major salivary glands. In J. G. Batsakis (Ed.), *Tumors of the head and neck: Clinical and pathological considerations* (1st ed., pp. 1–37). Baltimore: Williams & Wilkins.

Blanck, C., Eneroth, C. M., Jakobsson, F., & Jakobsson, P. A. (1967). Adenoid cystic CA of the parotid gland. *Acta Radiologica: Therapy, Physics, Biology, 6,* 177–181.

Buckwalter, J. A., Thomas, C. G., & Freeman, J. B. (1975). Is childhood thyroid cancer a lethal disease? *Annals of Surgery, 181,* 632–639.

Castro, E. B., Huvos, A. G., Strong, E. W., & Foot, F. W. (1972). Tumors of the major salivary glands in children. *Cancer, 29,* 312–317.

Clark, R., Rosen, I., & Lapierriere, N. (1982). Malignant tumors of the head and neck in a young population. *American Journal of Surgery, 144,* 459–464.

Cunningham, M. J., Myers, E. S., & Bluestone, C. D. (1987). Malignant tumors of the head and neck in children: A twenty-year review. *International Journal of Pediatric Otorhinolaryngology, 13,* 279–280.

DeKeyser, L. F. M. , & Van Herle, A. J. (1985). Differentiated thyroid cancer in children. *Head Neck Surgery, 8,* 100–114.

Eneroth, C. M., Hamberger, C. A., & Jakobsson, P. A. (1966). Malignancy of acinic cell carcinoma. *Annals of Otology, Rhinology and Laryngology, 75,* 780–792.

Fernandez, C., Cangir, A., Samaan, N., et al. (1976). Nasopharyngeal carcinoma in children. *Cancer, 37,* 2787–2795.

Foote, F. W., & Frazell, E. L. (1953). Tumors of the major salivary glands. *Cancer, 6,* 1065–1133.

Goepfert, H., Dichtel, W. J., & Samaan, N. (1984). Thyroid cancer in children and teenagers. *Archives of Otolaryngology—Head and Neck Surgery, 110,* 72–75.

Gorlin, J. B., & Sallan, S. E. (1990). Thyroid cancer in children. *Endocrinology and Metabolism Clinic of North America, 19,* 649–662.

Jaques, D. A., Krolls, S. O., & Chambers, R. G. (1976). Parotid tumors in children. *American Journal of Surgery, 132,* 469–471.

Kennedy, T. L. (1989). Cystic hygroma-lymphangioma: A rare and still unclear entity. *Laryngoscope, 99* (Suppl. 49), 1–10.

Kim, T. H., McLaren, N., Alvarado, C. S., et al. (1989). Adjuvant chemotherapy for advanced nasopharyngeal carcinoma in childhood. *Cancer, 63,* 1922–1925.

Millman, B., & Pellitteri, P. K. (1995). Thyroid carcinoma in children and adolescents. *Archives of Otolaryngology—Head Neck Surgery, 121,* 1261–1264.

Naegele, R. F., Champion, J., Murphy, S., et al. (1982). Nasopharyngeal carcinoma in American children: Epstein-Barr virus-specific antibody titer and prognosis. *International Journal of Cancer, 29,* 209–212.

Novick, M., Gard, D. A., Hardy, S. B., et al. (1977). Burn scar carcinoma: A report and analysis of 46 cases. *Journal of Trauma, 17,* 809–812.

Ohlms, L. A., McGill, T., & Nealy, G. (1994). Malignant laryngeal tumors in children: A 15-year experience with four patients. *Annals of Otology, Rhinology and Laryngology, 103,* 686–692.

Pager, S., & McClatchey, K. (1981). Carcinoma of the nasopharynx in childhood. *Otolaryngology—Head and Neck Surgery, 89,* 555–562.

Pao, W. J., Hustu, H. O., Douglass, K. C., et al. (1989). Pediatric nasopharyngeal carcinoma in long-term follow-up of 29 patients. *International Journal of Radiation Oncology, Biology, Physics, 17,* 299–305.

Rush, B. F., Jr., Chambers, R. G., & Rovitch, M. M. (1963). Cancer of the head and neck in children. *Surgery, 53,* 270–284.

Schuller, D. E., & McCabe, B. F. (1977). Salivary gland neoplasms in children. *Otolaryngology Clinics of North America, 10,* 399–412.

Shikhani, A. H., & Johns, M. E. (1988). Tumors of the major salivary glands in children. *Head and Neck Surgery,* 257–263.

Stewart, F. W., Foote, F. W., & Becker, W. F. (1945). Mucoepidermoid tumors of salivary glands. *Annals of Surgery, 122,* 820–844.

Sutow, W., & Montague, E. (1967). Pediatric tumors. In W. MacComb & G. Fletcher (Eds.), *Cancer of the head and neck* (pp. 428–446). Baltimore: Williams & Wilkins.

Weiland, L. (1985). Nasopharyngeal carcinoma. In L. Barnes (Ed.), *Surgical pathology of the head and neck* (pp. 453–466). New York: Marcel Dekker.

Winship, T., & Rosvoll, R.V. (1970). Thyroid carcinoma in children: Final report on a 20-year study. *Clinical Proceedings—Children's Hospital of the District of Columbia, 26,* 327–349.

Withers, E. H., & Rosenfeld, L. (1979). Long-term experience with childhood thyroid carcinoma. *Journal of Pediatric Surgery, 14,* 332–338.

Zohar, Y., Strauss, M., & Laurian, N. (1986). Adolescent vs. adult thyroid carcinoma. *Laryngoscope, 96,* 555–559.

15

Neoplasms of Bone and Cartilage Including Fibro-osseous Lesions

Thomas L. Kennedy, M.D., F.A.C.S.

MALIGNANT LESIONS

Osteogenic Sarcoma

Osteogenic sarcoma is a rare lesion in the craniofacial region of a young child, occurring most commonly in the mandible. Although this tumor is one of the most common malignant bony growths of the skeletal system outside the facial area, its incidence in the jaws has been reported at 0.07 per 100,000 per year in the U.S.A. (Batsakis, 1974a). The average age at which this neoplasm occurs in the head and neck is about 30 years, which is 10 years older than the peak age for this lesion elsewhere. Males seem to predominate, as in other locations, but not at the same high percentage. The most frequent locations include the body of the mandible and the alveolar ridge of the maxilla. A mass related to the jaws is the most common initial complaint. Other signs and symptoms include loosening of the teeth with periapical involvement, numbness from injury to the mental nerve, trismus, and nasal blockage. Diagnosis is suggested by the radiological appearance, which can be blastic or lytic in type, but frequently produces a classical "sun-ray" pattern (Batsakis, 1974a). A CT scan and panorex are helpful in evaluating the roentgenographic appearance.

The histological picture is variable with malignant supportive tissue manifesting the ability to form osteoid and osseous intercellular structures (Figure 15–1). Although the pathology of the neoplasm does not determine its biological behavior, the location in the mandible does and carries with it a better prognosis, nearly three times the survival of lesions found in the maxilla (Garrington, Scofield, Cornyn, & Hooker, 1967). Radical surgical removal is the recommended treatment for these neoplasms. Metastases spread in a hematogenous way and usually spread first to the lungs. Neck metastases are less frequent than in other head and neck malignancies but, if present at the time of surgery, warrant a neck dissection. The overall survival figures for these tumors in the jaws are higher than for extrafacial tumors and have been recorded from 21.5% to 35% in some studies (Batsakis, 1974a). It still, however, is a very deadly malignant growth in the pediatric population.

Chondrosarcoma

Cartilaginous tumors in the head and neck are rare tumors in general and become reportable cases when they present in the pediatric age. In a report of nonepithelial tumors of the nasopharynx and paranasal regions, 100 malignant tumors were identified with 17 cartilaginous neoplasms (Fu & Perzin, 1974). Ten of these represented chondrosarcomas with four patients under the age of 16 years and one that was only 20 months old. The malignant potential of these tumors is partially related to the site of origin, with the midfacial regions and jaw carrying the worst prognosis. Aside from the mandible, maxilla, nasal, and paranasal locations, this lesion also occurs in the larynx with an age range from 40 to 60 (Batsakis, 1974b). As previously mentioned, there are reports of these lesions in much younger individuals, but they are uncommon. In the larynx, the growth seems to take on an appearance of a

163

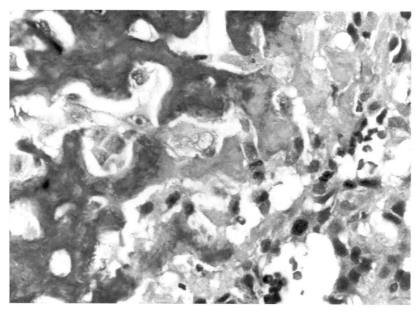

Figure 15–1. Osteogenic sarcoma histopathology. (Courtesy of A. Garbes, M.D.)

more benign process and, in fact, the histology and the biologic behavior may also favor this diagnosis. Some authors, however, feel that all laryngeal cartilage lesions should be considered malignant and treated as such.

The origin of chondrosarcomas is unknown. They have been associated with Paget's disease, fibrous dysplasia, and irradiation. Because of their preference for the anterior maxilla and posterior mandible, an origin from cartilage remnants of the nasal capsule and Meckel's cartilage has been suggested (Batsakis, 1974a). This theory lacks support from most authors who report on these lesions. Contrary to this neoplasm outside the head and neck, chondrosarcomas of the mandible and midface are painless masses that expand facial bones causing deformities, loosening of teeth, nasal obstruction, and epistaxis. Laryngeal growths usually present late with a mass, hoarseness, or difficulty with breathing. These lesions are usually seen only in the adult population.

The radiologic appearance can be variable with no real diagnostic characteristics. Most jaw lesions reveal a radiolucency with evidence of bone destruction. Widening of the periodontal membrane space, a cotton wool appearance within areas of bone erosion, and a sunburst radiologic picture have all been described. Pathologic diagnosis for this malignancy can be a challenge when distinguishing this lesion from a benign chondroma (Figure 15–2). Diagnostic pathologic criteria were described by Lichtenstein and Jaffe (1943), but the malignant aggressiveness of this tumor would be better established by a combination of the history, the location, the x-ray studies, and the histology. Treatment is surgical excision with good margins, and radiation has been added following surgery with improved re-

sults. Recurrences are common, however, and local extension with encroachment on vital structures leads to death.

BENIGN LESIONS

Osteoma

An osteoma is a slow-growing benign lesion that is composed of mature bone and various amounts of surrounding stroma. These lesions are sometimes confused with exostosis, which are overgrowths of normal bone and not true osteomas. Three types of osteomas have been described, based on the bone and stroma histology: osteoma spongiosum, durum, and eburneum. As the names imply, the bone density increases in these different lesions. These benign neoplasms are rare, but do occur in the facial bones and jaws more commonly than in other parts of the body. When these lesions show up in the pediatric age group, it usually is in adolescence, with the average range in all groups from 15 to 40 years of age.

The origin of osteomas is unknown; but as with many bony growths, trauma and infection are thought to play a role. Others feel that this tumor really represents a form of an osseous hamartoma. The presenting symptom is clinically almost always a mass. Sometimes these lesions are found incidentally on x-ray of the sinuses. When they arise in the sinuses, they more commonly present with pain and/or frontoethmoid obstruction due to their likely location at the frontoethmoid suture line (Figure 15–3). Diagnosis is easily made by their appearance on radiograph. Differential diagnosis would include exostosis, other ossifying tumors, and

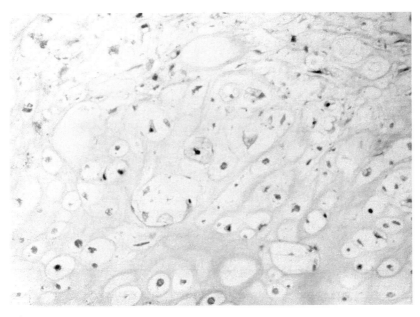

Figure 15–2. Chondrosarcoma histopathology. (Courtesy of A. Garbes, M.D.)

Gardner's syndrome. Gardner's is an inherited disease characterized by multiple fibromas, osteomas, cysts, and intestinal polyposis (Rayne, 1968). It is important for the otolaryngologist to be aware of this disease process, as these polyps have a 40% chance of malignancy and the patient's first presentation may be an osteoma. Treatment for osteomas is surgical excision when they are symptomatic, with the majority requiring no treatment at all.

Chondroma

Chondromas are similar in location, origin, and presentation to what was discussed under chondrosarcomas. In fact, it is sometimes very difficult to determine the malignant potential of these lesions on the basis of just their histology. Chondromas occur in the facial bones, jaws, and the larynx. In the facial areas they may arise at the base of skull, nasopharynx, nasal cavity, and paranasal sinuses. In the pediatric population these neoplasms are extremely uncommon, but, when they do occur, it is in the regions of the midface and mandible. Treatment is surgical excision, with recurrences more commonly seen in the lesions of the mandible and maxilla.

Fibrous Dysplasia

Fibrous dysplasia is a disease process that presents itself in the first and second decades of life. It has been classified on the basis of bone involvement into three groups: monostotic, polyostotic, and disseminated (Beleval & Schneider, 1953). This discussion is limited

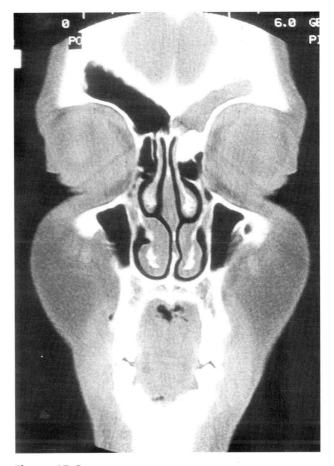

Figure 15–3. CT scan showing an osteoma obstructing the frontal sinus.

to those lesions that show their greatest activity in early childhood and stop growing once past the age of adolescence. Although fibrous dysplasia is felt to be a developmental lesion, a history of trauma is so common as to suggest a possible stimulating effect. It has a higher incidence in females and is slightly more common in black individuals. The origin comes from osseous metaplasia of the medullary bone. The pathology varies depending on the activity of the bony lesion. During the active period, there are numerous cells in mitosis, a moderate stroma, and islands of abnormal and coarse bone. As the disease becomes more mature, the mitosis decreases and the stroma and bone components become more stable and fixed.

Because the maxilla is the most common location for these fibrous lesions, facial asymmetry is the first presenting sign. This is followed by encroachment around the posterior upper teeth and, occasionally, proptosis of the eye. Loosening of the teeth, pain, and tenderness rarely occur. There are three types of x-ray findings: diffuse sclerosing with enlargement, lytic with expansion of the cortex, and the large unilocular form. The best evaluation can be obtained with a CT scan from which excellent reconstructions of the facial bones can now be reproduced (Figure 15–4). These 3-D reconstructions have greatly added in planning and carrying out surgical treatment. The treatment for this disease is surgery when needed and it usually is carried out for cosmetic or functional reasons. A large majority will require partial resection to treat the deformity until the disease process becomes mature and stops growing. Malignant potential for this neoplasm is small and may be related to prior radiotherapy. Long-term observation is recommended to look for any acute change in growth, which might indicate sarcomatous transformation.

Giant Cell Lesions

The true giant cell tumor is extremely rare and occurs in patients over 20 years of age, making it an un-

likely neoplasm in the pediatric age group. A giant cell reparative granuloma, on the other hand, can present in the younger age group, but is not a true neoplasm. The reparative granuloma can be one of two types, peripheral or central (Jaffe, 1953). The peripheral giant cell granuloma is four times more common than the central and is found on the gingiva or alveolar mucosa of the mandible more often than the maxilla. The surface is sometimes ulcerative and bleeds. Age of onset is usually over 20 years, as compared to the central type, which is seen in those between the ages of 10 and 20. The central type is endosteal and also more likely to occur in the mandible than in the maxilla. Central lesions predominate in males, whereas peripheral lesions are more commonly seen in females. Clinically, the peripheral granulomas are seen on the gingiva and can cause bleeding with injury. The intrabony lesions are seen on x-ray of the teeth and usually are a result of tooth extraction. The histology is composed of fibroblasts and vascular mesenchymal connective tissue that is a reparative response to injury to the underlying tooth elements. Both forms of the giant cell granuloma are treated with surgical excision or curettage. Malignant transformation has not been found to occur.

Giant cell tumors are separate from granulomas and are true neoplastic growths. The histology is dominated by giant cells, they seldom occur in the face or skull, they show little inflammatory or hemorrhagic change, and they are usually found in adults. They can, however, become confused with other giant cell lesions like a reparative granuloma, a brown tumor of hyperparathyroidism, and Paget's disease. Treatment requires complete surgical removal to prevent recurrences.

Myxoma

A myxoma is a lesion described in bone as well as soft tissue and behaves in a similar fashion in both locations. The myxomas of bone occur exclusively in the jaws, with the mandible as the most common site. These growths are thought to arise from the mesenchyme of the tooth germ and are, therefore, felt to be of odontogenic origin (Pindborg, 1965). The histology also reveals the presence of cells resembling dental origin. These lesions are found in young patients with an age range from 10 to 29. The presenting symptoms include facial deformity with swelling around the jaws, malocclusion, and loosening of teeth. Diagnosis is suggested by x-ray evidence of multilocular cysts and thinning of the bony cortex with areas of destruction indicating invasion of the overlying tissue. The masses are soft and the cut surface reveals a shiny, gelatinous appearance that lacks any true capsule around the lesion. Because of the absence of a capsule, these neoplasms in-

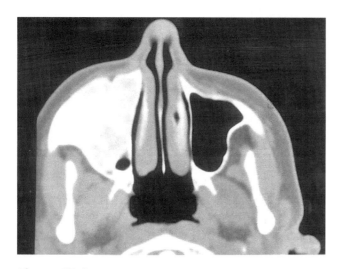

Figure 15–4. CT scan of fibrous dysplasia in a young child.

vade surrounding tissue and make surgical removal difficult. Surgery is the main treatment with recurrences as high as 25% (Whitman, Stewart, Stoopack, & Jerrold, 1971).

Ossifying Fibroma

Ossifying fibroma is a fibro-osseous lesion of bone that arises from cells within the periodontal ligament. It therefore is found in tooth-bearing areas and is most commonly seen in the mandible. Because of its dental origin and its fibrous component, it has been described with other names such as cementoma, periapical osteofibroma, and juvenile active ossifying fibroma. These lesions are more common in females and usually occur in the second, third, and fourth decades. Four stages of the maturation of ossifying fibroma were described by Billing and Ringertz (1946): osteoid or soft fibroma stage, moderate mature stage, osteoma or mature stage, and the well-differentiated or eburnifying stage. These growths present clinically as nonpainful expanding lesions of the jaws. The radiologic picture depends on the stage of disease and, therefore, may show a lytic, cystic, or dense appearance. Most will show radiolucent circumscribed margins. These growths are noticed in the mandible before they reach massive size, but can present at 4 cm or larger. Pathologic tissue is a mixture of fibrous and calcified components. The stroma is a loose, vascular, reticular fibrous connective tissue with multiple calcified globules. Treatment for these ossifying lesions is surgical excision and may involve a radical approach in the juvenile type with its more aggressive behavior. Although recurrences do develop, the results of treatment are good for most ossifying fibromas.

Aneurysmal Bone Cyst

Aneurysmal bone cysts (ABCs) are rare benign lesions that are seen more than 70% of the time in the long bones and vertebral column with very few cases reported in the craniofacial regions (Giddings, Kennedy, Knipe, Levine, & Smith, 1989). This nonneoplastic lesion was first described in 1893 by Van Arsdale, but it was Jaffe and Lichtenstein who gave it the name aneurysmal cyst (Jaffe, 1950; Lichtenstein, 1950; Van Arsdale, 1893), which they later changed to ABC in 1950. Most lesions in the head and neck area occur in the jaws, with the mandible affected 55% of the time and the maxilla 45% of the time. It occurs slightly more commonly in females and the average age appears to be around 17 years old (Giddings et al., 1987). The majority present at or before 20 years of age. The etiology of these cycts is unknown, but, as with other bony lesions, trauma has been suggested and the lesion may be a re-

action to a subperiosteal hematoma. A high percentage of these bony lesions are associated with other bone growths including chondroblastoma, ossifying fibroma, and others. Clinical symptoms of swelling around the jaw with developing malocclusion are the first complaints. Although the lesion expands and erodes bone, there is always a thin shell of bone around the mass. X-ray appearance reveals a cystic, expansile, soap bubble mass within the body or ramus of the mandible (Figure 15–5). Both CT and MRI scans are helpful to show the extent of the lesion. The histology reveals fibrous, tissue compressing blood-filled spaces. Cells making up the mass include multinucleated giant cells, osteoclast type, and fibroblasts. The cut surface of a gross specimen reveals a thin-walled, large cystic mass with cavernous spaces filled with blood.

The treatment for ABC is surgical excision and immediate reconstruction for lesions in the mandible and maxilla. Other forms of therapy have been tried with less success, including radiotherapy, curettage, and cryotherapy. Recurrence rates were very high in cases treated with curettage, and radiation treatment lost favor because of the reported cases of radiation-induced sarcomas (Giddings et al., 1987). Cryotherapy seemed to work better than curettage but has its limitation in areas like the mandible, where closely positioned vital structure may be significantly affected by this technique. In general, when these unusual lesions appear, the diagnosis is difficult and the initial impression is that of a malignant bony tumor. A biopsy is needed to try to confirm its benign nature so that surgical removal is complete, but not overly aggressive. Excellent results can be obtained by proper planning and reconstruction of the defect when it arises in the craniofacial bones.

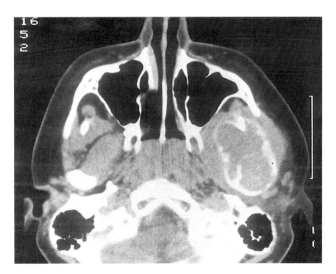

Figure 15–5. CT scan showing the typical appearance of a mandibular aneurysmal bone cyst.

References

Batsakis, J. G. (1974a). Non-odontogenic tumors of the jaws. In J. G. Batsakis (Ed.), *Tumors of the head and neck: Clinical and pathological considerations* (pp. 289–319). Baltimore: Williams & Wilkins.

Batsakis, J. G. (1974b). Neoplasms of the larynx. In J. G. Batsakis (Ed.), *Tumors of the head and neck: Clinical and pathological considerations* (pp. 135–154). Baltimore: Williams & Wilkins.

Beleval, G. S., & Schneider, R. W. (1953, July). Fibrous dysplasia of bone. *Cleveland Clinic Quarterly, 21*, 158–168.

Billing, L., & Ringerty, N. (1946). Fibro-osteoma: A pathologico-anatomical and roentgenological study. *Acta Radiology, 27*, 129–152.

Fu, U. S., & Perzin, K. H. (1974). Nonepithelial tumors of the nasal cavity, paranasal sinuses, and nasopharynx: A clinicopathologic study. *Cancer, 34*, 453–463.

Garrington, G. E., Scofield, H. H., Cornyn, J., & Hooker, S. P. (1967). Osteosarcoma of the jaws: Analysis of 56 cases. *Cancer, 20*, 377–391.

Giddings, N. A., Kennedy, T. L., Knipe, K. L., Levine, H. L., & Smith, J. D. (1989). Aneurysmal bone cyst of the mandible. *Archives of Otolaryngology—Head and Neck Surgery, 115*, 865–870.

Jaffe, H. L. (1950). Aneurysmal bone cyst. *Bulletin of the Hospital for Joint Diseases, 11*, 3–13.

Jaffe, H. L. (1953). Giant cell reparative granuloma, traumatic bone cyst, and fibroma (fibro-osseous) dysplasia of the jaw bones. *Oral Surgery, 6*, 159–175.

Lichtenstein, L. (1950). Aneurysmal bone cyst: A pathologic entity commonly mistaken for giant cell tumor and occasionally for hemangioma and osteogenic sarcoma. *Cancer, 3*, 279–289.

Lichtenstein, L., & Jaffe, H. L. (1943). Chondrosarcoma of bone. *American Journal of Pathology, 19*, 553–589.

Pindborg, J. J. (1965). Tumors of the jaw (benign and malignant). In R. N. Tiecke (Ed.), *Oral pathology* (pp. 287–290). New York: McGraw-Hill.

Rayne, J. (1968). Gardner's syndrome. *British Journal of Oral Surgery, 6*, 11–17.

Van Arsdale, W. W. (1893). Ossifying haematoma. *Annals of Surgery, 18*, 8–17.

Whitman, R. A., Stewart, S., Stoopack, J. G., & Jerrold, T. L. (1971). Myxoma of the mandible: Report of a case. *Journal of Oral Surgery, 29*, 63–70.

16

Recurrent Respiratory Papillomatosis

Craig S. Derkay, M.D.

Recurrent respiratory papillomatosis (RRP) is the most common benign neoplasm of the larynx among children (Jones & Myers, 1985). It is also the second most common cause of childhood hoarseness (Fearon & MacRae, 1976; Morgan & Zitsch, 1986), and is often difficult to treat because of its tendency to recur and spread throughout the respiratory tract. Although it most often involves the larynx, RRP may involve the entire aerodigestive tract. The course of the disease is variable with some patients experiencing spontaneous remission and others suffering from aggressive papillomatous growth requiring multiple surgical procedures over many years. The clinical course is unpredictable with malignant transformation possible in chronic invasive papillomatosis. RRP may have its clinical onset during either childhood or adulthood. Two distinct forms are generally recognized: a "juvenile" or aggressive form and an "adult" or less aggressive form. The aggressive form, although most common in children, also can occur in adults.

In most pediatric series, RRP is diagnosed between 2 and 3 years of age; with a delay in diagnosis from the time of onset of symptoms averaging about 1 year (Kashima et al., 1992). Seventy-five percent of the children are diagnosed before their fifth birthday (Cohn, Kos, Taber, & Adam, 1981). It is estimated that between 1500 and 2500 new cases of childhood-onset disease occur in the U.S.A. each year. The incidence among children in the U.S. is estimated at 4.3 per 100,000 children, translating into more than 15,000 surgical procedures at a cost of greater than $100 million per year (Derkay, 1995). Anecdotal observations suggest that most patients are firstborn, have young, primigravid mothers, and come from families of low socioeconomic status (Derkay, 1995; Mounts, Kashima, & Shah, 1992).

The most common symptoms of RRP are related to airway obstruction. It is not uncommon for children to be initially misdiagnosed as having asthma, croup, or chronic bronchitis. The hallmark of RRP in children is the triad of relentlessly progressive hoarseness, stridor, and respiratory distress. Though hoarseness in children tends to be overlooked or at least accepted until it reaches a certain level of severity, any infant or young child with symptoms of voice change, along with obstructive airway symptoms or recurrent croup, warrants laryngoscopy to rule out neoplasia, of which RRP is the most common lesion.

ETIOLOGY

Before the 1990s, the human papillomavirus (HPV) had been suspected, but not confirmed, as the causative agent in RRP. This uncertainty arose from an inability to culture the virus *in vitro*, and from the failure to consistently demonstrate viral particles in papilloma lesions using electron microscopy or HPV antibodies. Now, through the use of viral probes, HPV DNA has been identified in virtually every papilloma lesion studied. The most common types identified in the airway are HPV 6 and HPV 11, the same types responsible for genital warts. Specific viral subtypes may be correlated with disease severity and clinical course (Mounts & Kashima, 1984). Almost 70 different types of HPV have been identified. An association between cervical HPV infection in the mother and the incidence of RRP has been well established (Kosko & Derkay, 1996). Initial evidence for this association was established by electron microscopy, immunocytochemistry, and Southern Blot technique. More recently, *in situ* hybridization and polymerase chain reaction (PCR) techniques have confirmed the presence of HPV types 6 and 11 in RRP (Kashima, Kessis, Mounts, & Shah, 1991). Furthermore, viral DNA has been detected in areas of "normal-appearing mucosa" adjacent to papilloma lesions, suggesting a possible explanation for the recurrence of the disease following thorough surgical removal (Rihkaren, Aaltonen, & Syranen, 1993; Steinberg, Topp, Schneider, & Abramson, 1983). HPV is a nonenveloped icosahedral capsid virus with a double-stranded circular DNA 7900 base pairs long. The present understanding is that HPV establishes itself in the basal layer, where viral DNA enters the cell, and elaborates RNA to produce viral proteins. In addition to HPV types 6 and 11, subtypes 16 and 18 have also been found in RRP lesions. HPV 16 is the most frequently detected HPV in the genital tract. It is only rarely seen in benign aerodigestive tract lesions but is detected in 5–20% of aerodigestive tract squamous carcinomas. In the aerodigestive tract, HPV frequently causes latent infection (i.e., viral DNA present in tissue but no evidence of clinical or histologic disease). Brandsma reported finding HPV DNA in 4% of random, clinically normal biopsies of the airway (Brandsma & Abramson, 1989). Adult-onset respiratory papillomas could reflect either activation of virus present since birth or an infection acquired in adolescence or adult life.

The universality of HPV in the lower genital tract rivals that of any other sexually transmitted disease in humans. It is estimated that at least 1 million cases of genital papillomas occur per year in the U.S.A. (Koutsky & Wolner-Hanssen, 1989). These most often manifest as condylomata acuminata involving the cervix, vulva, or other anogenital sites in women, or involving the penis of male sexual partners of affected women. HPV has been noted to be present in the genital tract of as many as 25% of all women of childbearing age worldwide (Reid, Laverty, Copplesen, Isarangkul, & Hills, 1982). Clinically apparent HPV infection has been noted in 1.5% to 5% of pregnant women in the U.S.A. (Bennett & Powell, 1987). As in RRP, HPV types 6 and 11 are the most common subtypes identified in cervical condylomata. Ten percent of sexually active men and women with no evidence of disease have been shown to have HPV identified on the penis or cervix by Southern Blot hybridization analysis, suggesting the presence of a latent infection (Koutsky & Wolner-Hanssen; 1989).

RRP lesions occur at anatomic sites in which ciliated and squamous epithelium are juxtaposed (Kashima, Mounts, Leventhal, & Hruban, 1993). Histologically, RRPs appear as pedunculated masses with fingerlike projections of nonkeratinized stratified squamous epithelium supported by a core of highly vascularized connective tissue stroma (Figure 16–1). The basal layer may be either normal or hyperplastic, and mitotic figures are generally limited to this layer. Cellular differentiation appears to be abnormal with altered expression and production of keratins. The degree of atypia may be a sign of premalignant tendency, although HPV types and subtypes do not strongly correlate with clinical outcomes (Mounts & Kashima, 1984). The most common sites for RRP are the limen vestibuli, the nasopharyngeal surface of the soft palate, the midzone of the laryngeal surface of the epiglottis, the upper and lower margins of the ventricle, the undersurface of the vocal folds, the carina, and at bronchial spurs. In tracheotomized patients, RRPs are often encountered at the stoma and in the midthoracic trachea, areas that might be considered iatrogenic squamociliary junc-

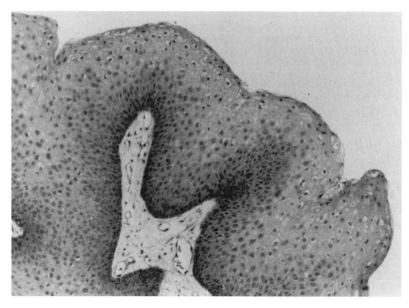

Figure 16–1. Low-power hematoxylin-eosin stain respiratory papilloma.

tions. Papilloma lesions may be sessile or pedunculated and often occur in irregular exophytic clusters (Figure 16–2). Typically, the lesions are pinkish to white in coloration. Iatrogenic implantation of papilloma may be preventible by avoiding injury to nondiseased squamous or ciliated epithelium adjacent to areas of frank papilloma. Ciliated epithelium undergoes squamous metaplasia when exposed to repeated trauma and is replaced with nonciliated epithelium that creates an iatrogenic squamociliary junction. It is postulated that an eddying flow of the mucous blanket at squamociliary junctions may concentrate infectious virus particles at these sites.

EPIDEMIOLOGY

RRP may affect people of any age with the youngest patient identified at 1 day of age and the oldest at 84 years old (Derkay, 1995). Childhood-onset RRP (arbitrarily defined as patients diagnosed at less than 12 years of age) is most often diagnosed between 2 and 3 years of age. Adult RRP peaks between the ages of 20 and 40 and has a slight male predilection; distribution among boys and girls is approximately equal (Fox, Kashima, Kurman, Lowry, & Steinberg, 1985). Childhood-onset RRP is more common and more aggressive than its adult counterpart. In a recent survey of practicing otolaryngologists in the U.S.A., half of the adults with RRPs had required fewer than five procedures over their lifetime compared with less than 25% of the children. Approximately equal percentages of children and adults (17% of children, 19% of adults) had very aggressive RRPs (defined as requiring more than 40 lifetime operations), although adults had more years to accumulate these operations (Derkay, 1995).

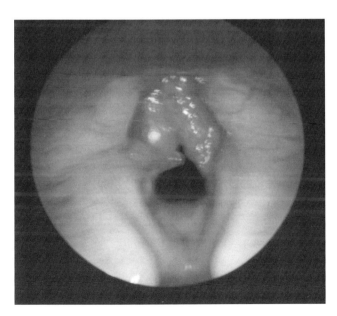

Figure 16–2. Sessile laryngeal papilloma.

The true incidence and prevalence of RRP is uncertain. In a Danish subpopulation incorporating 50% of the population of that country, the incidence of laryngeal papillomatosis was 3.84 cases per 100,000 (Lindeberg & Elbrond, 1991). The rate among children was 3.62 per 100,000, whereas adult-onset cases occurred at a rate of 3.94 per 100,000. These figures are comparable with those found in a recent U.S.A. survey, which estimated an incidence in the pediatric population of 4.3 per 100,000 children and 1.8 per 100,000 adults. This translates into roughly 2,300 new pediatric cases per year in the U.S.A. (Derkay, 1995).

The precise mode of HPV transmission remains unclear. Several studies have convincingly linked childhood-onset RRP to mothers with genital HPV infections, while circumstantial evidence suggests that adult disease may be associated with oral-genital contact. Cook et al. (1973) reported an association of juvenile laryngeal papillomatosis with maternal condylomata at the time of delivery. Strong, Vaughn, Healy, Cooperbrand, and Clemente (1976) reported that 50% of their patients younger than age 5 years were born to mothers with genital warts at the time of delivery and Quick, Kryzek, Walt, and Faras (1980) reported that 60% of children with laryngeal papillomatosis were born to mothers who had genital warts at the time of delivery. Hallden and Majmudar (1986) found that 54% of children with laryngeal papillomatosis were born to mothers who had genital warts. Condylomatas in the male sexual partners were not recorded in any of these studies, and subclinical disease was not detected or investigated.

Retrospective studies and a recent prospective study confirmed that HPV may be passed by vertical transmission from mother to child (Bennett & Powell, 1987; Smith, Johnson, Pignatari, Cripe, & Turek, 1991). In addition, a report by Kashima et al. (1992) found that patients with childhood-onset were more likely to be firstborn and vaginally delivered than control patients of similar age. This finding was collaborated by the anecdotal observations in a survey of otolaryngologists in the U.S. (Derkay, 1995). Kashima hypothesized that primigravid mothers are more likely to have a long second stage of labor and that the prolonged exposure to the virus leads to a higher risk of infection in the firstborn child. They also suggested that newly acquired genital HPV lesions are more likely to shed virus than long-standing lesions; this, they believe, may explain the higher incidence of papilloma disease observed among the offspring of young mothers of low socioeconomic status, the same group that is most likely to acquire sexually transmitted diseases such as HPV. Despite the apparent close association between maternal condylomata and the development of RRP, few children exposed to genital warts at birth actually develop clinical symptoms (Shah et al., 1986). It is not well understood why RRPs develop in so few children whose mothers have condylomata. The most likely method of maternal-fetal HPV transmission is direct contact in the birth canal (Kosko & Derkay; 1996). This would explain the clinical observation that most children in whom RRPs develop are vaginally delivered to mothers with a history of genital condylomatas. Although HPV could be recovered from the nasopharyngeal secretions of 47% of infants exposed to HPV in the birth canal (Sedlacek et al., 1989), the number of infants expected to manifest evidence of RRP is only a small fraction of this. Clearly, other factors (patient immunity, timing, length and volume of virus exposure, and local trauma) must be important determinants of development of RRP.

An occasional child with RRP has been delivered by cesarean section. Shah et al. (1986) reported that only 1% of 109 childhood-onset RRP cases reviewed gave a history of birth by cesarean section before rupture of uterine membranes. Even though cesarean section would seem to reduce the risk of transmission of the disease, this procedure is associated with a higher morbidity and mortality for the mother and a much higher economic cost than elective vaginal delivery. Shah estimates that the risk of a child contracting the disease from a mother who has an active condylomatous lesion and delivers vaginally to be only about 1 in 400. The characteristics that differentiate this one child from the other 399 are elusive. In light of the uncertainty surrounding intrapartum exposure, there is presently insufficient evidence to support delivery by cesarean section in all pregnant women with condylomata (Kosko & Derkay, 1996). Reports of neonatal papillomatosis suggest that, in at least some cases, development of the disease may occur *in utero*. Because cesarean section still does not prevent the development of papilloma disease in all cases, a better understanding of the risk factors associated with RRP is needed before the efficacy of cesarean delivery in preventing papilloma disease can be fully assessed.

CLINICAL FEATURES

The most common presenting feature of RRP in children is some degree of dysphonia. Unfortunately, changes in voice may go unnoticed, particularly in young children. Stridor is often the second clinical symptom to develop, beginning as an inspiratory noise and becoming biphasic with progression of the disease. Less commonly, chronic cough, recurrent pneumonia, failure to thrive, dyspnea, dysphagia, and acute life-threatening events may be the presenting symptoms. The duration of symptoms prior to diagnosis varies. Not uncommonly, a mistaken diagnosis of asthma, croup, allergies, vocal nodules, or bronchitis is entertained before a definitive diagnosis is made. When death occurs, it is usually associated with a complication of frequent surgical procedures or caused by respiratory failure due to distal disease progression. RRP presenting in the

neonatal period is thought to be a negative prognostic factor with a greater likelihood for mortality and need for tracheotomy (Chipps, McClurg, Freidman, & Adams, 1990; Cole, Myer, & Cotton, 1989; Leventhal et al., 1988). Because of the rarity of RRP and the slowly progressive nature of the disease, some cases may go unrecognized until respiratory distress results from papillomas obstructing the airway. The result is a relatively high need for tracheotomy to be performed in these children. Tracheotomy was necessary at some point in the management of 14% of children reported in two independent series, whereas its frequency among adults with RRP was estimated at about 6% (Derkay, 1995; Lindeberg & Elbrond, 1989). It has been suggested that tracheotomy may activate or spread disease lower in the respiratory tract. Cole et al. (1989) reported that tracheal papillomas developed in half of their tracheotomy patients and that, despite attempts to avoid this procedure, 21% of their patients still require a long-term tracheotomy. Prolonged tracheotomy and the presence of subglottic papilloma at the time of tracheotomy have been associated with an increased risk of distal tracheal spread. Most authors agree that tracheotomy is a procedure to be avoided unless absolutely necessary. When a tracheotomy is unavoidable, decannulation should be considered as soon as the disease is effectively managed with endoscopic techniques.

Children with bronchopulmonary dysplasia (BPD) who require prolonged endotracheal intubation may also be at increased risk for development of RRP (Chipps et al, 1990). Through interruption of the continuous respiratory mucosal surface, an endotracheal tube may have the same role in the mechanical dissemination/implantation of RRP as tracheotomy. Extralaryngeal spread of respiratory papillomas has been identified in approximately 30% of children and 16% of adults with RRP. The most frequent sites of extralaryngeal spread were, in order of frequency, the oral cavity, trachea, and bronchi (Derkay, 1995). A possible link between RRP and immunedeficiency states has also been observed. Children and adults with AIDS, with congenital immunedeficiencies, or on immune suppression after organ transplantation have been identified with RRP (Derkay, 1995).

Malignant transformation of RRP into squamous cell carcinoma has been documented in several case reports. A total of 26 patients were identified as having progressed to squamous cell carcinoma in the Task Force survey (Derkay, 1995). Lindeberg and Elbrond (1989) recorded three RRP patients with neoplastic progression. Interestingly, all three had received prior radiotherapy and two were heavy smokers, suggesting that these may be important cofactors for malignant transformation. Lie et al. (1994) reported on seven cases of laryngeal carcinomas and one patient with spread of papilloma to the bronchial tree who developed a bronchial carcinoma. The mean time between onset of papilloma and diagnosis of carcinoma was 24 years. In addition to smoking and irradiation, bleomycin was thought to be an important cofactor in this series.

PATIENT ASSESSMENT

History

Persistent or progressive stridor and dysphonia, with the possible development of respiratory distress, are the most consistent signs and symptoms of RRP in children. In the absence of severe respiratory distress, a careful history should be obtained. Information regarding the time of onset of symptoms, possible airway trauma including a history of previous intubation, and characteristics of the cry are obviously important. Hoarseness, although a common and often benign clinical complaint in young children, always indicates some abnormality of structure or function. Because of the precision of laryngeal mechanics, hoarseness may result from a remarkably small lesion and thus be an early sign in the course of a disease process. On the other hand, if the lesion's origin is remote from the vocal cords, hoarseness may present as a late sign. Although histologically the same lesion, a papilloma that produces hoarseness in one patient may produce stridor and obstruction in another, depending on the size and location of the lesion. The quality of the voice change may give only limited clues to its etiology while other characteristics such as age of onset, rate of progression, associated infection, history of trauma or surgery, and the presence of respiratory or cardiac distress may be of much greater significance. A low-pitched, coarse, fluttering voice suggests a subglottic lesion, whereas a high-pitched, cracking voice, aphonia, or a breathy voice suggests a glottic lesion. Associated high-pitched stridor also suggests a glottic or subglottic lesion. Although stridor that has been present since birth is more often associated with laryngomalacia, subglottic stenosis, vocal cord paralysis, or a vascular ring, it should be realized that neonates can also present with papillomatosis. Associated symptoms such as feeding difficulties, allergic symptoms, vocal abuse, and the presence of hereditary congenital anomalies may help sort RRP from alternative diagnoses, including vocal fold nodules, vocal fold paralysis, subglottic cysts, subglottic hemangioma, and subglottic stenosis. In the absence of any history suggesting these lesions, review of the perinatal period may reveal a history of maternal or paternal condylomata. If the onset of stridor and dysphonia is gradual and progressive over weeks or months, then neoplastic growth compromising the airway must be considered and investigated. Papillomas of the larynx usually do not become symptomatic before 6 months of age. In contrast, subglottic hemangiomas typically appear between 1 and 3 months of age with 85% present by 6 months. Additionally, 50% of children with subglottic hemangiomas will have an associated skin hemangioma. Certainly not every child with a hoarse voice or cry merits investigation beyond an assessment of the symptom. However, in the presence of hoarseness with respiratory distress, tachypnea, decreased air entry, tachycardia, cyanosis, dysphagia, chronic cough, failure to thrive, recurrent pneumonia, or dysphagia, the larynx must be visualized and a firm diagnosis of the cause of hoarseness must be made. Any child with slowly progressive hoarseness merits investigation and the clinician should not wait until total aphonia or airway problems occur. Additionally, the child with rapidly progressive stridor and hoarseness or aphonia in the absence of obvious infectious etiology should raise a high degree of suspicion for an aspirated foreign body warranting urgent intervention.

Physical Examination

Children presenting with symptoms consistent with RRP must undergo a thorough and organized physical examination. The child's respiratory rate and degree of distress must first be assessed. The physician should observe the child for tachypnea or the onset of fatigue that may indicate impending respiratory collapse. The child should be observed for flaring of the nasal alae and the use of accessory neck or chest muscles. Increasing cyanosis and air hunger may cause the child to sit with the neck hyperextended in an attempt to improve airflow. If a child is gravely ill, additional examination should not be undertaken outside the OR, the emergency room, or the intensive care unit, where resuscitation equipment for intubation of the airway, endoscopic evaluation, and possible tracheotomy are readily available. In the stable, well-oxygenated child additional examination can proceed. The most important part of the examination is auscultation with the aid of a stethoscope. The physician should listen over the nose, open mouth, neck, and chest to help localize the probable site of the respiratory obstruction. This author prefers to pull the bell off of the stethoscope and listen over these areas with the open tube. The respiratory cycle, which is normally composed of a shorter inspiratory phase and a longer expiratory phase, should then be observed. Stridor of a laryngeal origin is most often musical and may begin as inspiratory, but will progress to biphasic with worsening airway narrowing. Infants with stridor should be placed in various positions to determine their effect on the stridor. A child with RRP would not be expected to demonstrate much change in the stridor with position change in contrast to infants with laryngomalacia, a vascular ring, or a mediastinal mass. Pulse oximetry can add an accurate quantitative analysis of the child's respiratory state. In the stable patient in whom asthma is high on the differential diagnosis, pulmonary function testing combined with arterial blood gas evaluation may also be helpful. Inspiratory and expiratory airflow in relation to lung volume can be assessed by means of a flow volume loop to assist the physician in localizing obstructions or restrictions of the airway.

Imaging

In the patient without airway distress, appropriate radiologic evaluation of the upper aerodigestive tract may proceed after a careful history and physical examination. Fluoroscopy with the use of barium contrast medium is the radiographic study of choice. This will allow evaluation of both the inspiratory and expiratory phases of respiration. It allows the physician to evaluate the contribution of GER or encroachment by an anomaly of the great vessels to the child's airway abnormality, as well as contributing to the possible diagnosis of foreign body or airway neoplasm. CT and MRI are rarely necessary, although they may be helpful in evaluating the mediastinum for masses or aberrant vessels. This author does not find ultrasound or nuclear medicine studies to have any value in diagnosing RRP.

Airway Endoscopy

The preoperative diagnosis of RRP is best made with a flexible fiberoptic nasopharyngoscope. Careful, sequential inspection of the pharynx, hypopharynx, larynx, and subglottis provides the critical information necessary to make the diagnosis of RRP and allows estimation of lumen size, vocal cord mobility, and the urgency of operative intervention. Advances in instrumentation of flexible nasopharyngoscopes have resulted in instruments as small as 1.9 mm in diameter that allow passage in even the smallest newborns. Even the smallest diameter scopes provide images that can be seen on a video monitor and recorded for later review. Topical decongestion and local anesthesia can be applied by spray, dropper, or pledget. Oxymetazoline is the decongestant of choice because of its lack of cardiac side effects. Either topical ponticaine or lidocaine may be used to enhance patient cooperation but their dosage must be critically monitored in the small infant to avoid cardiotoxicity. It has been found that visualization with the flexible nasopharyngoscope is far superior to that obtained with indirect mirror laryngoscopy in young children. Patient cooperation, however, is required even with good topical anesthesia. In infants, this is not a large issue because they can easily be restrained in a sitting-up position in the parent's or nurse's lap for evaluation. Likewise, most children over 6 or 7 years of age can be "talked into" cooperating for the examination. It is the intermediate age group, between 1 and 6 years of age, who may be the most difficult to examine, taxing the patience and skill of even the most experienced clinicians. Although dynamic evaluation is best appreciated when children are spontaneously breathing, endo-

scopy in the OR under anesthesia is warranted in any child suspected to have RRP who cannot be fully examined in the outpatient setting.

Preoperative Preparation

The gold standard for endoscopic diagnosis of RRP is still operative-direct laryngoscopy. This can be performed with or without general anesthesia in the neonate but requires a general anesthetic for older infants and children. It is ideally performed in the OR where resuscitation equipment, small endotracheal tubes, and a tracheotomy set are readily available. Cooperation among the surgeon, anesthesiologist, and OR staff is imperative in the examination of the upper airway in children. In the child suspected, but not confirmed, of having RRP, a consent should be obtained for direct laryngoscopy, bronchoscopy, biopsy, possible use of the CO_2 laser for vaporization, and possible tracheotomy. Children newly diagnosed with RRP warrant a substantial time commitment on the part of the otolaryngologist in order to provide the family with a frank and open discussion of the disease and its management. Support groups such as the Recurrent Respiratory Papilloma Foundation (609-890-0502) can be a tremendous resource to the families for information and support. Most RRP patients require frequent office visits and endoscopic procedures after the initial diagnosis is made in order to establish the aggressiveness of their disease. They are encouraged to return to the office or call as often as necessary while family members and the healthcare team both get a feel for the child's symptoms and level of distress and the rapidity of regrowth of papillomas. Since RRP frequently results in the need for recurring, periodic therapies, it behooves the physician to start his or her relationship with the child and family on the right foot. If this is the child's first surgery, the physician should discuss all aspects of the surgery, as well as the possibility of laser complications and the need for tracheotomy. Once the child's diagnosis is established, many families benefit from the ability to network with other papilloma patients in their community. This is best arranged through the otolaryngologist's practice, when feasible.

Before the child enters the operating suite, the surgeon, anesthesiologist, and OR team must select the proper-sized endotracheal tubes, laryngoscopes, and bronchoscopes and ascertain that all ancillary equipment, including telescopes, light cords, suction tips, and forceps, are available and properly functioning. The surgeon, along with the OR team, should check that all equipment used for the procedure, including the surgical microscope with appropriate size lens, the laser unit, the micromanipulator, filtered suction, and smoke evacuation units, are all functioning properly. In our institution, the surgeon personally checks the laser for beam alignment by test-firing it prior to the child entering the room. Laser safety is carefully monitored in our institution by the laser safety committee. This includes a laser safety officer, a physician for each specialty that uses the laser, nurses from the OR, a hospital administrator, and a biomedical engineer. All OR personnel are required to wear eye protection whenever working around the laser. Specially designed laser masks are worn by OR personnel during the surgery to prevent the inhalation of viral particles liberated during the laser procedure.

Before the institution of any anesthesia, the surgeon should discuss the pathology with the anesthesiologist. Additionally, the staff within the OR should also be informed of the surgeon's concerns so that appropriate instrumentation is ready. Intraoperative teamwork is enhanced with the availability of video monitors during the operation, as this allows the entire OR staff to follow the operation as it progresses. Dialogue between the surgeon and the anesthesiologist continues throughout the procedure regarding the current status of ventilation, the amount of bleeding encountered, the motion of the vocal folds, the timing of laser use in conjunction with respiration, and the concentration of oxygen in the anesthesia mix. The ultimate decision about the technique of anesthesia should be shared between the anesthesiologist and the surgeon when utilizing an endotracheal tube. The smallest possible laser-safe endotracheal tube that allows for adequate ventilation should be used. If a cuffed tube is necessary, then the cuff should be filled with saline so that, if it is inadvertently struck by the laser beam, the saline acts as a heat sink and fire extinguisher. Some surgeons prefer to use methylene blue-colorized saline to provide an additional warning in case the cuff is penetrated. The laser-ignited airway explosion is a shocking emergency. Prompt, appropriate management is facilitated if the OR team has previously rehearsed and discussed this potential disaster (Schramm, Mattox, & Stool, 1981).

OPERATIVE PROCEDURE

No single modality has consistently been shown to be effective in eradication of RRP. The current standard of care is surgical therapy with a goal of complete removal of papillomas with preservation of normal structures. In patients in whom anterior or posterior commissure disease or highly aggressive papillomas are present, the goal may be subtotal removal with clearing of the airway. Although the CO_2 laser allows for precision of surgery and excellent hemostasis, multiple procedures are often necessary. It is advisable to debulk as much disease as possible while preserving normal morphology and anatomy and preventing the complications of subglottic and glottic stenosis, web formation, and a diminished airway. Frequent interval laser laryngoscopies are recommended to attempt to avoid tracheotomy and to permit the child to develop

good phonation with preservation of normal vocal cord anatomy.

The CO_2 laser has been favored over cold instruments in the treatment of RRP involving the larynx, pharynx, upper trachea, and nasal and oral cavities (Derkay, 1995). When coupled to an operating microscope, the laser vaporizes the lesions with precision causing minimal bleeding. When used with a no-touch technique, it minimizes damage to the vocal cords and limits scarring. The CO_2 laser has an emission wave length of 10,600 nm and converts light to thermal energy. It provides a controlled destruction of tissues with vaporization of water. It also cauterizes tissue surfaces. The smoke plume contains water vapor and destroyed tissue material. Although the CO_2 laser is the most commonly used laser for RRP in the larynx, the KTP/532 as well as the argon laser could also be used. The newest generation of laser microspot micromanipulator enables the surgeon to utilize a spot size of 250 microns at 400-mm focal length and 160 microns at 250-mm focal length (Ossoff, Werkhaven, Reif, & Abraham, 1991). The 710 Accuspot Sharplan laser is our current choice for managing RRP of the larynx. This unit allows direct visualization of the surgical target with elimination of the parallax problem inherent in earlier models. We utilize the Accuspot in the defocused mode to initially debulk papilloma, then focus the 250-micron spot size to excise papilloma from potentially tricky areas such as near the anterior and/or posterior commissure and along the true vocal folds. We may combine its use with a subglottiscope for removal of papilloma in the subglottic trachea (Ossoff, Tucker, & Werkhaven, 1991).

The majority of children with RRP require repeated laser surgeries with a median of 7 operative procedures in Lindeberg and Elbrond's (1989) series and 13 operations in Morgan and Zitsch's (1986) series. It is helpful when tracking the progression of a child's disease, communicating to other surgeons, and treating patients in a protocol format to have a surgical scoring system to assess severity and clinical course of RRP disease. Kashima (1985) has devised a relatively simple format that was utilized during the Alfa-n-1 interferon multi-institutional trial. Other scoring systems have been in use at University of Alabama, Birmingham, Children's National Medical Center, and a computerized system is currently being devised at the Centers for Disease Control for application with the National Registry (B. Wiatrak, G. Zalzal, W. Reeves, personal communication). Because there is currently no therapeutic regimen that reliably eradicates the HPV, when there is a question about whether papilloma in an area needs to be removed, it is prudent to accept leaving some residual papilloma rather than risk damage to normal tissue and producing excessive scarring. Even with the removal of all clinically evident papilloma, latent virus may remain in adjacent tissue, which may explain the recurrent nature of RRP. Therefore, the aim of therapy in extensive disease should be to reduce the tumor burden, decrease the spread of disease, create a safe and patent airway, improve voice quality, and increase the time interval between surgical procedures. Staged papilloma removal for disease in the anterior commissure is appropriate to prevent the apposition of two raw mucosal surfaces. The surgeon who is not aware of injury to deeper tissue layers with injudicious laser usage may encounter unacceptable scarring and subsequent abnormal vocal fold function. Inappropriate and aggressive use of the laser may also cause injury to nonaffected tissues and create an environment suitable for implantation of viral particles. Use of the CO_2 laser can also result in delayed local tissue damage, which may be related to the total number of laser surgeries and the severity of RRP disease.

After informed consent has been obtained from the appropriate family members, including a discussion regarding potential laser complications, the child is brought back into an OR that has been prepared and inspected by the surgeon and the laser team. When performing surgery for RRP, it is advisable to have an experienced team of OR nurses who are familiar with the sequence in which equipment is used and have been instructed in the proper use of the laser. In our facility we also have a laser safety team and provide yearly updates for the OR staff to ensure everyone's familiarity with the equipment and its potential complications. All of our pediatric anesthesiologists are familiar and comfortable with microlaryngoscopy laser surgery in children. However, in a nonchildren's hospital or nonacademic setting if there are only one or two anesthesiologists experienced with these techniques, they should be exclusively utilized whenever possible. This type of surgery is not well suited to the novice surgeon, anesthesiologist, or OR nurse. It is our practice to insist that the attending anesthesiologist be present and hands-on involved with all critical portions of the surgical procedure, including induction, securing of the endotracheal tube, positioning of the patient, changing of anesthesia techniques from a laser-safe tube to apnea technique, and extubation.

In our facility, the laser team consists of a scrub nurse, a circulating nurse, and a laser nurse. The laser is the responsibility of the laser nurse, allowing the circulator and scrub nurse to concentrate on their duties. All OR personnel are equipped with micropore laser filtration masks and approved goggles (Figure 16–3). The room is set up in advance with a suspension microlaryngoscope (Lindholm), a full set of Parson's laryngoscopes, two appropriately sized ventilating bronchoscopes, and a 7200A and 8700A Hopkins Rod telescope (Figure 16–4). A microscope with a 400-mm lens is fitted with the AccuSpot 710 micromanipulator. An assortment of suctions, alligators, cup forceps, and light cords, as well as a pack of neuro-patties and topical neosynephrine, are also standard. An endoscopy video cart equipped with color TV monitor, VCR, 3-chip camera, and xenon light source are also utilized (Figure 16–5). Still photography through the endoscope is also

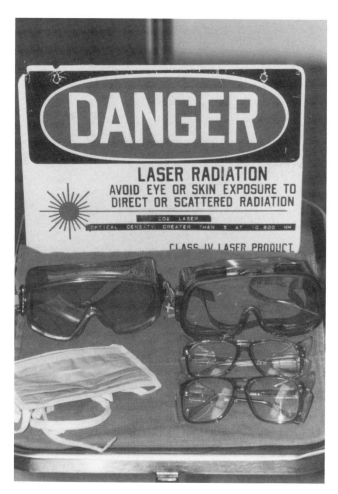

Figure 16–3. OSHA-approved safety goggles and high-filter masks.

available as needed. Additionally, a pediatric tracheotomy set is brought into the room, although the pack is not opened.

The surgical sequence begins with the mask induction utilizing halothane and the establishment of intravenous access. Dexamethasone at .5 mg/kg and cefazolin at 20 mg/kg are preoperatively routinely administered. The larynx is exposed utilizing the Parson's laryngoscope attached to 6 liters/minute of oxygen flow through its insufflation port, and the vocal folds are then sprayed with 2% lidocaine utilizing a syringe attached to a Cass needle. A diagnostic laryngoscopy is then performed utilizing the 7200A telescope under video control to assess the degree of papilloma disease and its encroachment on the laryngeal airway. Depending on the extent of disease, the child's history, and the interval since the last endoscopy, a full tracheoscopy and bronchoscopy may also be performed. Again, depending on the child's level of preoperative and operative distress, the surgeon may choose to perform this maneuver either with the 7200A telescope (if there is a low likelihood of discovering distal disease) or with an appropriate size ventilating bronchoscope (if there is high likelihood of discovering distal disease).

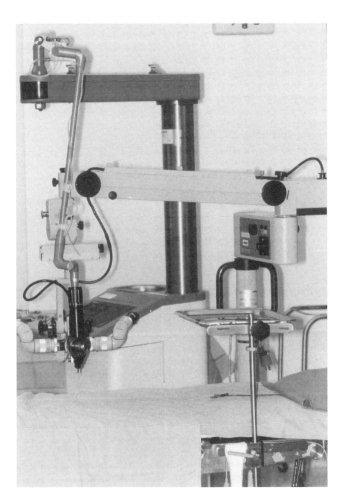

Figure 16–4. Operative setup for laser microsurgery.

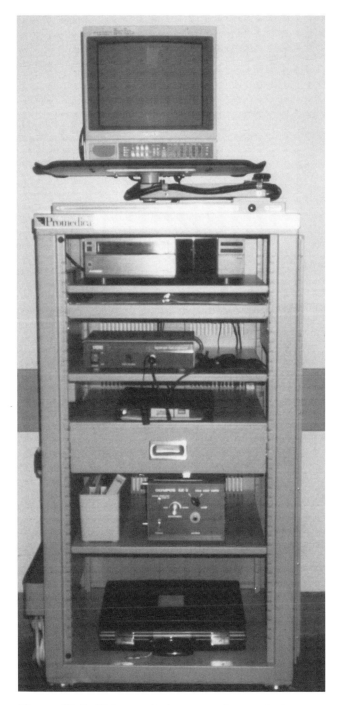

Figure 16–5. Video cart for intraoperative monitoring.

Still photography with the 8700A telescope is then performed at this stage, if desirable. If no distal disease is present, then the patient is intubated by the surgeon with a laser-safe tube (metal Xomed-Treace) of the smallest caliber that will allow the anesthesiologist adequate ventilation. Once the airway has been secured with the endotracheal tube, then the anesthesiologist is given the option to administer muscle relaxants. As an alternative, the child may be maintained on propofol. It should be stressed that no muscle relaxants are administered until the surgeon has assessed the degree of laryngeal obstruction and ascertained that the airway has been secured. This precaution serves to prevent the situation in which the child has lost his or her respiratory drive or obstructs his or her airway with papilloma and/or blood or mucus, precipitating hypoxia and a possible laryngospasm. Once the airway has been secured, the endotracheal tube is taped in place with a single piece of tape (allowing the surgeon easy access for removal of the endotracheal tube in the case of an airway fire) and the child is suspended for microlaryngoscopy with the Lindholm microlaryngoscope. We prefer to suspend the Lindholm either to a Mayo stand attached to the OR table or to a suspension platform

fashioned from Plexiglass (Matt, 1993). These two devices allow the microsuspension system to be moved along with the patient and allow angulation of the laryngoscope over a 120-degree range. The child's eyes are then protected against any stray laser beam exposure with moist saline-soaked gauze eye pads. Lubricant is placed in the eyes and the operative field is draped with moistened towels. OR personnel are all equipped with ocular protection, including side shields, and a sign is posted outside the OR warning that a laser procedure is occurring. A spare set of safety glasses is left outside the door for OR personnel who wish to come inside the room while the laser is in operation. Special laser masks with extremely small pores are worn to minimize exposure to the laser plume. A high-volume smoke evacuator is attached to one port of the Lindholm to collect the laser plume. A second suction attached to the smoke evacuator is utilized by the surgeon. By this point, the inspired FIO_2 delivered to the patient should be as close to a room-air mixture as possible. The laser is ideally not utilized until the oxygen in the mixture is between 26% and 30%. In selected circumstances, it may be warranted to proceed with an FIO_2 at or below 40%. These precautions are taken to minimize the possibility of a laser-induced endotracheal tube fire.

As an initial procedure, a microcup forceps is utilized to obtain a biopsy specimen from the bulkiest portion of papilloma. We utilize the AccuSpot laser at initial settings of 4 watts power, 0.1-second intervals, and repeat mode. Bulky papilloma is handled by defocusing the laser. Moistened neuro-patties are placed in the subglottis to decrease the air leak and to provide a backstop for errant laser shots. These must be kept moist as they too can act as a source of combustion. With the laser refocused, lesions are gradually vaporized to the level of the mucosa, avoiding entry into Reinke's space and the deeper vocalis muscle. I prefer using low-power settings to limit thermal injury to the surrounding tissue, although this does result in longer operating time. A small-caliber suction device is kept close to the laser impact site to remove the hot steam of vaporization and to remove eschar. Neuro-patties soaked in neosynphrine are also utilized for removal of eschar and debris as well as hemostasis. The blunt tip of the suction can also be used as a probe and retractor of the false fold, or to roll the true fold for exposure of the subglottic region. Care is taken to avoid injuring the anterior commissure, and at least 1 mm of untreated mucosa should be left in this region so that a web does not develop during the healing period (Figure 16–6). Similar considerations are taken for the posterior commissure. We normally begin the procedure with removal of papillomas in the supraglottic larynx, followed by the anterior half of both true vocal folds. If disease has been noted in the posterior half of the glottis or in the subglottic region, then we have found that the endotracheal tube obstructs exposure to these areas of the operative field and we seek an alternative means of anesthesia. We prefer an apneic technique in which the endotracheal tube is intermittently removed and work is performed while the patient's oxygen saturation is monitored. Another alternative would be spontaneous ventilation, although we find increased circulation of anesthesia gases with this technique to be an undesirable side effect. Once a decision is made to go apneic, the anesthesiologist increases the FIO_2 to 100%. The child is extubated though not unsuspended from the microlaryngoscope, and the smoke evacuation port of the Lindholm is disconnected; oxygen tubing connected to this port is allowed to

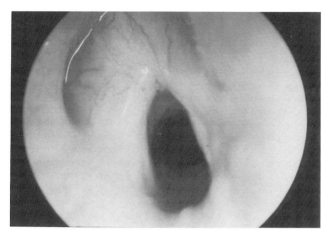

Figure 16–6. Acquired anterior commissure web.

flow 6 liters per minute of O_2. While utilizing an apneic technique, the laser initially is used for 90- to 120-second intervals; and the child reintubated with a polyvinyl chloride endotracheal tube directly through the microlaryngoscope, utilizing a stylet to stiffen the tube and improve the angulation. The CO_2 and O_2 levels are closely monitored and the length of "laser-on" time is appropriately adjusted. Typically, the child is reoxygenated for the same period of time that he or she was apneic before proceeding with the next cycle. At the end of the case, the child is reintubated with a standard endotracheal tube utilizing a Selinger technique to avoid any difficulty in reestablishing the airway on removal of the Lindholm microlaryngoscope. The child is then extubated only when fully awake. High humidity and, occasionally, racemic epinephrine are administered postoperatively in the recovery room. The patient is then closely monitored for several hours prior to discharge. Often, an overnight stay in a monitored bed unit is necessary. As a general rule, the more extensive the papilloma disease and the more compromised the airway, the more important it is for the child to be postoperatively monitored in an intensive care unit. Additional doses of steroids can be administered at 6-hour intervals if needed, while continuous pulse oximetry is mandatory.

Another anesthetic alternative is the use of jet ventilation for microsurgery of the larynx. Jet ventilation eliminates the potential fire hazard of the endotracheal tube and allows good visualization of the vocal folds. A limitation of this technique is the possibility of transmission of HPV particles into the distal airway. The jet cannula can be placed either above or below the vocal folds and each has its own particular benefit. We prefer placement of the cannula proximal to the end of the laryngoscope to decrease the risk of possible pneumothorax or pneumomediastinum. With large laryngeal lesions, narrowed airways, and ball-valve lesions, there may develop a high degree of outflow obstruction, which could lead to increased intrathoracic pressure and a subsequent pneumothorax. This may also result if there is inadequate muscle relaxation. Jet ventilation also requires constant communication between the operating surgeon and the anesthesiologist. Excessive mucosal drying and damage can occur as can insufflation of air into the stomach with gastric distention. As mentioned, there is also the potential risk of disseminating papilloma or blood into the tracheobronchial tree.

Postoperative Care

Children with stable papilloma disease requiring fewer than four laser procedures per year and whose parents reliably bring them in before showing signs of respiratory distress can be monitored at home with commercially available infant home intercom-type monitors (Fischer-Price). Those with rapidly reforming papillomas and those whose parents wait until the child is in distress before seeking medical attention may warrant home pulse oximetry with frequent home health visits. Children with RRP are encouraged to return to the office or call as often as necessary. We give parents carte blanche within our practice and explain to them that their children have a special problem that allows them access to speak with the doctors and nurses and to show up unexpectedly whenever they feel their child is in need. We have yet to experience a family that has abused this privilege. On the contrary, it has enhanced their trust in the healthcare team and has avoided urgent and emergent laser procedures.

Children with RRP are regularly followed up in the office, and flexible fiberoptic laryngoscopy in the office is utilized to monitor disease progression. Speech and language therapy are offered early in the course of the disease and used liberally. Control of other medical factors such as GER and asthma is also aggressively pursued. All papilloma families are put in touch with the Recurrent Respiratory Papilloma Foundation Support Group. Many have found this a tremendous resource for information and support. We have made local arrangements to network papilloma families in our community with good feedback from the participating families.

ADJUVANT TREATMENT MODALITIES

Although surgical management remains the mainstay of therapy for RRP, ultimately as many as 10% of patients with the disease will require some form of adjuvant therapy. The most widely adopted criteria for initiating adjuvant therapy are a surgery requirement of more than four procedures per year, distal multisite spread of disease, and/or rapid regrowth of papilloma disease with airway compromise. The most commonly recommended adjuvant therapy is α-interferon (Derkay, 1995). The exact mechanism by which interferon elicits its response is unknown (Cantell, 1995). It appears to

modulate host immune response by increasing production of a protein kinase and endonuclease, which inhibits viral protein synthesis. Interferons are a class of proteins manufactured by cells in response to a variety of stimuli, including viral infection. The enzymes that are produced block the viral replication of RNA and DNA and alter cell membranes to make them less susceptible to viral penetration. Common interferon side effects fall into two categories: acute reactions (fever and generalized flulike symptoms, chills, headache, myalgias, and nausea that seem to decrease with prolonged therapy) and chronic reactions (decrease in the growth rate of the child, elevation of liver transaminase levels, leukopenia, and febrile seizures). Thrombocytopenia has been reported, as have rashes, dry skin, alopecia, generalized pruritus, and fatigue. Acetaminophen has been found to be effective to relieve the fevers, and interferon injections are best tolerated at bedtime. Interferon produced by recombinant DNA techniques appears to have fewer side effects and better efficacy than blood bank-harvested interferon (Zemer et al., 1985).

Several large multi-institutional studies regarding interferon have arrived at seemingly conflicting conclusions regarding its efficacy. Healy et al. (1988) reported on 123 patients who received 2 million units/M^2 of α-interferon 3 days per week for 12 months and achieved a significant response that was not sustained at one-year follow-up. At this dosage, interferon seemed to control disease in the first 3 to 6 months of treatment but the effectiveness was questionable after 6 months of therapy. Leventhal et al. (1991) reported on 66 patients who received 5 million units/M^2 given initially on a daily basis for 1 month and then three times a week for 6 months with sustained or repeated responses in the majority of patients. Of the 66, 22 had a complete remission and 25 had partial remission with a median duration of 550 days. They also found that a response could be reintroduced after a period of nontreatment with interferon. Based on their study, Leventhal et al. recommend a 6-month trial of interferon if surgery is required every 2 to 3 months for a year.

Photodynamic therapy (PDT) in the treatment of RRP has been studied extensively at Long Island Jewish by Abramson et al. (1992) and by Shikowitz, Steinberg, and Abramson (1986). PDT is based on the transfer of energy to a photosensitive drug. The most common drug utilized is dihematoporphyrin ether (DHE), which has a tendency to concentrate within papillomas more so than in surrounding normal tissue. The ideal photosensitive drug would absorb light and transfer light and energy to triplet oxygen. This then converts it to a highly toxic singlet oxygen which is retained in tumor tissue longer than in normal tissue. Patients are typically treated with 2.5 mg/kg intravenous DHE prior to photoactivation with an argon pump dye laser. The use of PDT and DHE shows a small but statistically significant decrease in RRP growth, especially in patients with the worst disease. The drawback of this therapy is that patients become markedly photosensitive for periods of time lasting 2 to 8 weeks. A new drug, m-tetra (hydroxyphenyl) chlorin has shown efficacy in HPV-induced tumors in rabbits with minimal tissue damage, and a clinical trial utilizing this drug is being planned.

Avidano and Singleton (1995) reported the University of Florida's experience with 34 patients with severe RRP requiring adjuvant therapy. All 34 were treated with α-1 interferon utilizing 5 million units/M² for 21 to 28 days followed by a maintenance dose three times a week for at least 6 months. Interferon was administered by subcutaneous injection and the drug was held for severe side effects and then restarted at a lower dosage. Forty-seven percent of patients achieved a complete response and 35% achieved a partial clinical response. Five of the nonresponders out of the original 34 were subsequently treated with cis-retinoic acid (Accutane). No clinical response was achieved with any of these patients. Three of the 34 patients with minimal response to both interferon and Accutane were subsequently treated with methotrexate. Methotrexate is an antimetabolite used in the treatment of neoplastic diseases. Its mechanism of action is through the inhibition of dihydrofolic acid reductase, blocking synthesis of purine nucleotides and thymidylate, thus interfering with DNA synthesis. Methotrexate acts best on rapidly proliferating cells and was shown in Avidano's series to have some effect in recalcitrant RRP cases. All three patients achieved a significant clinical response, but none had a complete response within 3 to 6 months of initiating methotrexate therapy.

Retinoids, which are analogues of vitamin A, have been evaluated in several small trials with inconsistent results. Bell, Hong, Itri, McDonald, and Strong (1988) used 100 mg/M²/day of oral 13 cis-retinoic acid (Accutane) in nine patients without success and with significant toxicity. Alberts, Coulthard, and Meyskens (1986) experienced more success using a dose of 0.5 mg to 2 mg/day. Eicher reported success in a single patient with aggressive disease (Eicher, Taylor-Cooley, & Donovan 1994). Trans-retinoic acid, a similar drug with less potential toxicity, is currently in experimental use at several sites.

Ribavirin is an antiviral drug used to treat respiratory syncytial virus (RSV) pneumonia in infants that has also shown some promise in the treatment of aggressive laryngeal papillomatosis. McGlennen, Adams, Lewis, Faras, and Ostrow (1993) reported its use in three adults and one infant at a daily dose of 23 mg/kg. The authors found a complete response in two of their patients and a partial response in the other two. Morrison, Kotecha, and Evans (1993) reported a single patient with extensive tracheobronchial tree papillomatosis who experienced remarkable regression of this disease on ribavirin without adverse reaction. These authors recommend further evaluation to define the

role of ribavirin in the treatment of RRP. Ribavirin is currently available only in aerosolized form and costs over $1,000/day to utilize.

Another antiviral treatment that has received interest in the treatment of RRP is acyclovir. Although the activity of acyclovir is dependent on the presence of virally encoded thymidine kinase, an enzyme that is not known to be encoded by papillomavirus, conflicting clinical results have been obtained in several small series. Theoretically, it would not be expected to have a positive effect. However, it has been postulated that perhaps acyclovir is most effective when there are codisease factors such as a simultaneous infection with herpes simplex virus. Lopez-Agado, Periez-Pinero, Betancor, Mendez, and Banales (1991) achieved complete remission in three patients on the drug. Endres, Burke, Bauman, and Smith (1994) observed significant reduction only in patients not previously treated with interferon; patients on interferon developed worsening disease. Morrison and Evans (1993) found no response to acyclovir in four patients with aggressive RRP.

Recent interest has focused on chemically pure indole-3-carbinol (I3C), which has been shown to inhibit papilloma formation in mice (Newfield, Goldsmith, Bradlow, & Auborn, 1993). This compound is found in high concentration in cruciferous vegetables such as cabbage, broccoli, and cauliflower. A small dietary study at Long Island Jewish (LIJ) Hospital showed promise, although there were concerns regarding how much active drug the patients were actually receiving. I3C is now available in pure chemical form and new trials are ongoing at LIJ, the University of Pittsburgh and the University of Tennessee. Preliminary data suggest a linear relationship between the ratio of estrogen metabolism pathways (2-hydroxylation: 16 α-hydroxylation) and the severity of RRP disease. Ratios less than 1 are associated with severe disease and those greater than 3 are associated with mild disease (Steinberg & Auborn, 1993). Efforts are currently underway to expedite FDA approval of I3C as an investigational drug.

It should be stressed that participation in national and regional protocols of adjuvant treatment modalities is essential for the scientific community to learn more about RRP. A national registry of patients with RRP is being formed through the cooperation of the National Institutes of Health and the Centers for Disease Control. This will aid in the identification of patients suitable for enrollment in multi-institutional studies of adjuvant therapies and will better define the risk factors for transmission of HPV and the cofactors that may determine the aggressiveness of RRP.

LASERS

The CO_2 laser is the mainstay of lasers in otolaryngology. It is the most widely used, well understood, and well studied of the medical lasers and can be used for incision, excision, and vaporization of tissue. It was the first laser to be used clinically in otolaryngology and the first to be used in laryngology by Strong and Jako (1976). Use of the CO_2 laser results in shallow and predictable tissue penetration with minimal edema. Its hemostatic capability is limited, however, to blood vessels not larger than capillaries (0.5 mm). The CO_2 beam can be focused to create a precise cut and defocused to produce coagulation of small blood vessels. The CO_2 cannot be transmitted through flexible fibers and is delivered through a somewhat awkward articulated mirror system. If used improperly with a large spot size (> .5 mm), continuous exposure, or high-power settings (> 10 watts), significant mucosal scarring, fibrosis, and poor voice quality can result. The CO_2 laser is well absorbed by most tissues of the body because of the high water content of soft tissues. Water molecules are excellent absorbers of the CO_2 wave length. This is in contrast to bone and cartilage, which contain minimal water and thus will not absorb CO_2 laser energy. Because the CO_2 wave length is invisible to the human eye, a helium neon aiming beam is necessary to allow the surgeon to visualize the area of intended application. The advantage of using a CO_2 laser is its superficial extent of injury on tissues and its excellent precision, especially with the microspot micromanipulator.

COMPLICATIONS

Laser fires can occur in the operating room due to impact of the laser beam on materials such as towels, cloth drapes, or anesthetic tubing. This may be preventable by always placing the laser on "standby" when not in use. The most serious complication of laser surgery is an endotracheal tube fire. In order for combustion to take place, a source of energy (the laser beam), an oxidizable material (the endotracheal tube), and oxygen must all be present. Laser-induced endotracheal tube fires can be avoided by eliminating flammable endotracheal tubes from the procedure or by utilizing jet ventilation, apneic, or spontaneous anesthesia techniques. If the use of a tube is deemed necessary, then a nonflammable metal endotracheal tube can be utilized. Contrary to previous authors, I do not recommend the use of red-rubber endotracheal tubes that have been wrapped with aluminum foil by the anesthesiologist. These run too high a risk of possible flammability if the wrapping is inexact. Whenever possible, a cuffless endotracheal tube is preferred. If a cuff is utilized, it should be protected with wet cottonoids or a metal platform. Studies have shown that the higher the oxygen concentration flowing through the endotracheal tube, the more likely an endotracheal tube fire will occur. Thus the anesthesiologist should ventilate the patient's lungs with the lowest possible oxygen concentration. In an effort to reduce excessive tissue damage, I recommend utilizing brief intervals of as little as

a fraction of a second between laser impacts (repeat instead of continuous mode) to allow dissipation of laser energy and spare the normal tissue. The laser and laryngoscope should be repositioned as frequently as necessary to gain adequate tissue access and visualization. Eschar on tissue that has been lasered should be removed because this tissue absorbs energy and transmits heat to the underlying tissue. Hemorrhage should be controlled with neuro-patties soaked in neosynephrine because blood will absorb laser energy and diminish the laser's effectiveness as well as obscure the anatomy. Circumferential lasering should be avoided as this will lead to cicatrix formation and stenosis. Laser plume should be removed for adequate visualization and because the plume itself may dissipate the CO_2 laser beam. Because HPV may be present in a latent state in adjacent tissue, errant lasering should be avoided to prevent reactivation of disease.

Corneal or retinal burns are possible from an acute exposure to the laser beam. This can occur secondary to direct impact of the laser beam on the eye or through indirect reflection off of surgical instruments. The operating room should be clearly marked whenever laser surgery is taking place and all entrances into the room should have additional appropriate eyewear protection located near the door so that OR personnel can use them when entering the room. Patients should have eye protection in the form of gauze eye pads that are taped in place and moistened with saline. The surgeon should wear protective glasses except when he/she is using the operating microscope.

A double layer of saline-saturated surgical sponges, towels, or lap pads is used to protect all exposed skin and mucous membranes of the patient outside the immediate surgical field. As previously mentioned, the laser should remain on standby mode whenever not in use. Because it is possible for the beam to reflect off the proximal rim of the laryngoscope when performing surgery, the patient's face is completely draped with saline-saturated surgical towels, thereby exposing only the proximal lumen of the laryngoscope.

Laser plume has the potential for carrying HPV particles and noxious substances. To date there has been no direct evidence that these particles have caused RRP in the operating surgeon or other OR personnel. However, plume and noxious fumes are irritating to the respiratory tract even if they do not contain infectious particles, and the use of a mechanical smoke evacuator with high-efficiency filters is recommended. Finger burns may occur during microlaryngeal surgery if the surgeon does not keep his or her hand out of the line of fire of the laser beam. Therefore, the surgeon should strive to keep his or her hand to the extreme side of the operative field.

The anterior commissure of the larynx has to be respected when using the laser. Failure to preserve mucosa on at least one side of the commissure will lead to an acquired glottic web. Subglottic stenosis may occur secondary to laser treatment of circumferential papillomas below the vocal folds. Vocal fold fibrosis may develop following laser surgery in which too much power for too long a period of time is delivered to the true vocal fold, resulting in partial vaporization of the vocalis muscle. Granulomas can form if the black carbonaceous debris is not removed from the operative site. Prolonged hypoxia and hypercarbia can occur with apneic techniques of anesthesia and can be avoided with close monitoring. Jet ventilation techniques can result in pneumothorax if there is significant outlet obstruction. Theoretically, jet ventilation may also result in the distal spread of papilloma disease down the tracheobronchial tree.

Adjuvant therapies using antiviral and antineoplastic drugs can also result in complications. Children placed on these medications are ideally entered into carefully controlled clinical protocols. When this is not possible, the known potential side effects of these medicines need to be monitored. For instance, children placed on α-interferon should have liver function studies, a complete blood count, urinalysis, and thyroid function studies obtained at the outset and repeated at least twice a year. It is often appropriate to involve the hematology/oncology or infectious disease subspecialists at your medical center to assist you with managing the potential complications of patients on adjuvant therapy.

The management of RRP that has spread distally in the tracheobronchial tree is both challenging and frustrating. The CO_2 laser can be coupled to a rigid bronchoscope via universal endoscopic coupler. Custom-designed laser bronchoscopes are now available with the universal endoscopic coupler. Alternatively, the KTP/ND:Yag laser can be utilized through a ventilating bronchoscope. Although the KTP and Yag lasers are more dependent on melanin or pigment for their absorption spectra, they can still be effective in controlling papillomas. The surgeon, however, must be aware that more tissue destruction is possible than with the CO_2 laser. The ND:Yag laser can also be utilized through a flexible fiberoptic bronchoscope. The surgeon should realize that the use of the KTP/Yag laser will require different eye protection for the OR personnel and the patient. Postoperative atelectasis is common after lasering of tracheal and bronchial papillomas, and aggressive chest physical therapy is needed postoperatively.

The parents of children who are in seeming remission from their papilloma disease and have developed anterior commissure webbing or subglottic stenosis may request reconstructive surgical therapy for these conditions. Although it may be tempting to embark on this repair, the surgeon must be aware and the family must be informed of the possibility of reactivating papilloma disease through the manipulation of this apparently normal tissue. In my opinion, whenever possible, laryngotracheal reconstruction and anterior commissure web repairs should be avoided.

Lastly, a comment needs to be made regarding the potential for litigation in RRP patients. This is a frustrating disease because of its often prolonged nature and there may be guilt on the parents' part regarding vertical transmission from parent to child. The American Academy of Pediatrics (1990) official statement on HPV disease specifically states that cesarean section is *not* indicated in the prevention of transmission of HPV from mother to child. A comprehensive review of this topic reached the same conclusion (Kosko & Derkay, 1996). In spite of this, lawsuits have been brought against obstetricians regarding the lack of provision of informed consent to parents regarding this disease process. From the otolaryngologist's standpoint, laser surgery for papilloma disease has many potential and even life-threatening complications associated with it. "An ounce of prevention" is the best strategy for avoiding these complications. Additionally, it is wise for the surgeon to establish rapport and a close relationship with the families of their patients with papilloma. Informed consent needs to be reviewed with each procedure and the families need to feel that they have access to the healthcare team should their child develop increasing respiratory effort.

Treating children with RRP can be very rewarding as we learn more about HPV. In the future, we will hopefully be more successful at reducing the morbidity and mortality of this disease process. The establishment of the national registry and coordinated efforts between basic scientists involved in human papillomavirus research and clinicians involved in the treatment of RRP should aid us in this endeavor.

References

Abramson, A. L., Shikowitz, M. J., Mullooly, V. M., Steinberg, B. M., Amella, C. A., & Rothstein, H. R. (1992). Clinical effects of photodynamic therapy on recurrent laryngeal papillomas. *Archives of Otolaryngology—Head and Neck Surgery, 118,* 25–29.

Alberts, D. S., Coulthard, S. W., & Meyskens, F. L. (1986). Regression of aggressive laryngeal papillomatosis with 13 cis-retinoic acid (Accutane). *Journal of Biological Response Modifiers, 5,* 124–128.

American Academy of Pediatrics/American College of Obstetrics and Gynecology. (1990). *Guidelines for perinatal care* (3rd ed., pp. 127–128). Elk Grove, IL: Authors.

Avidano, M. A., & Singleton, G. T. (1995) Adjuvant drug strategies in the treatment of recurrent respiratory papillomatosis. *Otolaryngology—Head and Neck Surgery, 112,* 197–202.

Bell, R., Hong, W. K., Itri, L. M., McDonald, G., & Strong, M. S. (1988). The use of cis-retinoic acid in recurrent respiratory papillomatosis of the larynx: A randomized pilot study. *American Journal of Otolaryngology, 9,* 161–164.

Bennett, R. S., & Powell, K. R. (1987). Human papillomavirus: Association between laryngeal papillomas and genital warts. *Pediatric Infectious Disease Journal, 6,* 229–232.

Brandsma J. L., Abramson A. L. (1989). Association of papillomavirus with cancers of the head and neck. *Archives of Otolaryngology—Head and Neck Surgery, 115,* 621–625.

Cantell, K. (1995). Development of antiviral therapy with alpha interferons: Promises, false hopes and accomplishments. *Annals of Medicine, 27,* 23–28.

Chipps, B. E., McClurg, F. L., Freidman, E. M., & Adams, G. L. (1990). Respiratory papillomas: Presentation before six months. *Pediatric Pulmonology, 9,* 125–130.

Cohn, A. M., Kos, J. T., Taber, L. H., & Adam, E. Recurring laryngeal papilloma. *American Journal of Otolaryngology, 2,* 129–5429.

Cole, R. R., Myer, C. M., & Cotton, R. T. (1989). Tracheotomy in children with recurrent respiratory papillomatosis. *Head and Neck, 11,* 226–230.

Cook, T. A., Brunchswig, J. P., Butel, J. S., Cohn, A. M., Goepfert, L. L., & Rawls, W. E. (1973). Laryngeal papilloma: Etiologic and therapeutic considerations. *Annals of Otology, Rhinology and Laryngology, 82,* 649–655.

Derkay, C. S. (1995) Task force on recurrent respiratory papillomas. *Archives of Otolaryngology—Head and Neck Surgery, 121,* 1386–1391.

Eicher, S. A., Taylor-Cooley, L. D, & Donovan, D. T. (1994). Isotretinoic therapy for recurrent respiratory papillomatosis. *Archives of Otolaryngology—Head and Neck Surgery, 120,* 405–409.

Endres, D. R., Burke, D., Bauman, N. M., & Smith, R. J. H. (1994). Acyclovir in the treatment of recurrent respiratory papillomatosis: A pilot study. *Annals of Otology, Rhinology and Laryngology, 103,* 301–305.

Fearon, B., & MacRae, D. (1976). Laryngeal papillomatosis in children, *Journal of Otolaryngology, 5,* 473–496.

Fox, C. F., Kashima, H. K., Kurman, R. J., Lowry, D. R., & Steinberg, B. M. (1985). Papillomaviruses: Biological and clinical implications. *Clinical Courier, 3,* 1–8.

Hallden, C., & Majmudar, B. (1986). The relationship between juvenile laryngeal papillomatosis and maternal condylomata acuminata. *Journal of Reproductive Medicine, 31,* 804–807.

Healy, G. B., Gelber, R. D., Trowbridge, A. I., Grundfast, K. M., Ruben, R. J., & Price, K. N. (1988). Treatment of recurrent respiratory papillomatosis with human leukocyte interferon: results of a multicenter randomized clinical trial. *The New England Journal of Medicine, 319,* 401–407.

Jones, S., & Myers, G. N. (1985). Benign neoplasms of the larynx. *The Otolaryngologic Clinics of North America, 17,* 151–178.

Kashima, H. K. (1985). Scoring system to assess severity and course in recurrent respiratory papillomatosis. In *Papilloma-viruses: Molecular and clinical aspects* (pp. 125–135). New York: Alan R. Liss.

Kashima, H. K., Kessis, T., Mounts, P., & Shah, K. (1991). Polymerase chain reaction identification of human papilloma virus DNA in CO_2 laser plume from recurrent respiratory papillomatosis. *Otolaryngology—Head and Neck Surgery, 104,* 191–195.

Kashima, H., Mounts, P., Leventhal, B., & Hruban, R. H. (1993). Sites of predilection in recurrent respiratory papillomatosis. *Annuals of Otology, Rhinology and Laryngology, 102,* 580–583.

Kashima, H. K., Shah, F., Lyles, A., Glackin, R., Muhammed, N., Turner, L., VanZandt, S., Whitt, S., & Shah, K. (1992). Factors in juvenile-onset and adult onset recurrent respiratory papillomas. *Laryngoscope, 102,* 9–13.

Kosko, J., & Derkay, C. S. (1996). Role of cesarean section in the prevention of recurrent respiratory papillomas: is there one? *International Journal of Pediatric Otorhinology, 35,* 31–38.

Koutsky, L. A., & Wolner-Hanssen, P. (1989). Genital papillomavirus infection: Current knowledge and future prospects. *Obstetrics and Gynecology Clinics of North America, 16,* 541–561.

Leventhal, B. G., Kashima, H. K., Mounts, P., Thurmond, I., Chapman, S., Buckley, S., Wold, D., & the Papilloma Study Group. (1991). Long-term response of recurrent respiratory papillomatosis to treatment with lymphoblastoid interferon alfa-n1. *The New England Journal of Medicine, 325,* 613–617.

Leventhal, B. G., Kashima, H. K., Weck, P. W., Mounts, P., et al. (1988). Randomized surgical adjuvant trial of interferon alpha-n-1 in recurrent papillomatosis. *Archives of Otolaryngology—Head and Neck Surgery, 114,* 1163–1169.

Lie, E. S., Engh, V., Boysen, M., Clausen, O. P. F., Kvernvold, H., Steversen, T. C., & Winter, F. (1994). Squamous cell carcinoma of the respiratory tract following laryngeal papillomatosis. *Acta Otolaryngologica, 114,* 209–212.

Lindeberg, H., & Elbrond, O. (1989). Laryngeal papillomas: Clinical aspects in a series of 231 patients. *Clinical Otolaryngology, 14,* 333–342.

Lindeberg, H., & Elbrond, O. (1991). Laryngeal papillomas: The epidemiology in a Danish population 1965–1984. *Clinical Otolaryngology, 15,* 125–131.

Lopez-Aguado, D., Perez-Pinero, B., Betancor, I., Mendez, A., & Banales, E. C. (1991). Acyclovir in the treatment of laryngeal papillomatosis. *International Journal of Pediatric Otorhinolaryngology, 21,* 269–274.

Matt, B. H. (1993). Suspension platform for stable microlaryngoscopy. *Otolaryngology—Head and Neck Surgery, 108,* 199–200.

McGlennen, R. C., Adams, G. L., Lewis, D. M., Faras, J. J., & Ostrow, R. S. (1993). Pilot trial of ribavirin for the treatment of laryngeal papillomatosis. *Head and Neck, 15,* 504–513.

Morgan, A. H., & Zitsch, R. P. (1986). Recurrent respiratory papillomatosis in children: a retrospective study of management and complications. *Ear, Nose and Throat Journal, 65,* 19–28.

Morrison, G. A., & Evans, J. N. (1993). Juvenile respiratory papillomatosis: Acyclovir reassessed. *International Journal of Pediatric Otorhinolaryngology, 26,* 193–197.

Morrison, G. A. J., Kotecha, B., & Evans, J. N. G. (1993). Ribavirin treatment for juvenile respiratory papillomatosis. *Journal of Laryngology and Otology, 107,* 423–426.

Mounts, P., & Kashima, H. (1984). Association of human papillomavirus subtype and clinical course in respiratory papillomatosis. *Laryngoscope, 94,* 28–33.

Mounts, P., Shah, K. V., & Kashima, H. (1982). Viral etiology of juvenile and adult onset squamous papilloma of the larynx, *Proceedings of the National Academy of Sciences of the United States of America, 79,* 5425–5429.

Newfield, L., Goldsmith, A., Bradlow, H. L., & Auborn, K. (1993). Estrogen metabolism and human papillomavirus-induced tumors of the larynx: Chemo-prophylaxis with Indole-3-Carbinol. *Anticancer Research, 13,* 337–341.

Ossoff, R. H., Tucker, J. A., & Werkhaven, J. A. (1991). Neonatal pediatric microsubglottiscope set. *Annals of Otology, Rhinology and Laryngology, 100,* 325–326.

Ossoff, R. H., Werkhaven, J. A., Reif, J., & Abraham, M. (1991). Advanced microspot microsland for the CO_2 laser. *Otolaryngology—Head and Neck Surgery, 105,* 411–414.

Quick, C. A., Kryzek, R. A., Walt, S. L., & Faras, A. J. (1980). Relationship between condylomata and laryngeal papillomata: clinical and molecular virological evidence. *Annals of Otology, Rhinology and Laryngology, 89,* 467–471.

Reid, R., Laverty, C. R., Copplesen, M., Isarangkul, W., & Hills, E. (1982). Non-condylomatous cervical wart virus infection. *Obstetrics and Gynecology, 55,* 476–482.

Rihkaren, H., Aaltonen, L. M., & Syranen, S. M. (1993). Human papillomavirus in laryngeal papillomas and in adjacent normal epithelium. *Clinical Otolaryngology, 18,* 470–474.

Schramm, V. I., Mattox, D. W., & Stool, S. E. (1981). Acute management of laser-ignited intra-tracheal explosion. *Laryngoscope, 91,* 1417–1426.

Sedlacek, T. V., Lindeheim, S., Elder, C., et al. (1989). Mechanism for human papillomavirus transmission at birth. *American Journal of Obsetetrics and Gynecology, 161,* 55–59.

Shah, K., Kashima, H., Polk, B. F., Shah, F., Abbey, H., & Abramson A. (1986). Rarity of caesarean delivery in cases of juvenile onset respiratory papillomatosis. *Obstetrics and Gynecology, 68,* 795–799.

Shikowitz, M. J., Steinberg, B. M., & Abramson, A. C. (1986). Hematoporphyrin derivative therapy of papillomas. *Archives of Otolaryngology—Head and Neck Surgery, 112,* 42–46.

Smith, E. M., Johnson, S. R., Pignatari, S., Cripe, T. P., & Turek, L. Perinatal vertical transmission of human papilloma virus and subsequent development of respiratory tract papillomatosis. *Annals of Otology, Rhinology and Laryngology, 100,* 479–483.

Steinberg, B. M., & Auborn, K. K. (1993). Papillomaviruses in head and neck disease: Pathophysiology and possible regulation. *Journal of Cellular Biochemistry Supplement, 17F,* 155–164.

Steinberg, B. M., Topp, W. C., Schneider, P. S., & Abramson, A. L. (1983). Laryngeal papillomavirus infection during clinical remission. *New England Journal of Medicine, 308*, 1261–1264.

Strong, M. S., & Jako, G. J., (1976). Recurrent respiratory papillomatosis: Management with the CO$_2$ laser. *Annals of Otology, Rhinology and Laryngology, 8*, 508–516.

Strong, M. S., Vaughan, C. W., Healy, G. B., Cooperband, S. R., & Clemente, M. C. A. P. (1976). Recurrent respiratory papillomatosis: Management with the CO$_2$ laser. *Annals of Otology, Rhinology and Laryngology, 85*, 508–516.

Zemer, H. P., Kley, W., Claros, A., et al. (1985). Recombinant interferon-alpha-2C in laryngeal papillomatosis: Preliminary results of a prospective mulicenter trial. *Oncology, 42*(Suppl. 1), 15–18.

17

Unusual Neoplasms

Phillip K. Pellitteri, D.O.

MALIGNANT TERATOMA

True teratomas contain tissue elements derived from all three germinal cell layers. Malignancy is suggested when cells are noted to be in an interimmature stage of differentiation. These tumors occur at an incidence of approximately 1 in 4000 live births with 7–9% localized to the head and neck region (Berry, Keeling, & Hilton, 1969). The incidence of malignancy occurring in teratomas is estimated to be approximately 20% (Grosfield & Billmire, 1985).

These tumors may be found in a number of head and neck locations, including the neck, nasopharynx, pharynx, orbit, and paranasal sinuses. Cervical teratoma presents as a mass in the neck and is usually present at birth. Symptoms are the result of compression resulting in upper airway obstruction leading to stridor and apnea (Figures 17–1, A and B). Dysphagia from esophageal compression may be seen. Affected infants have an increased incidence of polyhydramnios, stillbirth, and prematurity. Plain radiographs of the neck indicate a soft tissue mass, which contains speckled calcifications in approximately 50% of patients and posteriorly displaces both the trachea and esophagus. Teratoma may be ultrasonographically differentiated from both a lymphangioma and congenital goiter in that it demonstrates mixed echogenicity. Cystic hygroma typically appears as a lobulated cystic structure extending to the mediastinum, whereas goiter appears solid.

Once the diagnosis of cervical teratoma is made, surgical excision to prevent airway obstruction is required. Significant morbidity may result from these procedures because of their bulk and proximity to vital structures. Malignant teratomas may develop after resection of a benign tumor and, accordingly, prolonged follow-up is required.

The nasopharynx represents another common location for teratomas, which arise from the superior and lateral walls. The dermoid cyst represents the most common teratoma in the nasopharynx, presenting as a "hairy" polyp in the nasal or oral cavity. Orbital teratomas are also present at birth, usually as massive unilateral proptosis. Most orbital teratomas are benign and require orbital exenteration (Gnepp, 1985).

Therapy for malignant teratomas in the head and neck consists primarily of surgical resection, if feasible, followed by multidrug chemotherapy. Unresectable or residual disease is usually treated by irradiation to the primary site. Initial response to therapy is almost uniformly good; however, 2-year disease-free survival rates decrease to approximately 50% (Grosfield & Billmire, 1985).

MALIGNANT MELANOMA

Melanoma is uncommon in older children and is rare in children less than 12 years of age. A number of congenital and hereditary syndromes associated with the development of melanoma in the pediatric population have been described. These include: hereditary cutaneous melanoma, dysplastic nevus syndrome, giant congenital nevus transformation, and generalized congenital metastatic malignant melanoma (Greene et al., 1985a, 1985b; Kopf et al., 1986; Skov-Jensen, Hastrup, & Lambrethsen, 1966).

Melanoma of the head and neck in children and adolescents is found most commonly on the face and, in

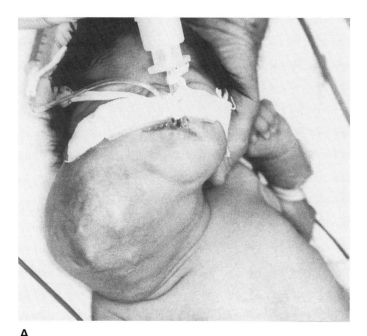
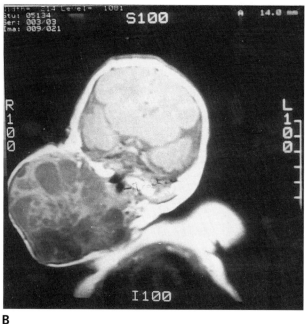

A   **B**

Figure 17–1. A. Malignant teratoma involving the cervical region and resulting in airway obstruction in a newborn infant. **B.** MRI of patient with lesion illustrated in Figure 17–1**A** demonstrating compression of trachea. (Courtesy of A. Seid, M.D.)

particular, the cheek. Discovery is usually prompted by the change in a lesion represented by increased size, bleeding episode, color change, or pruritic reaction. Regional lymphatic metastases are frequently clinically present.

The diagnosis is made by biopsy and subsequently should be followed by a thorough systemic evaluation to rule out distant metastasis. Once this work-up is completed, surgical resection is indicated with the approach individualized for each child in accordance with principles established for adults. The most useful staging criteria are those of Clark (depth of tissue invasion) and Breslow (tumor thickness) with reference to prognosis. Tumor thickness has been correlated with recurrence and survival, and depth of invasion of the primary tumor has been correlated with survival only (Clark et al., 1975; Koh, 1991).

The margin of resection at surgery depends on tumor stage, depth of invasion, and location. For lesions less than 1–2 mm thick, a margin of 1 cm circumferentially is sufficient, whereas tumors with greater thickness require a margin of 3 cm. Regional disease, if clinically present, should be surgically addressed by parotidectomy and neck dissection. The role of prophylactic elective neck dissection in the absence of clinically palpable lymph nodes is not well defined. The utility of chemotherapy and immunotherapy is also undetermined. Survival generally depends on the anatomic location; the status of the regional lymph; and, in older children, the depth of tumor invasion. When all sites are considered, survival for malignant melanoma in children approximates 40–50%.

DESMOID TUMOR

Desmoid tumors, also known as fibromatosis, are fibrous neoplasms of uncertain etiology that are intermediate in their biologic characteristics and behavior between benign fibrous growth and fibrosarcoma. They behave in a more aggressive fashion than the former benign tumors by invading local surrounding structures and recurring after resections; however, unlike fibrosarcoma, desmoid tumors have no predilection for metastasis.

Desmoid tumor, although an uncommon disease in children, forms an important intermediary in the spectrum of fibrous tissue tumors. Various entities compose the spectrum of fibrous growths found in children with a convenient classification proposed by Enzinger and Weiss (1983). This group may be divided into tumors that are found in both adults and children and tumors that are peculiar to infants and children. The former group may be subdivided into superficial and deep types. The superficial category is categorized by slow growth, small size, and superficial tissue level of involvement. The deep group tends to be faster growing and of larger size, an example of which is extraabdominal fibromatosis.

Because of the relatively rare occurrence in children, precise data regarding the incidence of desmoid tumors occurring in this population are difficult to obtain. One large series reported that desmoid comprised 2.2% of all benign soft tissue tumors (Schmidt & Harms, 1985). Half of these patients were younger than 5 years of age, with a male to female ratio of 1.36:1. When all types are considered, the tumor is indeed rare, with an estimated incidence of two to four cases per million patients per year. Desmoid lesions of the head and neck are even less common and are associated with a high recurrence rate, estimated to be between 20–70% following excision.

Histologically, desmoid tumors appear benign and have been categorized with the fibromatoses as a group of benign tumors formed by proliferating fibroblastic tissue (Figure 17–2). The etiology of desmoid tumors is unknown. Several factors have been proposed as playing a role in the initiation of tumors and modifying growth characteristics, but none have been strongly supported.

Tumors involving the head and neck region most commonly present in the cervical and supraclavicular regions, usually as an asymptomatic mass that is firm, solid, and nontender on palpation. Symptom onset heralds the encroachment of the tumor mass on vital structures such as large vessels, sensory nerves (i.e., brachial plexus), and the airway. The soft tissues of the face and oral cavity are less commonly involved but these tumors may occur in the orbit, cheek, and tongue musculature. Desmoid tumors of the head and neck, in general, occur in younger patients (Fasching, Saleh, & Woods, 1988).

With few exceptions, aggressive surgical wide resection with adequate margins provides the best opportunity for cure. The natural history of untreated tumors, in general, is slow, relentless growth with invasion of adjacent structures. Resection of head and neck tumors may be formidable (Figure 17–3), depending on the tumor location, but should provide for a clear margin of tissue with the least functional morbidity. The use of adjuvant modes of therapy, such as radiation and chemotherapy, poses a problem in the growing child. Recurrent disease should be managed by surgical resection where feasible and where considerable morbidity may be avoided. The effectiveness of radiotherapy is controversial, but its use should be reserved for older children with residual or unresectable disease or in younger children for whom further resection cannot be performed. Chemotherapeutic effectiveness is equally unproven. Agents that have shown activity with the lesion include dactinomycin, doxorubicin, and theophylline (Goepfert et al., 1982).

Desmoid tumors in the head and neck occurring in children usually occur after initial resection. The anatomic structure of the neck allows this aggressive infiltrating lesion to involve vital structures, often precluding the removal of tumor with an adequate margin of normal tissue or without incurring severe functional morbidity. The long-term prognosis for lesions occurring in younger patients has been variably reported but, in general, seems poorer in children with head and neck lesions. Aggressive resection in an effort to obtain as wide a margin of uninvolved surrounding tissue as possible is clearly the single most important determinant of a successful outcome (Figures 17–4 and 17–5).

CHORDOMA

Chordoma is an uncommon neoplasm arising from remnants of embryonic notochord, predominantly in the spheno-occipital and sacrococcygeal regions. It is a slow-growing neoplasm which is rarely found to metastasize. The malignant potential of this tumor lies in its locations of origin, its unrelenting and destructive growth, and its demonstration of a high recurrence rate. Approximately half of all chordomas originate in the spheno-occipital region, where they account for less than 0.5% of nasopharyngeal tumors and less than 1% of CNS tumors (Krespi, Levine, & Oppenheimer, 1986). A slight male to female predominance (3:2) is noted for this lesion with the exception being the chondroid type, which favors females (Heffelfinger et al., 1973; Spoden, Baaested, & Warren, 1980). Chordoma is a very rare lesion in children despite its origin within embryonic notochord.

Grossly, these tumors are gelatinous, lobulated, semitranslucent, and gray (Figure 17–6). They give the

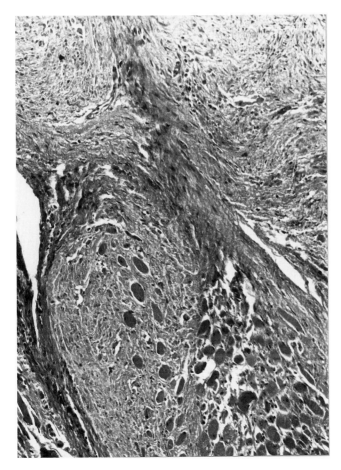

Figure 17–2. Desmoid tumor (fibromatosis). Note bland appearing fibroproliferative tissue. (Courtesy of A. Garbes, M.D.)

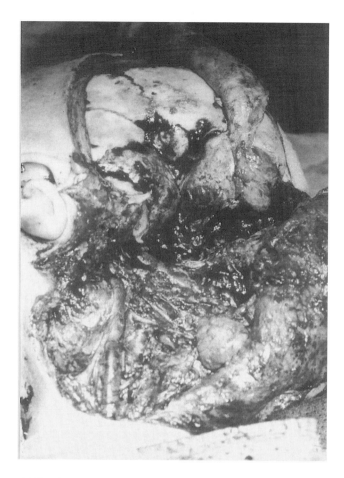

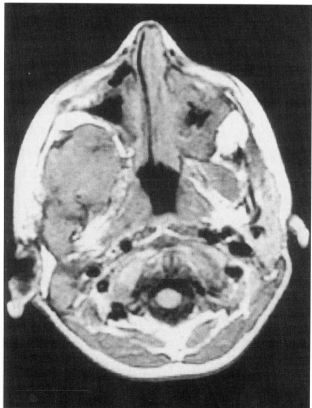

Figure 17–4. Preoperative MRI showing patient in Figure 17–3 with lesion involving the infratemporal fossa.

Figure 17–3. Intraoperative photograph illustrating resection of a large desmoid neoplasm involving the anterolateral cranial base in a 10-year-old child. Note exposed temporal fossa dura superiorly and spinal accessory nerve crossing internal jugular vein inferiorly.

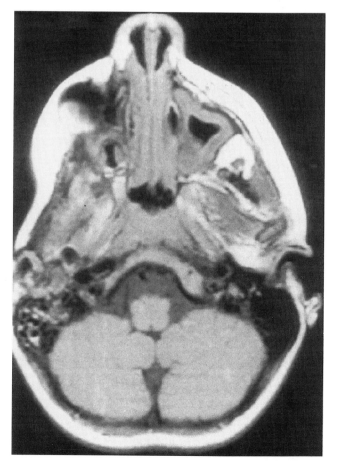

Figure 17–5. Postoperative MRI of patient in Figure 17–3 showing area of resection with soft tissue reconstruction of infratemporal fossa using myogenous free flap.

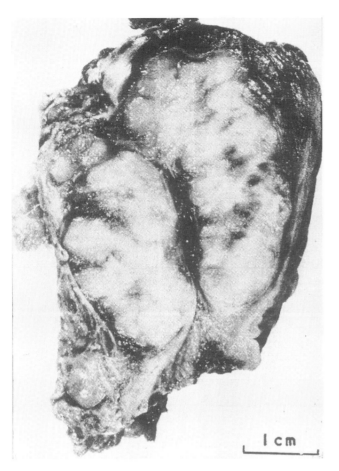

Figure 17–6. Gross specimen of clival chordoma.

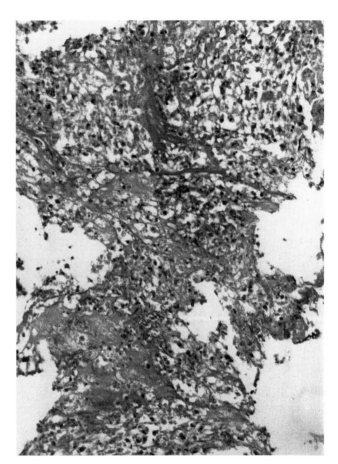

Figure 17–7. Histopathology of tumor pictured in Figure 17–6 demonstrating characteristic "foamy" appearing physaliferous cells. (Courtesy of A. Garbes, M.D.)

appearance of being encapsulated with encroaching margins into the soft tissue and, at times, against dura and brain parenchyma. Their margins of involvement in bone are less demarcated and more infiltrative (Heffelfinger et al., 1973). Histologically, the tumors are noted to be surrounded by a pseudocapsule composed of fibrous bands, which also form septi within the tumor mass. The characteristic cellular feature of the chordoma is marked by the presence of physaliferous cells containing varied amounts of intracytoplasmic mucin (Figure 17–7) (Batsakis, 1974). Mitotic activity and pleomorphism are usually not striking and belie the malignant potential of these lesions (Heffelfinger et al., 1973). Two varieties of chordoma have been identified based on the degree of chondroid features present. Those with a significant chondroid component demonstrated features resembling either chondrosarcoma or chondroma (Heffelfinger et al., 1973). The stroma of the chondroid-type chordomas resembled hyalin cartilage with neoplastic cells and lacuna. These features are admixed in a variable amount with typical histological characteristics of chordoma.

Chordomas are slow-growing and locally invasive. Signs and symptoms of spheno-occipital lesions are reflected by specific sites of tumor extension, such as cellar, paracellar, and clival invasion. The most common

presenting symptom is diplopia, usually the result of sixth cranial nerve palsy, which occurs in about 90% of these lesions (Spoden et al., 1980). Additional symptoms reflect involvement of other cranial nerves; and in nearly 90% of spheno-occipital tumors, a nasopharyngeal mass is present. Because the tumor originates in spheno-occipital synchondroses within the clivus, the mass presents as a downward extension from this site.

Most patients will show osseus destruction of the midline skull base from an expansile osteolytic lesion within the clivus on imaging with CT scans. Calcifications within the tumor are seen more commonly with the chondroid type (Batsakis, 1980). MRI will demonstrate the degree of intracranial involvement and whether or not brain parenchymal invasion is present (Figure 17–8). A tissue diagnosis is obtained through transoral or transnasal biopsy. Cerebral angiography to determine the location of potentially displaced internal carotid arteries is necessary prior to any attempt at resection.

The treatment of chordoma centers on surgical resection. The area of involvement at the skull base and the proximity of vital structures almost uniformly makes complete resection impossible. Postoperative radiotherapy should be administered, as incomplete resection

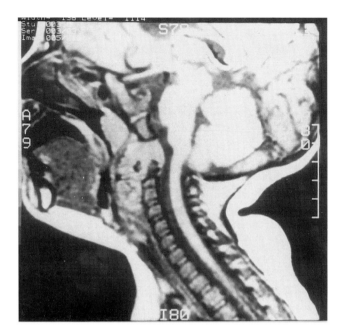

Figure 17–8. Sagittal MRI demonstrating a large chordoma involving the clivus of a young child.

results in recurrence within a 3-year period. Surgical approaches include those usually employed to reach the midline and anterolateral skull base, some of which are the transoral, transcervical-transmandibular, and craniofacial disassembly procedures.

In general, the prognosis for children with chordoma is not appreciably different than that for adults. Mean survival is approximately 7 years with a 5-year disease-free survival rate of only 10%. The chondroid type has been associated with a better prognosis in terms of disease-free survival. A large Mayo Clinic series found that the average survival of patients with typical chordoma was about 4 years compared with approximately 16 years for those with the chondroid variety (Heffelfinger et al., 1973). The usual cause of death was as a result of local recurrence with significant intracranial extension.

GRANULAR CELL TUMOR

The granular cell tumor is a benign neoplasm of uncertain origin most commonly found in the upper aerodigestive tract. The tumor has been assigned a plethora of names in order to characterize it, including Abrikossoff's tumor, granular cell myoblastoma, granular cell neurofibroma, myoblastic myoma, and congenital epulis, to name several. The large number of names indicates the tumor's uncertain histogenesis.

Two types of granular cell tumor have been identified in humans. The first, congenital epulis, occurs in newborns as a submucosal mass along the alveolar ridge. The tumor is found in the maxilla more often

than in the mandible, but both may occur concurrently. It is approximately eight times more frequent in females than in males (Batsakis, 1979). Most lesions undergo spontaneous regression; surgical excision is recommended for lesions that do not spontaneously resolve.

The second type of granular cell neoplasm occurs primarily in young adult patients. It is found more frequently in females and in black patients. The tumor is found most frequently in the tongue as a submucosal, well-circumscribed nodule, but may occur in any upper aerodigestive tract site, including the larynx, trachea, and bronchus. Wide local excision is the treatment of choice and is usually adequate in preventing recurrence.

References

Batsakis, J. G. (1974). *Tumors of the head and neck* (pp. 266–284). Baltimore: Williams & Wilkins.

Batsakis, J. G. (1979). Tumors of the peripheral nervous system. In J. G. Batsakis (Ed.), *Tumors of the head and neck: Clinical and pathological considerations* (2nd ed.). Baltimore: Williams & Wilkins.

Batsakis, J. G. (1980). The pathology of head and neck tumors: Neoplasms of cartilage, bone and the notochord. *Head and Neck Surgery, 3,* 43–57.

Berry, C., Keeling, J., & Hilton, C. (1969). Teratoma in infancy and childhood: A review of 91 cases. *Journal of Pathology, 98,* 241–250.

Clark, W. H., Jr., Ainsworth, A. M., Bernandino, E. A., et al. (1975). The developmental biology of primary human malignant melanoma. *Seminars in Oncology, 2,* 83–88.

Enzinger, F. M., & Weiss, S. W. (1983). Fibromatoses. In S. E. Harshberger (Ed.), *Soft tissue tumors* (pp. 45–70). St. Louis: C. V. Mosby.

Fasching, M. C., Saleh, J., & Woods, J. E. (1988). Thyroid tumors of the head and neck. *American Journal of Surgery, 156,* 327–331.

Gnepp, D. (1985). Teratoid neoplasms of the head and neck. In L. Barnes (Ed.), *Surgical pathology of the head and neck* (pp. 1411–1433). New York: Marcel Dekker.

Goepfert, H., Cangir, A., Ayala, A. G., et al. (1982). Chemotherapy of locally aggressive head and neck tumors in the pediatric age group. *American Journal of Surgery, 44,* 437–444.

Greene, M. H., Clark, W. H., Jr., Tucker, M. A., et al. (1985a). Acquired precursors of cutaneous malignant melanoma: The familial dysplastic nevus syndrome. *New England Journal of Medicine, 312,* 91–93.

Greene, M. H., Clark, W. H., Jr., Tucker, M. A, et al. (1985b). High risk of malignant melanoma in melanoma-prone families with dysplastic nevi. *Annals of Internal Medicine, 102,* 458–462.

Grosfield, J., & Billmire, D. (1985). Teratomas in infancy and childhood. *Current Problems in Cancer, 9,* 1–10.

Heffelfinger, M. J., Dahlin, D. C., MacCarty, C. S., et al. (1973). Chordomas and cartilaginous tumors at the skull base. *Cancer, 32,* 410–420.

Koh, H. K. (1991). Cutaneous melanoma. *New England Journal of Medicine, 325,* 171–182.

Kopf, A. W., Hellman, L. J., Rogers, G. S., et al. (1986). Familial malignant melanoma. *JAMA, 256,* 1915–1918.

Krespi, Y. P., Levine, T. M., & Oppenheimer, R. (1986). Skull base chordomas. *Otolaryngologic Clinics of North America, 19,* 797–804.

Schmidt, D., & Harms, D. (1985). Fibromatosis of infancy and children—histology, ultrastructure and clinicopathologic correlation. *Zeitschrift für Kinderchirurgie, 40,* 40–46.

Skov-Jensen, T., Hastrup, J., & Lambrethsen, S. (1966). Malignant melanoma in children. *Cancer, 19,* 620–631.

Spoden, J. E., Baaested, R. M., & Warren, E. D. (1980). Chondroid chordoma: Case report and literature review. *Annals of Otology, 89,* 279–285.

18

Pediatric Maxillofacial Trauma: Dental, Dentoalveolar, Mandibular, and LeFort Type 1 Injuries

Micheal E. Lessin, B.S.D., D.D.S., Thomas J. Bitterly, M.D., F.A.C.S., Joseph G. DeSantis, M.D., and Thomas L. Kennedy, M.D., F.A.C.S.

The topic of this chapter, pediatric maxillofacial trauma, is of worldwide interest, yet the incidence of significant maxillofacial trauma in the pediatric population averages only 5% to 10% of all reported major maxillofacial injuries. The incidence of significant facial trauma increases during the teenage years with male to female ratios of approximately 3:1. The sources of trauma reported are significant and are preventable in many cases. The major etiologies listed are: motor vehicle-related injury (passenger, pedestrian, and driver), bicycle injuries (individual injuries or bicycle vs. motor vehicle), falls, sports-related injury, personal altercations, dog bites, horse kicks, and other sources. Incidences of maxillofacial injury attributed to child abuse are not reported as significant, but must be suspected and reported when suspected (Amaratunga, 1988; Guven, 1992; Hardt & Gottsauner, 1993; Harrington, Eberhart, & Knapp, 1988; Infante Cossio et al., 1994; Kaban, 1993; Lindquist, Sorsa, & Santavirta, 1986; Posnick, Wells, & Pron, 1993; Tanaka et al., 1993; Thoren et al., 1992).

Experience of practitioners of the various specialties treating pediatric maxillofacial injuries varies between significant numbers and experience at various centers to the individual practitioner who is infrequently called upon to treat such cases. The latter circumstance may not be in the patient's best interest. In addition, while major experience may be had in treating adult injuries and general principles always apply, the particular differences which occur in treating pediatric injuries lie in the great variations in age and body habitus encountered from infancy, toddler stage, adolescent

stage to teenage, and finally adult. This is perhaps further complicated by faster bone healing in the younger patient and by the different stages of tooth development and presence of deciduous vs. mixed vs. adult dentition (Kaban, 1990b).

This chapter has contributions from four specialists, representing only three of the many possible specialties that may be called on to treat pediatric maxillofacial injuries. This helps to make the point that teamwork, proper utilization of consultants, and, perhaps, experience only serve to make the treatment of pediatric maxillofacial injuries more successful in final outcomes related to form, function, and cosmesis. Subjects discussed in this chapter include treatment of:

1. Pediatric dental, dentoalveolar, mandibular, and maxillary injuries.
2. Pediatric midface injuries.
3. Pediatric soft tissue injuries.
4. Pediatric laryngeal injuries.

ADVANCED TRAUMA LIFE SUPPORT

While this chapter will not discuss many of the specifics, it must be clearly understood that the principles of pediatric and adult advanced trauma life support (Committee on Trauma, 1993) must be embraced and practiced as appropriate, particularly in the multisystems injured patient. A specially trained trauma team in the emergency unit of the hospital may be in charge of the emergency treatment and overall care of the multisystems trauma patient in the hospital. If the hospital system is organized into those who treat major trauma vs. those who do not, the seriously injured should be transported to the trauma center as soon as possible. Traditional airway maintenance and support either with appropriate positioning, tongue extension, nasopharyngeal or oral airway, or oral tracheal intubation must be considered in addition to supplemental oxygen. Breathing may be spontaneous or assisted, dependent on the condition of the patient, with hyperventilation indicated for the comatose or neurologically impaired patient so often encountered. Fluid resuscitation with crystalloid or blood products must be initiated in the seriously injured with intravenous or intraosseous access and flow rates dependent on body size and weight of the patient, as well as age. Cervical spine and chest x-rays will be ordered for the seriously injured and must be carefully reviewed. Primary and secondary system evaluation will proceed with particular emphasis on neurological status, chest, abdominal injury, and extremity injury.

Other than measures to stop life-threatening hemorrhage, including packing to stop severe nasal bleeding, hemostatic clamping of pumping vessels, and gross suturing or bandaging of gaping wounds, emergency treatment of maxillofacial injuries is not always a part of the initial trauma management. Following resuscitation and stabilization of the multisystems injured patient, more definitive evaluation of the maxillofacial injuries becomes possible and more practical. If the patient must be emergently treated in the OR because of concomitant injuries, the initial evaluation and treatment may be first done under these circumstances and may not necessarily be as thorough or complete as desired. Further radiological evaluation and treatment may be necessary after initial recovery.

For the patient without multisystem injury, initial evaluation and treatment may proceed more emergently as may be appropriate. However, it is wise for the treating practitioner to review the total patient prior to initiating care of the localized area to ensure a gross injury has not been coincidentally missed. For example, a fall from a bicycle directly to the chin should include evaluation of the cervical spine to ensure the odontoid process is intact while the chin laceration and condylar fracture may be obvious in a 12-year-old.

PEDIATRIC DENTAL, DENTAL ALVEOLAR, MANDIBULAR, AND MAXILLARY INJURIES

Clinical Evaluation

Although this section is devoted to evaluation and treatment of dental, dentoalveolar, mandibular, and maxillary injuries, it is impossible to discuss the examination of these structures without discussing the complete extraoral and intraoral examination. It may certainly be difficult to perform a thorough exam in the young pediatric patient secondary to pain, fear, or unusual swelling, which may make it difficult for the patient to see or speak. A calm, reassuring voice and gentle manner, along with a simple explanation of what has happened and what the examiner is going to do, is necessary prior to attempting the examination. The presence of a parent nearby or holding a hand can be quite helpful with the right parent. If the parent is obstructive or hysterical, it may be necessary to remove the parent from the immediate vicinity.

A complete bimanual exam, checking for integrity of the facial bone and mandibular structures, is the goal. The examiner should intraorally and extraorally check for crepitus, loss of continuity, or step-off. Mobility of fragments, as well as sensory and/or motor deficits or differences, should be noted without inflicting unnecessary trauma. Loose, chipped teeth as well as avulsed or partially avulsed teeth should be noted and recorded. The pharynx must be inspected in the case of traumatically absent teeth, unless they are accounted for. If still unaccounted for, the trachea, bronchi, lungs, esophagus, and stomach must be later radiologically studied to locate the tooth or fragments or confirm their absence. Dental malocclusion must be suspect, as well as limited jaw opening, pain on function, or deviation on opening or closing. Intraoral or extraoral ecchymosis or laceration should be further evaluated for fracture in the area. A midline palatal blood clot may indicate a midpalatal fracture, and the clot should not be suctioned away at this time for fear of reinitiating severe bleeding. Simple lacerations of the soft palate area may also profusely bleed at this time if manipulated, and these should be left alone until definitive care is to be delivered. At times it is practical to perform temporary reduction of severely mobile or displaced fractures in the tooth-bearing areas of the maxilla or mandible with simple finger reduction and temporary circumdental bridle wire (with or without individual interdental wires of 25-, 26-, or 28-gauge surgical steel wire). Simple local anesthetic technique can be used to facilitate such minor treatment and will do much to reduce pain and bleeding, particularly in the mandibular body, parasymphyseal, or symphyseal area, as well as in the maxillary midline or cuspid-bicuspid, cuspid-deciduous molar region, and will allow the examination and radiological evaluation to proceed better.

If possible, the ear canals should be examined for canal laceration or hemotympanum. In the case of canal laceration, the examiner must suspect trauma from a condyle perforating the canal as well as potential condyle fracture. Hemotympanum as well as postauricular ecchymosis (Battle's sign) must be suspect for basilar skull fracture.

Extraocular motions must be evaluated, as well as pupillary size, reaction, and vision, but severe periorbital ecchymosis and swelling may prevent this. An immediate ophthalmological consultation should then be requested to further assist in evaluation of the globe and retinal structures. Simple swelling may not prohibit the examination, but gross swelling or the presence of hyphema mandates an immediate consultation.

Examination of the nasal area may demonstrate crepitus or displacement with or without open laceration. While infants and toddlers have relative hypertelorism and telecanthus due to their nasal development and epicanthal folds, more severe telecanthus and nasal-orbital crepitus may indicate some form of naso-orbital-ethmoidal (NOE) injury. NOE injury and traumatic telecanthus must be suspected in the adolescent or teenager with these findings. Intranasal examination with speculum and good lighting may reveal intranasal laceration or cartilaginous septum displacement. Septal hematoma, which in itself requires more immediate treatment such as aspiration and nasal packing, may appear as a bluish, tense painful swelling along the septum. The pediatric patient with clinical signs of serious midface trauma may have a CSF leak from the nose, which may be difficult to discern amid the bloody and mucous secretions. The use of filter paper to perform a ring test may be helpful in diagnosis as well as using a glucose test strip applied to the secretion pool. If CSF is suspected, packing of the nares should be avoided unless severe hemorrhage is present.

In certain types of deacceleration injury or kicks to the neck from human or animal sources, or even from severe dog bite to the area, bruising to the anterior neck, hoarse voice, or evidence of laryngeal edema is an acute problem that may indicate laryngeal fracture. This requires immediate treatment and will be discussed later in another section.

Following as complete an examination as possible, a list of findings should be recorded and a clinical impression should be formulated. The use of diagrammatic supplementation, as possible, to record lacerations types and lengths or other significant findings is always helpful. The clinical evaluation may now be followed by appropriate radiographic studies.

Radiographic Evaluation

To further assist in the diagnosis and treatment of maxillofacial bone and tooth injuries, appropriate radiographic studies should be ordered dependent on the urgency of need, the state of cooperation of the patient, and above all the stability of the patient in regard to other injuries. It is certainly inappropriate to demand multiple immediate esoteric radiographs in a nonstable patient or in a patient who does not require immediate definitive treatment.

For the cooperative toddler, adolescent, or teenager with simple, obvious injury to the mandible, zygoma, maxilla, or nasal bones, plane films can be quite informative and perhaps all that is necessary. A facial

series should have a good quality Waters view to demonstrate the bony orbits and zygoma and maxillary areas. A quality posteroanterior view of the mandible to show the mandibular angle, body, and symphysis area; a modified Towne's view to project the mandibular condyles; and left and right lateral oblique mandibular views can offer significant information to the diagnostician. Open and closed temporomandibular joint views are unnecessary and usually offer nothing to trauma diagnosis. Additionally, if available, a quality panographic or orthopanographic survey can offer much information as to condyle position, as well as fracture to the mandibular angle, and body and parasymphysis region (Figure 18–1).

Dental injury, mandibular symphyseal, or maxillary midline injuries may necessitate dental periapical radiographs or mandibular or maxillary occlusal radiographs to better delineate the injury (Figure 18–1). In the patient with complex or multisystem injuries these films may be difficult to obtain, although some facilities have portable dental x-ray units available so that films may be taken in the emergency unit, OR, or intensive care units.

For the uncooperative, or unconscious and intubated patient, or the patient with multiple suspected facial and mandibular fractures, the CT scan can certainly offer much more information with less x-ray exposure and in less time. If possible, axial images from frontal area to hyoid area at no more than 5-mm cuts can reveal practically all injuries in this orientation (Figure 18–1). Supplemental coronal images are also most helpful and at times essential in the diagnosis of complex injuries in these patients. The newer rapid sequence scanners can offer these studies in just minutes, and if necessary, finer cuts of the orbits (3 mm) can be produced. In addition, the newer 3-D imaging programs can produce scans with even more helpful information to assist in the treatment of patients with multiple facial fractures. There is no doubt that in the appropriate patient, the CT scan in axial and coronal images is the gold standard (Kaban, 1993).

Treatment Planning

Using the information obtained from the clinical examination and appropriate radiographic studies, a treatment plan may be formulated. Simple injuries in an otherwise healthy and stable patient may be treated within the emergency department or private office. Some patients, because of the severity of the injury complex or simply because of lack of cooperation, may be best treated in an OR. Whether the patient can be treated as an outpatient or as an inpatient is again dependent on the patient and the injuries to be treated. A decision must also be made as to whether or not immediate treatment is required or if treatment is to be delayed.

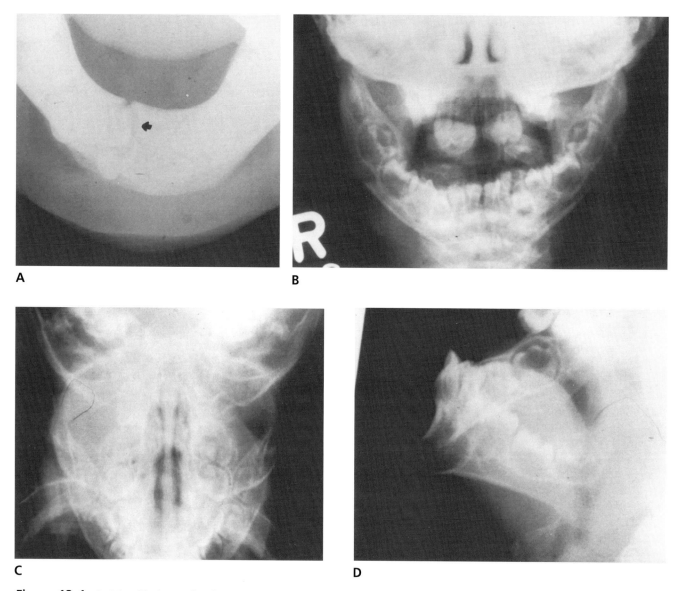

Figure 18–1. A. Mandibular occlusal x-ray, demonstrating symphyseal fracture in young child (*arrow*). **B**. Mandibular posteroanterior x-ray best demonstrates fractures of angle and body. **C**. Towne's view of mandibular condyle is necessary to evaluate for condylar fractures. This x-ray depicts bilateral extracapsular fractures with medial displacement. **D**. Lateral oblique view of mandible is most helpful to evaluate the mandibular body and angle. Right and left obliques are necessary.   *continued*

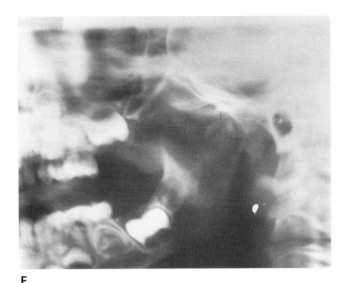

E

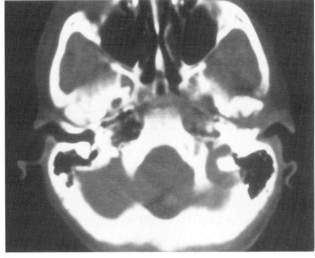

F

Figure 18–1. *(continued)* **E.** Panographic x-ray is extremely valuable in overall evaluation of the mandible and is essentially a tomographic view. This particular close-up view of a panographic film clearly shows a left condylar fracture. **F.** CT view in axial plane demonstrates bilateral condylar fractures. Coronal views, if possible to obtain, are also helpful diagnostically, particularly in condylar and midface fractures.

In general, patients with injuries requiring intraoral and extraoral care, such as closed reduction with arch bars and primary closure of perioral lacerations, should have the intraoral treatment completed first and then closure of the lacerations including closure of mucous membrane in through-and-through lacerations from an inside-out approach. After mucous membrane closure, extraoral closure would proceed for deeper muscular layers, subcuticular layers, and finally skin. The concept that oral wounds are dirty and should not be closed is invalid because of the prolific vasculature and potential for healing as well as the availability of appropriate antibiotic drugs. In a similar methodology, multiple fractures of the mandible, maxilla, or midface that affect the dental occlusion should be planned for treatment so that the jaws are placed into appropriate maxillomandibular fixation prior to accomplishing open reduction of the mandible if indicated, and then of the superior midfacial, zygomatic, and maxillary fractures, if indicated. In other words, the patient should be considered for treatment from a "bottom-up," teeth, mandible, midface approach, as well as an inside-out approach to assist in ensuring a functional as well as a cosmetic result (Figure 18–2).

Pediatric Anatomical Considerations

The space occupied by the cranium in the infant and young child, as compared to the older child and adolescent, is significantly greater than the midface and mandible. This tends to protect the midface and mandible from significant bony injury in infants and young children, while making the cranial vault and frontal area more prone to injury. As the child grows and matures, the midface and mandible tend to equally share with the cranial vault; consequently, the injury distribution changes significantly. The density of the maxilla and nasofrontal area is significantly greater in the infant and child because of lack of development of the accessory and paranasal sinuses. In addition, this denser space is filled with developing and erupting deciduous and permanent teeth (Crockett, Mungo, & Thompson, 1989; Posnick, 1992).

The mandibular condyle, which serves as a growth center in the infant and child, tends to have a thin bony cortex and increased cancellous bone, which makes it more prone to injury. However, the injuries in this age group tend to be more green-sticked or bending-type injuries rather than the distinct fracture or dislocation-type injuries found in older adolescents, teenagers, and adults. The remarkable healing and regenerative capacity of the condyle as well as other mandibular areas and facial bones means that fractures usually heal quicker in this group, and in general need to be treated within 7 days for a better result. In general, when dealing with closed reduction and maxillomandibular fixation, the main treatment considerations in maxillary and mandibular injuries in infants and children, the period of fixation needs to be no more than 1–3 weeks because of rapid bone healing (Kaban, 1990b; Posnick, 1992; Turvey & Kendell, 1991).

In dealing with the dentition, the short root-crown ratio of deciduous teeth, unfavorable crown anatomy of deciduous teeth, degree of root resorption of deciduous teeth, incomplete root development of newly erupted permanent teeth and associated tooth mobility, the state

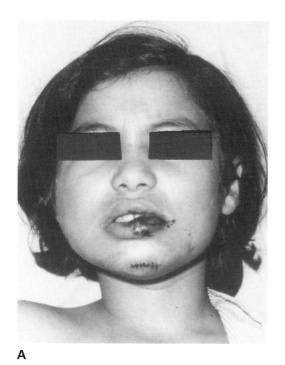

A

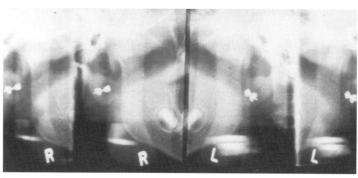

B

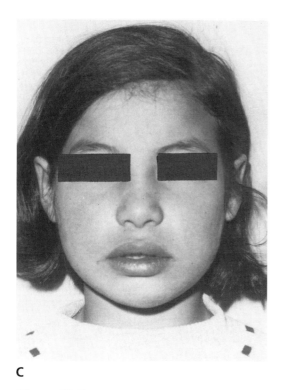

C

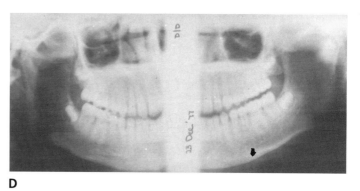

D

Figure 18–2. A. Frontal photograph of a 14-year-old girl injured when she fell off her bicycle. Obvious chin laceration has been repaired while ignoring the bilateral preauricular edema, malocclusion, and inability to function. **B.** Bilateral open and closed panographic views clearly show left and right low condylar fracture. **C.** Frontal photograph post closed reduction for 10 days and control of occlusion with elastics applied to arch bars and postmobilization physical therapy for 6 weeks to regain full mandibular movement, while preserving the dental occlusion. **D.** Posttreatment panographic film shows excellent healing and bilateral recontouring of the condyles.

of repair of the dentition, and the presence of developing tooth buds in both jaws are factors that must be dealt with on an individual patient basis to provide proper therapy. In short, the infant, child, and younger adolescent each has special individualized treatment considerations that set them apart from the older adolescent, teenager, and adult patients with facial injuries (Kaban, 1990b; Posnick, 1992).

Tooth Fracture, Tooth Avulsion, and Dentoalveolar Fracture

The prominence of the maxillary and mandibular anterior teeth within the dental arches of the infant, child, and younger adolescent make these teeth most prone for trauma. Injury may exist as individual tooth trauma or to multiple teeth. Blunt trauma to teeth may result in compressive injury to the apex of the tooth, so that even if the tooth is minimally mobilized, necrosis of the nerve and vasculature entering the tooth can occur in an immediate or delayed fashion, which leads to eventual tooth abscess. Injuries leading to fracture of tooth substance can also lead to the same sort of problem. Fractures horizontally or obliquely into the tooth pulp are evidenced by exposure of the vasculature and bleeding and pain. This is a true dental emergency situation and, if possible, warrants immediate dental consultation. The decision to place a sedative dental restoration, vs. pulpal extirpation or mummification techniques, is best made by the dentist based on multiple factors including whether the tooth is deciduous or permanent, state of repair, and hygiene of the dentition. Fractures occurring vertically into the root may not be repairable and may require extraction. Unfortunately, at times economic factors may play a role in the decision-making process.

Total avulsion of maxillary or mandibular teeth is not uncommon in the pediatric patient. In fact, this sort of injury represents the greatest hard tissue injury to the pediatric population, but generally is not included in the statistical reviews published for facial injuries because so many of these injuries are treated in the private offices of general dentists, pediatric dentists, and oral and maxillofacial surgeons (Harrington et al., 1988; Perez et al., 1991). If possible, instruction should be given to the patient or the individual accompanying the patient to find the avulsed tooth and replace it within the socket if possible and, if not possible, to place it in the buccal vestibule of the patient or the escort. These are the best options available if any hope of success in reimplanting the tooth or teeth is to be expected. Placing the tooth in a container of milk or saline is more favorable than rinsing the tooth off in tap water and transporting it in tap water or transporting it dry. According to Andreasen (1981), the literature demonstrates that success of reimplantation is not affected if the tooth is placed in the vestibule of the patient vs. some other individual. What is critical is the time from avulsion or disarticulation to reimplantation, with the best statistical result obtained in patients undergoing reimplantation within 1 hour of injury.

Consideration must be also given as to whether the deciduous tooth should be reimplanted. The age of the child, the stage of root resorption, and cooperation are all factors to be considered. Generally, reimplantation and stabilization of deciduous teeth is not critical to the health and development of the succedaneous permanent tooth (Andreasen, 1981) Once the decision is made to reimplant the tooth, it should be expeditiously done. Local anesthesia may be administered although it may not be necessary; the socket is gently suctioned and irrigation of dirt or other debris is performed with normal saline. Minor gingival laceration associated with the socket need not be repaired, but more extensive gingival injury should be repaired as possible.

The tooth or teeth are finger-repositioned into the socket and an acid etched acrylic and wire splint is applied to stabilize the tooth to adjoining teeth on either side (Figures 18–3 and 18–4). The occlusion is checked and a periapical dental radiograph taken to check position. Absolute repositioning is not necessary for success. The splint is left in place for 10 to 14 days and then

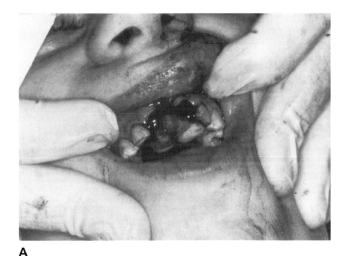 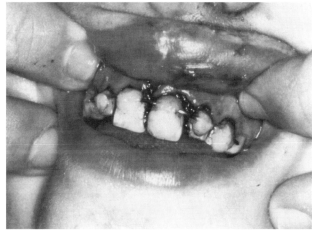

A **B**

Figure 18–3. A. Eighteen-year-old with avulsion of teeth 8 and 9 (maxillary central incisors) and gingival laceration. **B.** Teeth 8 and 9 have been finger positioned and splinted with a nonactive wire and resin composite restoration material.

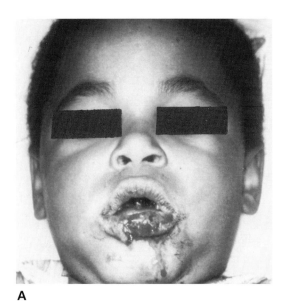

A

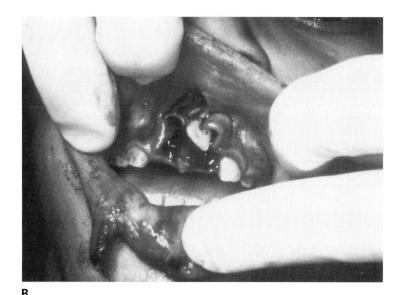

B

Figure 18–4. A. Nine-year-old male injured in a skateboard accident has suffered lower lip laceration and avulsion of tooth 8 (maxillary right permanent incisor) and partial avulsion (exarticulation) of tooth 9 (maxillary left permanent incisor). Tooth 8 was not recovered from the accident scene. **B.** Intraoral photo shows displacement of tooth 9 and fractured alveolus of tooth 8 area, as well as gingival laceration associated with this injury. **C.** Close-up view demonstrating repositioned tooth 9 and wire splint used for stabilization. Gingival tissues were repaired secondarily, and then the lip was properly repaired.

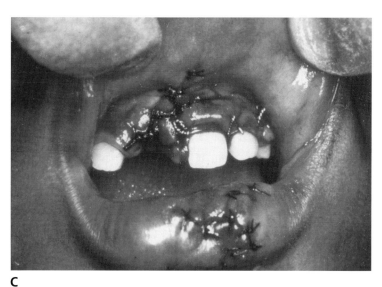

C

carefully removed. While some mobility is present at this time, there should be enough stability for the tooth to remain in light function. Again, per Andreasen (1981), longer maintenance of the splint has not been shown to be beneficial, and in fact is more deleterious, leading to rapid root resorption. The avulsed permanent incisor or cuspid with an open or incompletely formed root stands an excellent chance of being maintained and revascularized and may not require endodontic procedures to maintain it. If endodontic root therapy is deemed necessary, it should be completed within 2 weeks following removal of the splint by a qualified dental practitioner.

Avulsed or partially avulsed or subluxated teeth then require long-term follow-up as nonvitality, which requires further therapy, may be discovered later. Although long-term maintenance of avulsed teeth has been reported, survival for 3 to 5 years must also be

considered a success. After reimplantation, consideration should be given to the state of tetanus immunization and antibiotic therapy. Tetanus booster or tetanus immune globulin may need to be considered, dependent upon the circumstances. Usually, penicillin for the nonallergic patient should also be considered and given for a period of 10 days.

While avulsion of teeth probably involves some fracture of the dental alveolus, larger segmental fracture and dislocation of tooth and bone is a more severe problem. It may also occur as an isolated injury or as part of a larger fracture complex. Treatment of these segmental injuries also involves relocation of the fracture segment as best as possible and splinting. In some cases, use of the acid etch wire splint may be preferable. In other cases, use of an arch bar ligated to adjacent teeth, as well as to the teeth in the dentoalveolar segment, is more available and will work in the same fashion. The arch bar may be prefabricated or handmade of wire ligature (Figure 18–5). Again, in the isolated pediatric injury, the splint should be maintained for only 10 to 14 days and then removed. Evaluation of the teeth for endodontic treatment should then be considered and appropriate dental referral should be made. In the patient with multiple maxillomandibular injuries requiring closed reduction, a dentoalveolar segment may be treated in this fashion as a part of the overall treatment. Timing of removal of maxillomandibular fixation appliances in these patients is usually consistent with the general principle that closed reduction in the child or adolescent usually is for only 1 to 3 weeks. In the teenager with more serious mandibular or maxillary or midface fractures, longer periods of closed reduction may be necessary, as with the adult patient, but the need for treatment of those injuries takes precedence over dental or dentoalveolar injuries (Kaban, 1990b).

Acrylic Splints

In some cases of dentoalveolar fracture, in fractures of the mandibular body or symphysis, or in cases of hemi Le Fort I type fractures or Le Fort fractures of the maxilla with a midpalatine split (particularly in infants and young children), it is preferable to take dental impressions after temporary repositioning and stabilization of the fragment and then fabricate a quick cure acrylic splint. If the surgeon is unable to temporarily reposition and stabilize the fragment, this may be done on the dental stone cast poured from the impressions. The area of the fracture is cut apart, repositioned into the proper relationship, and waxed into place. The acrylic splint is then fabricated and inserted. Dependent upon the patient, the splint may be an occlusal-lingual splint, an occlusal-palatal splint, or simply a lingual or palatal splint, and may be secured with circummandibular

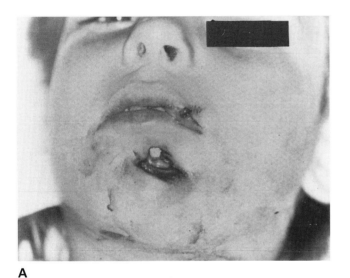

A

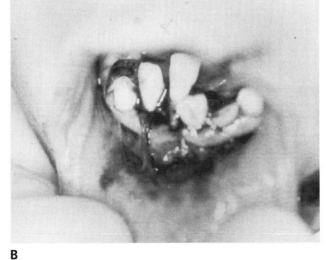

B

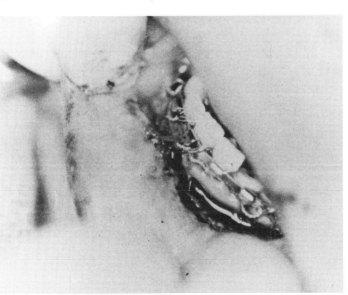

C

Figure 18–5. **A.** Ten-year-old sustained through-and-through laceration of infralabial area and open comminuted fracture of anterior mandibular alveolus. Note tooth exposed through laceration. **B.** Multiple displaced teeth are present. **C.** Teeth have been repositioned and fixated with arch bar and circumdental wires. Laceration was then appropriately repaired in layers, including oral mucosa of vestibule.

wires, circumdental wires, transalveolar wires, piriform aperture, or circumzygomatic suspension wires, or combinations (Figure 18–6). In some cases, consideration must be given to sedation or general anesthesia to obtain the impressions as well as to insert the splint. In any event, these splints are superb and can eliminate the need for consideration of maxillomandibular fixation in certain fractures.

Fractures of the Mandibular Body, Parasymphysis, and Symphysis

The common thread among the fractures to be discussed in this section is that they all occur in tooth-bearing regions of the lower jaw, whether or not the teeth have erupted or whether deciduous, mixed, or permanent dentition is present. Certainly, if any fracture extra-

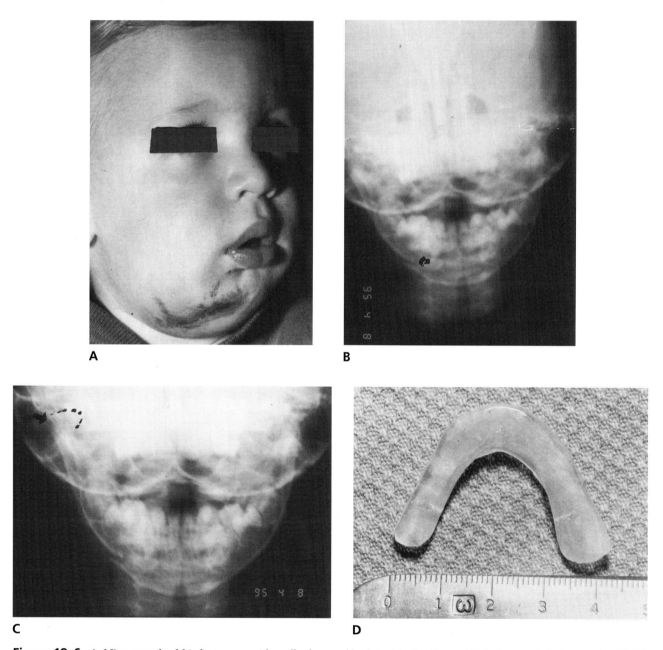

Figure 18–6. A. Nine-month-old infant was accidentally dropped by his older brother while being carried downstairs. Child has visible signs of trauma to the right jaw, including ecchymosis and swelling. Child was fussy and unable to eat well. **B.** PA mandible film demonstrates displaced fracture of right mandibular body. **C.** Towne's view shows fracture of right mandibular condyle with medial displacement as well as the body fracture. **D.** While infant was anesthetized in OR, maxillary and mandibular dental impressions were obtained and a "quick cure" autopolymerizing acrylic resin splint was fabricated for reduction of the body fracture. The splint was designed to occlude with the maxillary teeth. *(continued)*

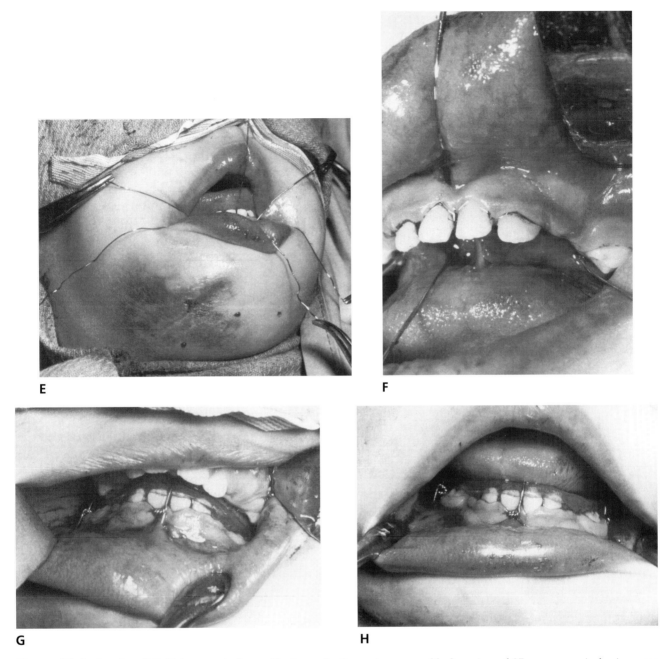

Figure 18–6. *(continued)* **E.** Using surgical mandibular awls, three circummandibular wires of 25-gauge surgical wire were passed. **F.** Close-up view shows the wire passing around the mandible lingual to labial. **G.** The occlusal lingual splint has been wired in place using the circummandibular wires, and provides adequate reduction and fixation to the right body fracture. The splint is indexed to the maxillary teeth in occlusion to provide guidance for closing of the jaw in an attempt to treat the condylar fracture with occlusal guidance and continued function. **H.** The splint allows the infant to function and not be placed into maxillomandibular fixation. The infant was able to feed more normally in this case. The splint was maintained for only 3 weeks and then removed.

orally communicates through the skin, it is recognized as an open fracture. What must be remembered, however, is that any fracture of the mandible or the maxilla that is directed through the periodontal ligament space adjacent to the tooth is also an open fracture. Consequently, antibiotic therapy should be considered in any open fracture, with a cephalosporin drug preferable for extraoral open fractures and penicillin-type

drugs if the intraoral open fracture is predominant. The old misconception that all teeth in the line of fracture must be removed must be changed. Teeth that have no bone support and are mobile should be removed. Teeth that are in such bad state of repair that they are nonrestorable or already abscessed should be removed as well. Teeth that are vertically fractured through the root also should be removed. However, impacted or erupting teeth in the line of fracture do not necessarily require removal unless they prohibit adequate reduction of the fracture (Kaban, 1990b). Teeth that are left in the line of fracture should be carefully watched, both clinically and radiographically, to ensure that healing proceeds and that an abscess or nonunion has not occurred because of the teeth. In treating severe open or comminuted fractures of the tooth-bearing areas, every attempt should be made not to sacrifice developing tooth germs just because they are seen. Care should be taken not to dislodge them with the suction or other instruments if possible.

In the infant and young child, as stated previously, closed reduction and short periods of maxillomandibular fixation are the rule rather than the exception. The use of splints, if available, will often eliminate the need for fixation. If not, then some sort of system must be applied to allow for maxillomandibular fixation for periods of 2 to 3 weeks maximum (Infante Cossio et al.,

1994) (Figure 18–7). Fortunately, fractures in infants are rare (Lustman & Milheim, 1994) but the occurrence rate of fractures requiring such therapy significantly increases in the toddler and young child. Toddlers and young children actually tolerate short periods of fixation quite well (Kaban, 1990b). Diets can be altered and supplements can be prescribed to get the child through this difficult period.

The surgeon treating these patients must be able to apply arch bars if necessary in spite of deciduous tooth form, loose teeth, or the mixed dentition. The use of 25- or 26-gauge surgical steel circumdental wires and circummandibular wires placed with surgical awls or large bore needles will help to secure the bars to these mandibular dentitions. Circumdental wires, transalveolar wires, and other suspension type wires such as piriform aperture wires will help to secure the bar to most maxillary dentitions as well. The teeth must be placed into the proper occlusal relationship using wear facets

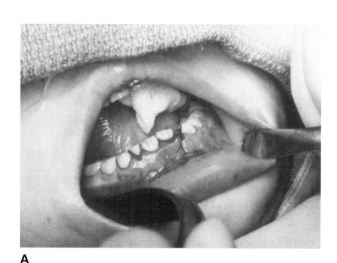

A

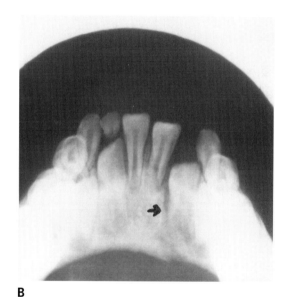

B

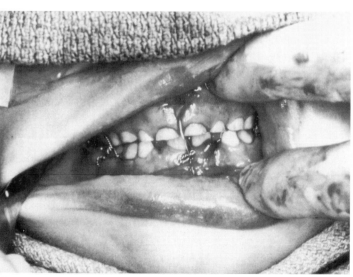

C

Figure 18–7. A. Eight-year-old with bilateral condyl fractures and fracture of mandibular symphyseal area. Operative intraoral view shows gingival mucosal laceration secondary to fracture in the area of unerupted tooth 23 (mandibular permanent left lateral incisor). **B.** Occlusal x-ray shows the symphyseal fracture in the area of unerupted tooth. **C.** Patient was treated with closed reduction using three maxillary transalveolar wires twisted together to provide a simple method of maxillomandibular fixation. Fixation was maintained for 3 weeks prior to initiating vigorous physical therapy consisting of range of motion exercises. The symphyseal fracture mandated the period of fixation in this child

and cuspal inclines as guides. The experience factor certainly comes into play here, and in some cases, the use of other consultants such as the oral and maxillofacial surgeon may be helpful to establish the proper occlusion. Additional wires are then used to ligate the maxilla to the mandible, thus the term maxillomandibular fixation. Other wire techniques such as Ivy loops or multiple eyelet wiring techniques may be utilized; both of these techniques also allow for maxillomandibular wires to be applied to establish the occlusion. Other wire techniques and devices are available and may be considered where appropriate.

Although closed reduction and short periods of fixation are a solid standard in the treatment of these injuries in the infant and young child or adolescent (Turvey & Kendell, 1991), there are indications for open reduction and the use of modified techniques of rigid fixation in certain fractures to allow the patient to function after operation. Patients with medical conditions that preclude maxillomandibular fixation, such as poorly controlled seizure disorder or profound mental retardation, or absolute aversion and inability to tolerate fixation, should be considered for open reduction (Beirne & Myall, 1994; Posnick, 1994; Zide & Kent, 1983). There are several key points to be emphasized, however.

At the time of operation, there is still a need to place the patient in appropriate maxillomandibular fixation with arch bars being preferable if possible. Almost all open reductions of the mandibular body and symphyseal region should be transorally performed as access is good and healing of extraoral incisions in the juvenile population is not as predictable as desired (Figure 18–8). The use of miniplates and unicortical screws applied at the inferior border or below developing teeth is preferable (Figure 18–9). The applied arch bar acts as a tension band at the level of the teeth. The use of direct wire techniques to provide reduction and fixation of fractures in these areas is an option but does not eliminate the need for maxillomandibular fixation, as the muscles acting on the areas are the same in the pediatric population as in the adults, and nonunion or fibrous union will be promoted without maxillomandibular fixation. Properly applied rigid fixation in these patients does not automatically have to be removed as it is well tolerated and does not necessarily interfere with growth and development. The use of rigid fixation techniques for the teenager with permanent dentition has the same indications as for the adult patient. The use of bicortical screws with compression plating systems or lag screw osteosynthesis techniques are applicable (Beirne & Myall, 1994; Posnick, 1994).

Fractures of the Mandibular Ramus and Angle

Fractures of the ramus and angle are not as prevalent in the infant and child. Closed reduction and max-

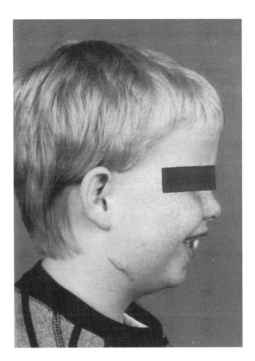

Figure 18–8. Lateral view photograph of an 8-year-old child who underwent costochondral graft procedure for treatment of hemifacial microsomia. Child had no condyle and short vertical ramus height with associated facial asymmetry. Unreliable and unpredictable healing of extraoral skin incisions in children lead to hypertrophic scarring as shown here. Later revision will be necessary.

illomandibular fixation techniques as described above are again the standard. If open reduction is entertained, well-designed and limited incision is preferable. If possible, a transoral technique is preferred. Percutaneous trochar use to apply screws is available and a rigid fixation technique may eliminate the need for any period of maxillomandibular fixation. A direct wire osteosynthesis technique with a short period of maxillomandibular fixation may be considered and will generally provide good results. Both direct wiring techniques and rigid fixation techniques have their advocates. At times, usage of a particular technique for this age group of patients may be based on no more than opinion or affection for a technique.

Fracture of the coronoid process is extremely rare in the pediatric population and requires no therapy except pain control, modified diet, and jaw mobility exercise.

Fractures of the Mandibular Condyle

As previously stated, the mandibular condyle is a growth center in the young patient and is also an extremely common area for fracture to occur in the pediatric patient (Amaratunga, 1987, 1988). For fractures that occur intracapsularly, no treatment other than pain control, modified diet, and exercise to prevent ankylosis within the joint is necessary if the occlusion can be

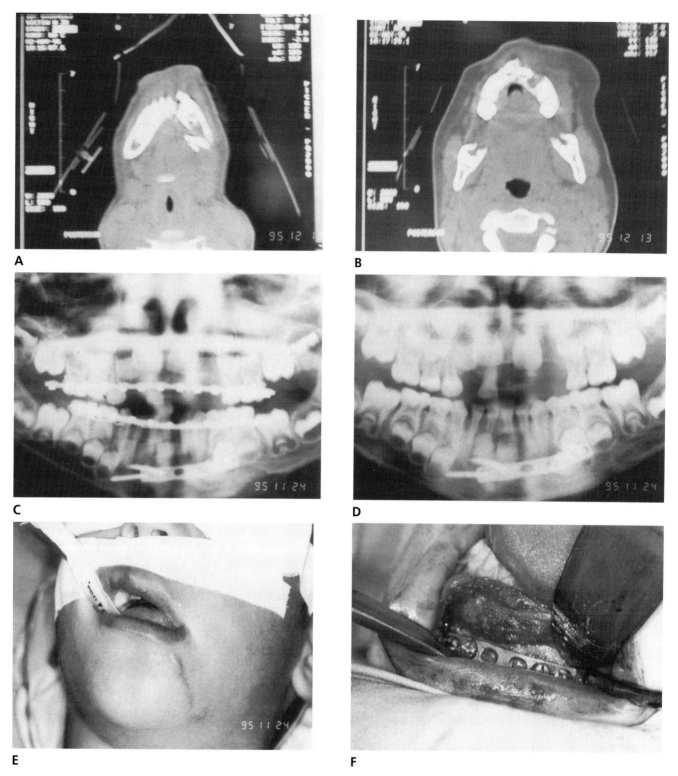

Figure 18–9. A. CT scan of 5-year-old male kicked by a horse. Child sustained open and comminuted fracture of left mandibular symphyseal area with complex through-and-through laceration of left lip and chin. CT shows displacement and comminution. **B.** Higher axial CT cuts through level of maxilla shows injury to left maxillary alveolus and avulsion of left lateral incisor. **C.** Child was taken to OR emergently and tracheostomy was performed. Maxillary and mandibular arch bars were applied for maxillomandibular fixation and open reduction of the symphysis was performed using 2.0 titanium plate and screws. No oral and maxillofacial surgery consultation was requested. While excellent reduction was achieved, the plate was placed too far superiorly and the screws are too close to the unerupted teeth and tooth buds. More inferior placement of the plate and screws, or perhaps a smaller plate and screws, or even wire osteosynthesis at the inferior border region would have been more appropriate. **D.** Panographic x-ray taken 6-months posttreatment shows excellent healing. Note the healing and recontouring of the left interior cortex area, which originally had been comminuted. The screws and plate are scheduled for removal. **E.** Intraoperative photo shows hypertrophic healing of scar from original injury 6 months prior. **F.** Intraoral lip vestibule incision was used to access the symphyseal region and plate.   *(continued)*

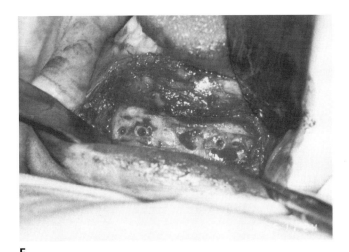

F

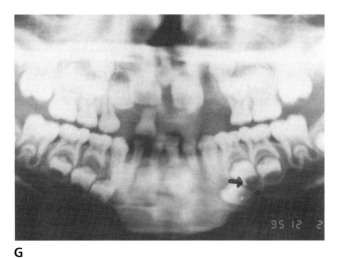

G

Figure 18–9. *(continued)* **G.** The plate and screws were removed without difficulty. The exposed bone demonstrated excellent union and healing. **H.** Panograph postremoval of the plate shows screw hole apparent *(arrow)* within the structure of the bud of tooth 21 (left permanent mandibular first bicuspid). The child requires long-term follow-up to evaluate the eruption of the teeth involved in the fracture site and those possibly injured by the screws.

maintained. If need be, a short period of maxillomandibular fixation may be necessary using the techniques previously described. After 7–10 days, the fixation may be removed and the patient may be started on an intensive supervised therapy program to insure reestablishment of normal function and maintenance of occlusion. At times, continued elastic guidance therapy may be necessary using the arch bars applied. Studies have confirmed the remarkable healing and regenerative capabilities of the child's condyle (Beekler & Walker, 1969; Dahlstrom, Kahnberg, & Lindahl, 1989; Infante Cossio et al., 1994; Tanaka et al., 1993). Even if the condylar head is dislocated, conservative treatment and strict postfixation physical therapy and follow-up will almost always lead to a satisfactory result (Figure 18–10). For condylar fractures that are extracapsular or in the condylar neck, the conservative therapy outlined will almost always produce good results, even in cases of bilateral fracture (Walker, 1994). While potential growth deformity is of concern, what is even more troublesome is the fibrous or bony ankylosis that may develop if the patient is kept in fixation too long or does not participate in an aggressive postfixation therapy program. Teenagers with condylar fractures do not necessarily return to normal as well as the child patient with dislocated fractures (Figures 18–11 and 18–12). Adults appear to adjust to the position established at the trauma with functional deficits such as severe deviation on jaw opening (Dahlstrom, Kahnberg, & Lindahl, 1989; Worsaae & Thorn, 1994). Zide and Kent (1983) and Zide (1989) have suggested a protocol of absolute indications for open reduction of condylar fractures for adults and children. Indications include:

1. Displacement of the condyle into the middle cranial fossa.

2. Inability to obtain adequate occlusion by closed reduction techniques.
3. Lateral extracapsular displacement of the condyle with cosmetic deformity.
4. Presence of a foreign body.

In addition, inability to open or close the mouth because of mechanical obstruction caused by the dislocated fragment should be considered an indication for open reduction (Zide, 1989). The conditions previously discussed as rationale for open reduction in other mandibular fractures such as seizure disorder, mental retardation, and inability to tolerate fixation are also applicable to condylar fractures (Zide & Kent, 1983). Because of the relative difficulty in performing such open reduction and the potential sequelae of facial nerve branch injury, we as surgeons are indeed fortunate that the relative numbers of these fractures in the pediatric population requiring open reduction is small. The controversy as to which technique is best, direct wire osteosynthesis vs. rigid fixation techniques vs. only approximate repositioning with no osteosynthesis necessary, remains unresolved (Boyne, 1989; Hall, 1994; Raveh, Vuillemin, & Ladrach, 1989) (Figures 18–12, 18–13, 18-14).

LeFort I Maxillary Fractures

The incidence of LeFort I type fractures in the pediatric population is relatively low. Again, the protection afforded by the large cranial vault and relative density of the bone due to lack of sinuses and presence of developing teeth contribute to this low frequency. If present, placement of maxillomandibular fixation devices and reestablishment of occlusion is the goal.

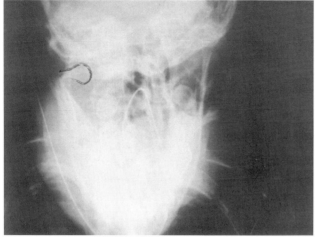

A

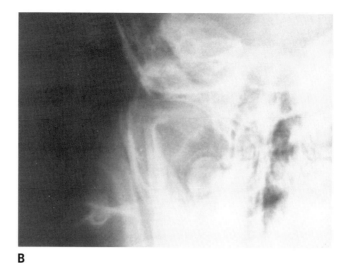

B

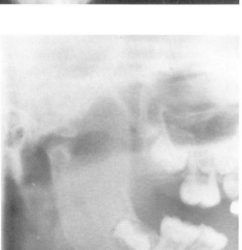

C

Figure 18–10. A. Towne's view shows fracture with medial placement of right condyle in an 8-year-old child. Child was treated with 7 days of maxillomandibular fixation and then allowed to function while using elastics applied to arch bars. After wearing the elastics day and night for 4 weeks, the child wore the elastics at night for an additional 8 weeks. **B.** Close-up view of right condyle showing extreme angulation of the fracture segment. **C.** Close-up panographic view of right condyle shows extensive remodeling 1 year postinjury. The patient was functioning well but requires long-term follow-up to ensure proper growth and development.

Additional skeletal suspension wires may be considered but are not usually necessary to treat just this injury (Kaban, 1990a). As previously mentioned, the patient with a hemi-LeFort I or division of the maxilla through the midpalatine suture may be a candidate for an acrylic palatal splint, as well as maxillomandibular fixation. If open reduction is considered necessary, the same consideration for the developing or nonerupted teeth as for mandibular fractures is imperative. Use of wire osteosynthesis for direct wiring techniques is appropriate along with up to 2 weeks of maxillomandibular fixation. Although there is little need for rigid fixation techniques for these injuries in this age group, there are microplating systems available such as the 1.0 mm or 1.3-mm plates or screws, which are more appropriate for this indication.

In the adolescent patient or teenager, the incidence of LeFort I fractures significantly increases. Open reduction, if considered, may be performed through an intraoral approach with an incision high in the maxillary vestibule from buttress to buttress. In this age group, the maxillary antra are usually well developed and require debridement of bone and blood during the

reduction procedure. Rigid fixation using plates and screws or direct wire osteosynthesis may be considered only after establishing the preinjury occlusion. Screw lengths in these cases is usually 5–6 mm with plate and screws varying from 1.3 mm to 2.0 mm in diameter and thickness. When using rigid fixation, which is extremely unforgiving of error, the dental occlusion must be tested by releasing the maxillomandibular fixation after application of the plates and screws and before incision closure (Beirne & Myall, 1994; Posnick, 1994). The use of wire osteosynthesis still has its applications and advocates but mandates a period of wire maxillomandibular fixation of 4 weeks in this patient age group.

CONCLUSION

A discussion of treatment of pediatric injuries to the teeth, dentoalveolar segment fractures, and fractures of the mandible and LeFort I fractures of the maxilla has been presented. Emphasis was placed on obtaining proper dental occlusion and the use of closed reduction and short-term maxillomandibular fixation.

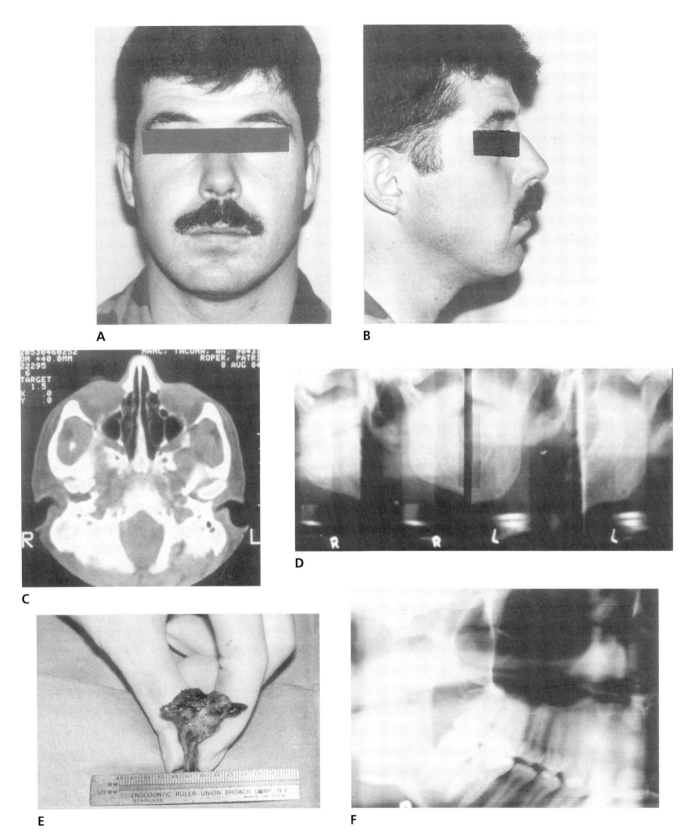

Figure 18–11. **A**. Frontal photograph of 25-year-old who was treated with closed reduction and conservative management for right condyle fracture at age 16. He continued to complain of pain on function. As expected, when he opens his mouth, he deviates to the right. **B.** Lateral view shows relatively normal facial profile and mandibular antero-posterior relationship. **C.** Axial CT shows distortion of right condylar head. **D.** Panographic view of condyles in open and closed position show differences in condylar morphology and more anterior translatory movement of the left condyle compared to the right. **E.** Condylectomy with immediate autogenous costochondral grafting was performed. On removal of the condyle, the obvious deformation was consistent with the preop x-rays and CT views. Teenagers and adults with similar injuries tend to show poorer healing and condylar reformation than children. **F.** Two years after grafting, the x-ray shows excellent healing and reconstitution of the TMJ.

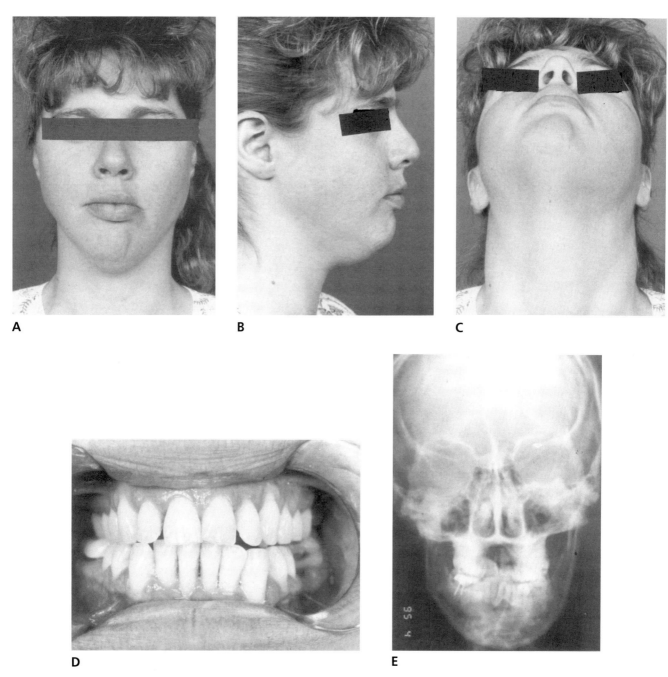

Figure 18–12. A. Frontal photo of 24-year-old female who suffered a right mandibular condyle fracture at age 12. She was treated at that time with maxillomandibular fixation for 4 weeks and then allowed to function. Note the facial asymmetry and left facial fullness as compared to the right. The right mandibular angle is at a higher level than the right. Also note chin deformity. **B.** Lateral photo demonstrates retrognathic tendency of the mandible. **C.** Dog's eye view confirms facial asymmetry associated with her injury. **D.** Intraoral view demonstrates that, while the maxillary and mandibular midlines are near coincident, there is some occlusal discrepancy and tendency for shift of the mandible to the injured right side. The occlusion is further compromised by periodontal disease and dental compensatory changes. **E.** PA cephalometric x-ray shows well the foreshortened right mandibular ramus, occlusal cant, and asymmetry.   (continued)

The indications for open reduction and application of rigid fixation techniques, as well as direct wire osteosynthesis use, were also presented. It is hoped that the surgeon using this reference will take the advice offered and will also consider use of appropriate consultants from other surgical specialties, as appropriate and available, to obtain the best possible result in form, function, and cosmesis with the minimal morbidity possible.

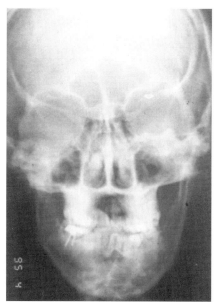
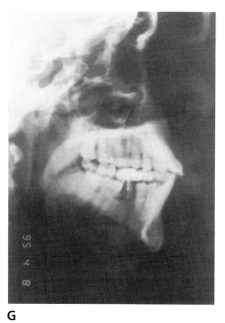

F   G

Figure 18–12. *(continued)* **F.** Lateral cephalometric view shows retrognathic posterior positioned mandible. **G.** Panographic view shows right condylar deformity and shortened ramus. The patient shows no condylar movement on her right clinically and deviates severely to her right with pain when she opens her mouth. She has apparent ankylosis and poor condylar reformation and maintenance of growth, perhaps secondary to an extended period of maxillomandibular fixation and lack of follow-up. Surgical correction would require periodontal and orthodontic therapy in preparation for LeFort I maxillary osteotomy to level the maxilla and a right costochondral graft and left sagittal split ramus osteotomy to correct the retrognathism and an associated genioplasty to correct the chin deformity.

References

Amaratunga, N. A. (1987). A study of condylar fractures in Sri Lankan patients with special reference to the recent views on treatment, healing, and sequelae. *British Journal of Oral and Maxillofacial Surgery, 25*, 391–397.

Amaratunga, N. A. (1988). Mandibular fractures in children—a study of clinical aspects, treatment needs, and complications. *Journal of Oral and Maxillofacial Surgery, 46*, 637–640.

Andreasen, J. O. (1981). Exarticulations. In J. O. Andreasen (Ed.), *Tramatic injuries of the teeth* (2nd ed., pp. 203–242). Philadelphia: W. B. Saunders.

Beekler, D. M., & Walker, R. V. (1969). Condyle fractures. *Journal of Oral Surgery, 27*, 563–564.

Beirne, O. R., & Myall, R. W. T. (1994). Rigid internal fixation in children. *Oral and Maxillofacial Surgery Clinics of North America, 6*, 153–167.

Boyne, P. J. (1989). Free grafting of traumatically displaced or resected mandibular condyles. *Journal of Oral and Maxillofacial Surgery, 47*, 228–232.

Committee on Trauma. (1993). *Advanced trauma life-support manual* (5th ed). Chicago: American College of Surgeons.

Crockett, D. M., Mungo, R. P., & Thompson, R. E. (1989). Maxillofacial trauma. *Pediatric Clinics of North America, 36*, 1471–1494.

Dahlstrom, L., Kahnberg, K. E., & Lindahl, L. (1989). 15 years followup on condyle fractures. *International Journal of Oral and Maxillofacial Surgery, 18*, 18–23.

Guven, O. (1992). Fractures of the maxillofacial region in children. *Journal of Cranio-Maxillo-Facial Surgery, 20*, 244–247.

Hall, M. B. (1994). Condylar fractures: Surgical management. *Journal of Oral and Maxillofacial Surgery, 52*, 1189–1192.

Hardt, N., & Gottsauner, A. (1993). The treatment of mandibular fractures in children. *Journal of Cranio-Maxillo-Facial Surgery, 21*, 214–219.

Harrington, M. S., Eberhart, A. B., & Knapp, J. F. (1988). Dentofacial trauma in children. *ASDC Journal of Dentistry for Children, 55*, 334–338.

Infante Cossio, P., Espin Galvez, F., & Guiterrez Perez, J. L. (1994). Mandibular fractures in children: A retrospective study of 99 fractures in 59 patients. *International Journal of Oral Maxillofacial Surgery, 23*, 329–331.

Kaban, L. B. (1990a). Facial trauma I: Midface fractures. In L. B. Kaban (Ed.), *Pediatric oral and maxillofacial surgery* (pp. 209–232). Philadelphia: W. B. Saunders.

Kaban, L. B. (1990b). Facial trauma II: Dentoalveolar injuries and mandibular fractures. In L. B. Kaban (Ed.), *Pediatric oral and maxillofacial surgery* (pp. 233–260). Philadelphia: W. B. Saunders.

Kaban, L. B. (1993). Diagnosis and management of fractures of the facial bones in children. *Journal of Oral and Maxillofacial Surgery, 51*, 722–729.

Lindquist, C., Sorsa, S., & Santavirta, S. (1986). Maxillofacial fractures sustained in bicycle accidents. *International Journal of Oral and Maxillofacial Surgery, 15*, 12–18.

Lustmann, J., & Milheim, I. (1994). Mandibular fractures in infants: Review of the literature and report of seven cases. *Journal of Oral and Maxillofacial Surgery, 52*, 240–245.

Perez, R., Berkowitz, R., & McIlveen, L. (1991). Dental trauma in children: A survey. *Endodontics and Dental Traumatology, 7*, 212–213.

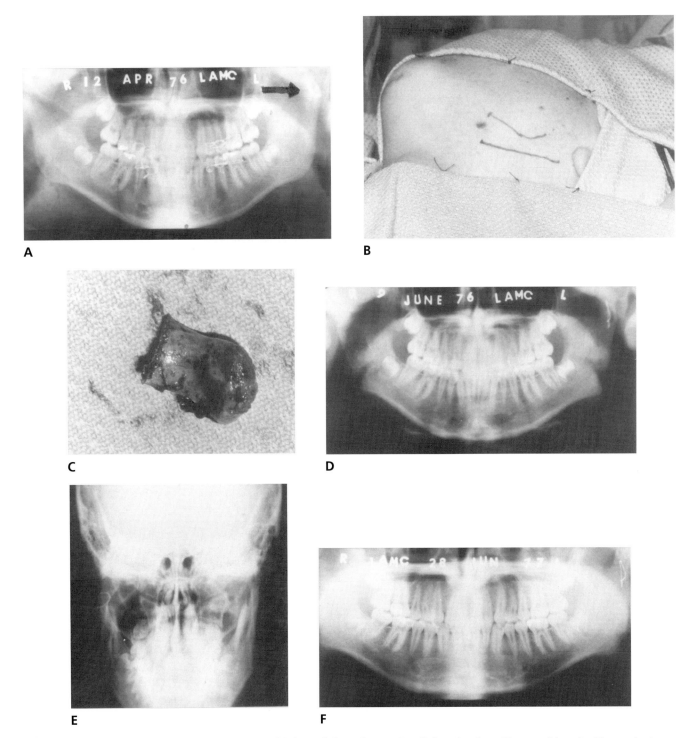

Figure 18–13. **A.** Panograph shows fracture of left condyle with anterior dislocation in a 15-year-old male. The patient was treated with closed reduction and immobilization for 7 days. He was then unable to function well or maintain his occlusion, and was scheduled for open reduction 2 weeks postinjury. **B.** Intraoperative photo demonstrates submandibular incision only planned for exposure. **C.** A wire placed at the mandibular angle allowed distraction of the ramus. The condyle literally fell out of the incision. **D.** Wire osteosynthesis of the condyle was achieved with relative ease. Maxillomandibular fixation was maintained for 4 weeks prior to mobilization and vigorous physical therapy. X-ray shows symmetry and maintenance of left ramus vertical height. **E.** AP x-ray shows relatively good position of the condyle with some mild medial inclination. **F.** Postoperative panograph at 14-month recall continues to show excellent condylar integrity with little resorption of the condylar free graft. Function continued to be excellent with little complaint of discomfort. Minimal deviation of the jaw to the left was evident on opening.

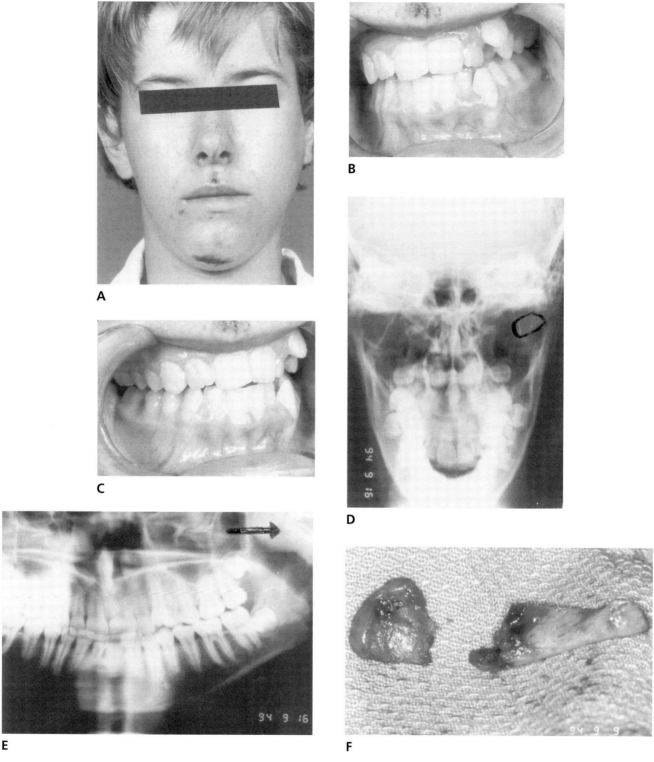

Figure 18–14. A. Thirteen-year-old girl injured when falling off her bike has obvious chin laceration, which was poorly repaired at a local emergency room. Although x-rays were taken, the left condylar fracture was missed in spite of left preauricular swelling and complaints of pain. The patient was contacted 48 hours later and informed of the fracture. **B.** Intraoral examination demonstrated malocclusion consistent with left condylar fracture. **C.** The right-sided occlusion showed shift to the left and the patient had considerable pain when functioning. **D.** The Towne's view definitively showed medial fracture dislocation of the left condyle. **E.** Close-up panographic view shows left condyle fracture with rotation of the fragment. **F.** The patient's treatment was complicated by her medical and social history. She had been the victim of repeated sexual abuse by her stepfather, had severe psychological problems, and was taking antiseizure medication, but still had seizures. These factors led to the decision to perform open reduction. A preauricular and modified Risdon submandibular approach were used. Osteotomy vertically of a portion of the distal ramus was performed and the segments removed because of inability to retrieve the original fracture segment (Boyne, 1989).

(continued)

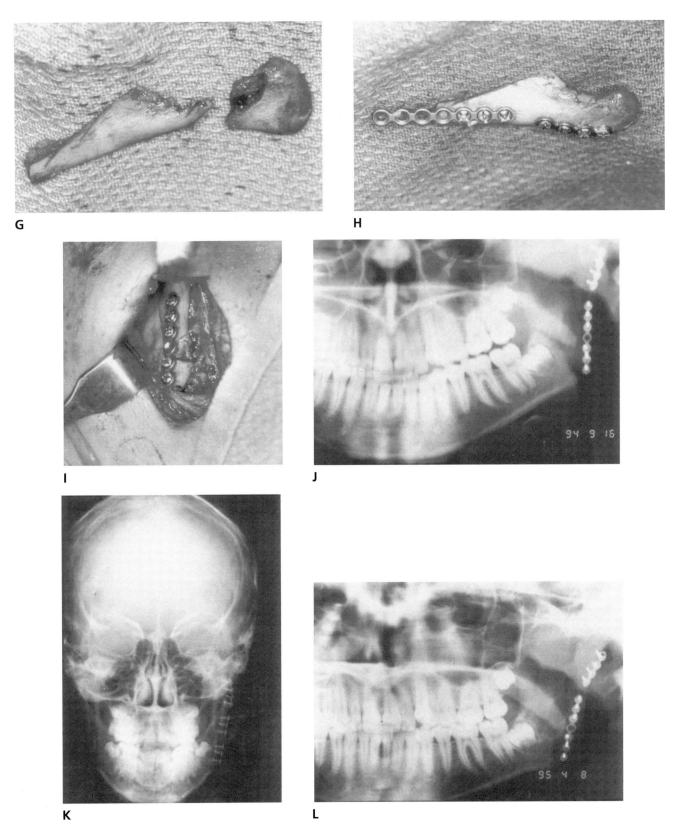

Figure 18–14. *(continued)* **G.** Additional view of the segments. **H.** The condyle is shown repositioned and fixated to the osteotomized segment using 2-mm titanium plate and screws. **I.** The condyle is showed fixated to the distal ramus with additional screws. **J.** Panographic film after removal of intraoral hardware. Patient was allowed to function immediately and after 14 days begun on jaw exercises to regain mobility. **K.** Posteroanterior mandibular x-ray shows condyle in position and rigid fixation intact. **L.** Six months later, excellent bony healing is seen. Some resorptive and adaptive changes are seen at the condyle fossa interface. The meniscus had not been sutured to the condyle at the time of operation, but was left as a soft tissue interface between the condyle and fossa.

(continued)

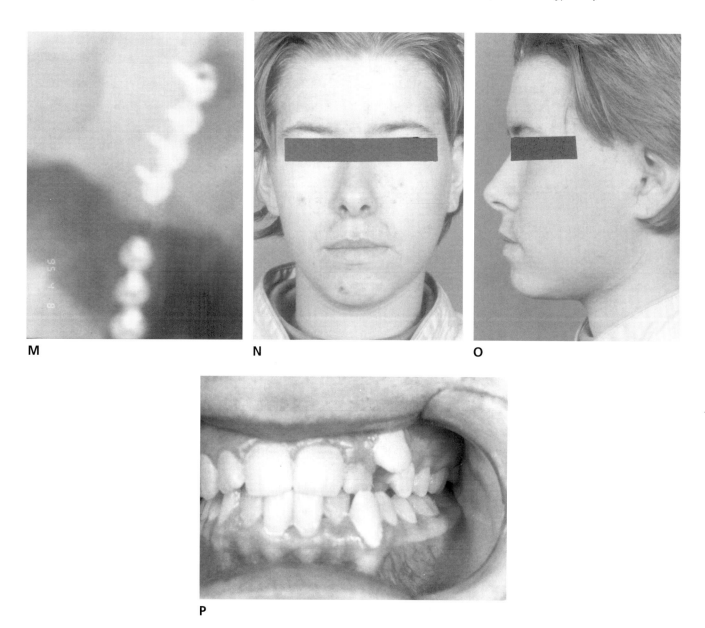

Figure 18–14. *(continued)* **M.** Close-up shows some bone loss at the superior screw-plate site. **N.** Postoperative facial view shows excellent maintenance of ramus height and symmetry. **O.** Lateral photo shows good scar healing and cosmesis of incisions. No facial nerve injury occurred as a result of incisions and exposure. **P.** Postoperative dental occlusion is normally abnormal for this girl, who was a candidate for orthodontic care prior to her injury.

Posnick, J. C. (1992). Diagnosis and management of pediatric craniomaxillofacial fractures. In L. J. Peterson (Ed.), *Principles of oral and maxillofacial surgery* (Vol. 1, pp. 623–640). Philadelphia: J. B. Lippincott.

Posnick, J. C. (1994). Craniomaxillofacial fractures in children. *Oral and Maxillofacial Surgery Clinics of North America, 6*, 169–210.

Posnick, J. C., Wells, M., & Pron, G. E. (1993). Pediatric facial fractures: Evolving patterns of treatment. *Journal of Oral and Maxillofacial Surgery, 51*, 836–844.

Raveh, J., Vuillemin, T., & Ladrach, K. (1989). Open reduction of the dislocated, fractured condylar process: Indication and surgical procedures. *Journal of Oral and Maxillofacial Surgery, 47*, 120–125.

Tanaka, N., Uchide, N., & Suzuki, K. (1993). Maxillofacial fractures in children. *Journal of Oral and Maxillofacial Surgery, 21*(7), 289–293.

Thoren, H., Lizuka, T., & Hallikainen, D. (1992). Different patterns of mandibular fractures in children. An analysis of 220 fractures in 157 patients. *Journal of Cranio-Maxillo-Facial Surgery, 20*(7), 292–296.

Turvey, T. A., & Kendell, B. (1991). Management of facial fractures in the growing patient. In R. J. Fonseca & R. V. Walker (Eds.), *Oral and maxillofacial trauma* (Vol. 2, pp. 722–753). Philadelphia: W. B. Saunders.

Walker, R. V. (1994). Condylar fractures: Nonsurgical management. *Journal of Oral and Maxillofacial Surgery, 52*, 1185–1188.

Worsaae, N., & Thorn, J. J. (1994). Surgical versus nonsurgical treatment of unilateral dislocated subcondylar fractures: A clinical study of 52 cases. *Journal of Oral and Maxillofacial Surgery, 52*, 353–360.

Zide, M. F. (1989). Open reduction of mandibular condyle fractures: Indication and technique. *Clinics in Plastic Surgery, 16*, 69–76.

Zide, M. F., & Kent, J. N. (1983). Indications for open reduction of mandibular condyle fractures. *Journal of Oral and Maxillofacial Surgery, 41*, 89–98.

19

Pediatric Midface Fractures

Joseph G. DeSantis, M.D.

MIDFACE FRACTURES IN CHILDREN

It is well established that the frequency of pediatric facial fractures is significantly less than adult facial fractures. It can be further stated that fractures of the midface in children, in particular, are even less common (Rowe, 1968; Tanaka et al., 1993). A low midface to cranium volume ratio, a high midface tooth to bone ratio, and the lack of pneumatization of the maxillary and frontal sinuses all likely contribute to this low incidence. In addition, the low occurrence of these injuries may, in part, be due to an underdiagnosis, as many midface fractures in children may be subclinical (Bartlett & DeLozier, 1992). The infrequency of pediatric midface fractures does insure that any practitioner's individual experience with these injuries is likely to be quite limited.

The basic principles dictating the proper treatment of adult midface fractures can be applied to the pediatric population. These precepts start with a comprehensive physical examination and radiologic evaluation. If surgery is indicated, a well-planned operative approach is undertaken, usually through multiple incisions, and requiring exacting reductions of the fractures and fixation with plates and screws. Pediatric facial fractures do, however, have unique aspects that render them different from adult fractures and must be considered during their treatment. The following will review the management of midface fractures with special regard to the peculiarities of the pediatric patient.

Nasal Fractures

A number of factors render the management of pediatric nasal fractures different from the adult.

Anatomically, a child's nose has a higher cartilage to bone ratio and has much less anterior projection. As a result, the pediatric nose is much less likely to be injured without injury to other facial structures (Stucker, Bryarly, & Shockley, 1984). In addition, the child's nose contains growth centers which, when damaged by either the injury or the treatment, may alter subsequent nasal growth (Precious, Delaire, & Hoffman, 1988).

Radiologic evaluation of a child's nasal bones is limited by the high proportion of cartilage. A physical examination remains the cornerstone of diagnosis in the pediatric nasal injury. Both internal and external examinations are mandatory and a general anesthetic may be required. Facial x-rays or a CT scan may be helpful in determining the presence of other fractures.

Cartilaginous nasal injury is more likely than bony injury in the child. The alar and upper lateral cartilages readily deform on impact and can withstand a considerable force with little damage. The most common injury to these structures is a dislocation of the upper lateral cartilages from the nasal bones (Koltai, 1993). This injury can often be appreciated on initial inspection, but becomes even more readily diagnosed after several days when the edema has decreased.

The most critical aspect in the initial evaluation of pediatric nasal trauma is determining whether a septal hematoma is present. Attachments between the septal cartilage and overlying mucoperichondrium may be torn with or without a septal fracture. Blood readily collects between these two structures. Any child having difficulty breathing through the nose after facial trauma must be suspected to have a septal hematoma. Internal examination will reveal a purple or blue bulge at the septum which is soft when probed with a cotton-tip applicator. A contralateral deflection of the septum may also be seen.

Immediate treatment of a septal hematoma is required. An undrained septal hematoma may become a fibrous mass, which permanently limits nasal breathing and can cause pressure necrosis of the septum, resulting in a saddle nose deformity. Needle aspiration of the hematoma can be utilized if the diagnosis is in question, but should not be used as a definitive treatment. Complete evacuation of the hematoma should be performed through an L-shaped incision in the mucoperichondrium with the horizontal component inferiorly placed to allow dependent drainage (Converse & Dingman, 1977).

Apart from the drainage of septal hematomas, the treatment of pediatric nasal injury does not need to be urgent. It is often prudent to allow edema associated with the trauma to resolve over several days before determining the need for surgical intervention. Elective delay beyond 1 week, however, is not advised as the reduction of the fractures will be more difficult and the ultimate result will possibly be adversely affected. Photographs taken prior to the injury can be helpful to the surgeon, as well as to the patient and family, in deciding the need for surgery.

The great majority of children who require surgery for nasal injuries can be treated with closed reduction (Stucker et al., 1984). Except in a very cooperative adolescent, pediatric nasal fractures should be reduced under a general anesthetic. The nasal bones and cartilages are repositioned through a combination of external and internal manipulation. The reduction is maintained by internal packing and an external splint. The Aquaplast Splint is lightweight and does not require external taping, making it well tolerated in the pediatric population. Alternatively, the more traditional plaster splint may be used. The splint is kept in place for 7 to 10 days.

Bone overgrowth, hypertrophic callus, and persistent cartilaginous displacement all may result in residual deformities even after the proper treatment of pediatric nasal trauma (Dufresne & Manson, 1990). Injury to the nasal growth centers may also contribute to a permanent nasal deformity (Grymer, Gutierrez, & Stoksted, 1985). The patient and the family should be made aware of the possible need for secondary surgery to correct these deformities. Secondary surgery following nasal trauma should be delayed until adolescence when possible to allow completion of nasal growth.

Zygomatic Fractures

The identification of displaced zygomatic fractures can be readily made on physical examination by a flattening of the malar eminence, which is typically accompanied by periorbital edema and ecchymosis (Figure 19–1). Tenderness and a palpable step-off can often be appreciated at the inferior orbital rim or in the area of the frontozygomatic suture. The older child may complain of hypesthesia of the cheek resulting from neurapraxia of the infraorbital nerve. A severely displaced zygomatic fracture may even impinge on the coracoid process of the mandible, resulting in malocclusion or inability to close the jaws.

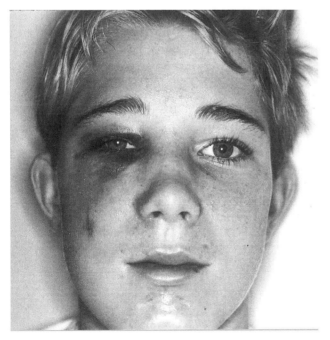

A

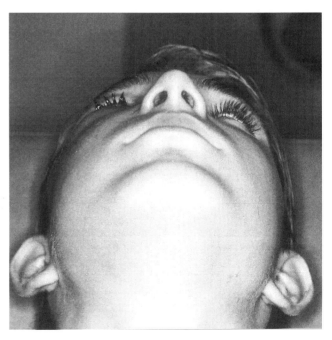

B

Figure 19-1. Clinical presentation of a right zygoma fracture. **A.** Periorbital edema and ecchymosis are apparent on the injured side. **B.** Flattening of the right malar eminence is noted even with edema.

A facial CT scan is always performed in a child suspected of having a zygomatic fracture (Figure 19–2). The extent of the displacement can be assessed, concomitant injuries can be ruled out, and the status of the orbital floor can be evaluated. Orbital floor fractures of varying severity usually accompany zygomatic fractures and can be best evaluated on coronal views. Information gained by the CT scan can help delineate whether reconstruction of the orbital floor will be necessary.

The decision to surgically treat a zygomatic fracture is based on the degree of malar displacement and the extent of the injury to the orbital floor. Edema may mask the true zygomatic depression or rotation, and an initial determination not to operate must be tempered by close observation as the edema resolves. Surgery should not be delayed beyond 7 days in the pediatric population, as bone healing occurs much earlier than in the adult, and efforts to reduce the fractures beyond 1 week may be significantly compromised. The malunited zygomatic fracture in the child can be especially difficult to correct secondarily (Manson et al., 1985; Manson, Hoopes, & Su, 1980).

Traditionally, the zygomatic fracture has been referred to as a tripod fracture, though this term underestimates the complexity of the injury. The fractured zygoma is actually separated from other facial bones at five areas: the frontozygomatic suture, the inferior orbital rim, the zygomatic arch, the lateral maxillary buttress, and the sphenoid bone. The anatomic alignment of three of these areas during surgical reduction insures that correct three-dimensional orientation of the zygoma has been achieved. This can be best accomplished through multiple surgical incisions. The infraorbital rim is approached through a conjunctival or subcilliary

incision, which also allows examination and reconstruction of the orbital floor. The frontozygomatic area can be visualized through a brow incision, an extension of the subcilliary incision, or, in the case of extensive fractures, through a bicoronal incision. Access to the lateral maxillary buttress is obtained via an intraoral superior buccal mucosa incision. The fractured zygoma is elevated and adequate reduction confirmed by direct visualization of alignment at the fracture sites (Figure 19–3). Fracture fixation utilizing plates and screws is performed at a minimum of two sites (Rinehart, Marsh, Hemmer, & Bresna, 1989). Additional fixation is required in severely comminuted or highly displaced fractures or fractures associated with significant soft tissue injury.

Orbital Floor Fractures

The orbital floor is the most fragile portion of the bony orbit. It may be fractured without a fracture of the inferior orbital rim, which is called a pure blowout fracture (Converse & Smith, 1957). The pure blowout fracture may result from an increase in intraorbital pressure which is transmitted to the weak floor, or it may occur when a force impacts on the inferior orbital rim and is transmitted to the floor (Fujino & Makino, 1980). The pure orbital blowout is typically seen in conjunction with a history of a direct single blow to the orbit as with a fist or a ball.

An impure blowout fracture has an associated fracture of the inferior orbital rim as seen with a zygoma fracture or a Le Fort II fracture. This injury is more often observed in motor vehicle accidents. In either case, the pediatric population is at less risk of orbital injury as the maxillary sinus is less developed and the orbital floor is comparatively stronger than in the adult.

The physical findings of an orbital floor fracture are related to the interaction between the fracture and the orbital contents. The inferior rectus muscle may become trapped in the fracture fragments preventing upward rotation of the globe (Figure 19–4). This can usually be demonstrated even in a younger child. In addition, an older child may complain of diplopia in an upward gaze. Enophthalmus may also be observed in conjunction with an orbital floor fracture. This results from the loss of orbital support together with the herniation of orbital contents through the defect in the orbital floor into the maxillary sinus. Enophthalmus may also result in diplopia.

Periorbital edema and ecchymosis, together with the mechanism of injury, should alert the clinician to the possibility of an orbital floor fracture. Examination of the globe and visual acuity are essential to determine if a direct injury to the eye has occurred (Figure 19–5). This can be difficult in the uncooperative child and consultation with ophthalmology is frequently obtained.

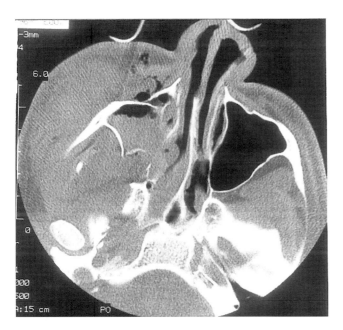

Figure 19-2. Axial CT scan view of fractured right zygoma. The malar bone is rotated and posteriorly displaced.

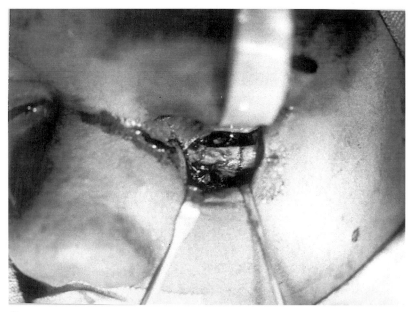

A

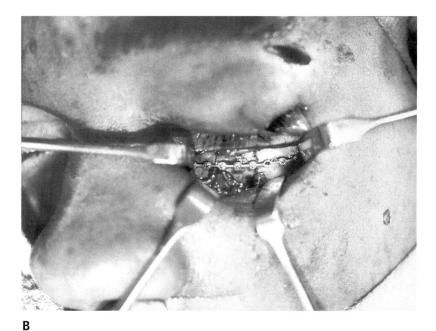

B

Figure 19-3. Open repair of a zygomatic fracture. **A.** The inferior orbital rim fractures are exposed and reduced through a subcilliary incision. **B.** The reduced fractures are fixated with plate and screws.

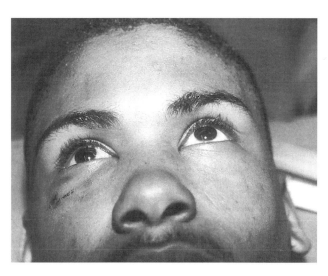

Figure 19-4. Clinical presentation of a right orbital floor fracture with trapping of the inferior rectus muscle and restriction of upward gaze on the injured side.

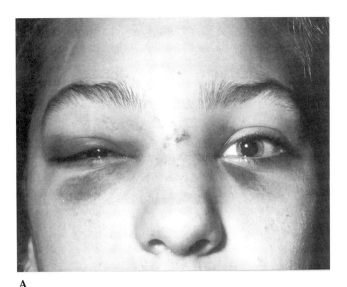

A

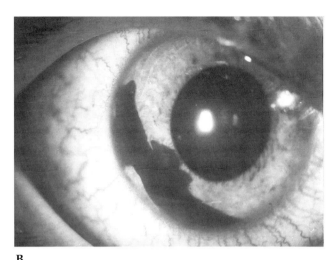

B

Figure 19-5. A. Clinical presentation of a child with an orbital floor fracture. **B.** Closer inspection of the globe re-veals hyphema, illustrating the importance of a complete examination of the eye.

Fractures of the orbital floor may be missed on plain facial films and a CT scan is mandatory in the child with a possible orbital floor fracture. Likewise, axial CT views may fail to delineate a floor fracture and coronal views are usually warranted (Figure 19-6).

Not all fractures of the orbital floor require surgery. The indications for orbital exploration and repair are as follows: (1) trapping of the inferior rectus muscle, (2) enophthalmus, (3) associated fractures requiring operative reduction and fixation, and (4) a large defect in the or-bital floor with herniation of orbital contents which may result in late enophthalmus. Diplopia may result from edema and hemorrhage of the intraorbital structures apart from a floor fracture and thus is not itself an indication for exploration (Putterman, Stevens, & Urist, 1974).

Orbital exploration is carried out through a con-junctival or subcilliary incision. Careful elevation of the orbital contents from the maxillary sinus is performed. Small defects in the orbital floor are treated with Gelfilm which is cut to cover the defect and fixed with a single absorbable stitch (Mermer & Orban, 1995). Larger defects are reconstructed with autologous bone grafts. Split cranial bone is the graft of choice (Figure 19–7), but other sites such as rib and iliac crest are also available. Particularly severe orbital floor fractures may require an orbital floor reconstruction plate usually cov-ered with a bone graft (Figure 19–8). Regardless of the method of orbital floor reconstruction, a forced duction test should be performed at the conclusion of the proce-dure to insure free movement of the globe (Figure 19–9). The sclera is grasped beneath the iris and the globe is gently rocked in all directions. Unrestricted movement that is similar to the contralateral side docu-ments that the extraocular muscles are free of the orbital floor.

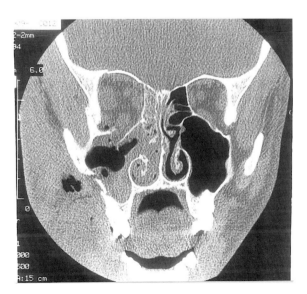

Figure 19-6. Coronal CT scan view of a right orbital floor fracture. This patient also sustained a right zygoma fracture as evidenced by the fractures at the frontozygomatic suture and the lateral maxillary wall. This patient also has a right orbital roof fracture.

Le Fort II and Le Fort III Fractures

The classic Le Fort fracture patterns are not typical-ly seen in the pediatric population (Dufresne & Manson, 1990). The underdevelopment of the maxillary sinus and the elasticity of the bones are likely major fac-tors contributing to this observation. Le Fort fractures involving half the facial skeleton, however, are relative-

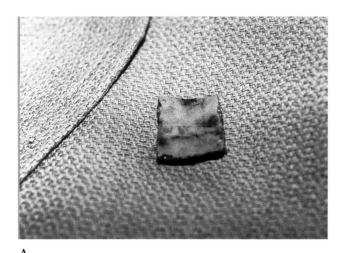

A

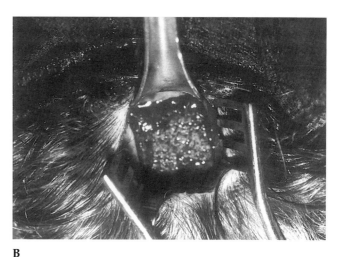

B

Figure 19-7. Split cranial bone graft harvest for orbital floor reconstruction. **A.** The split cranial bone graft prior to implantation is shown. **B.** The donor site may be exposed through a limited scalp incision.

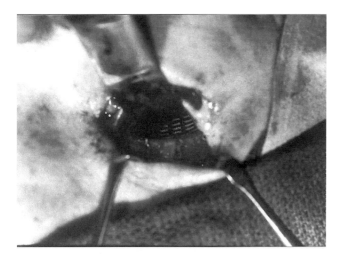

Figure 19-8. A titanium plate is used to reconstruct the orbital floor. Plate reconstruction is usually reserved for very large defects and typically covered with a split cranial bone graft.

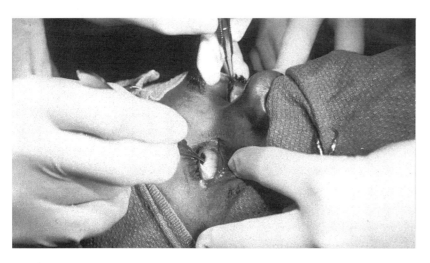

Figure 19-9. A forced reduction test is performed by grasping the sclera with fine forceps and gently rocking the globe. Unrestricted, symmetrical movement following orbital floor reconstruction insures that the orbital contents are not trapped by the repair.

ly more common in children due to an incompletely fused bony palate. The palate must be routinely examined in all children with facial trauma to rule out a possible sagittal split of the palate.

Le Fort fractures can be demonstrated on physical examination by grasping the maxilla and noting free movement of the midface. The level of the fracture can often be assessed by this maneuver. A CT scan is obtained to fully delineate the fracture, examine the orbital floors, and rule out other bony facial injuries.

The most crucial aspect in the treatment of Le Fort fractures is realignment of the dental occlusion, and the establishment of occlusion should be the first step in the reduction of these fractures. Methods of mandibular maxillary fixation, such as arch bar placement, often utilized in the adult, may not be satisfactory in the child with primary or mixed dentition. The low-profile conical shaped primary teeth may not be adequate for wiring, particularly if there is reabsorption of the deciduous roots. The fabrication of a dental splint, ideally made from dental impressions, can reestablish occlusion in these cases.

Once dental occlusion has been restored, fractures are exposed and reduced. Le Fort II fractures can be exposed through intraoral buccal incisions and subcilliary or conjunctival incisions. A bicoronal incision placed posterior to the hairline allows exposure of both the frontozygomatic area and the nasoethmoid area in Le Fort III fractures. The bicoronal incision also allows the harvest of cranial bone grafts if indicated. In general, immediate bone grafting should be utilized for bony defects greater than 5 mm (Manson et al., 1985). Alternative bone donor sites such as rib and iliac crest may also be considered, but undergo a greater degree of reabsorption as compared with cranial bone grafts (Zin & Whitaker, 1983).

Ideally, Le Fort fracture reduction is followed by plate and screw fixation. This form of internal rigid fixation allows removal of mandibular maxillary fixation before leaving the OR, a distinct advantage in the pediatric population with respect to feeding and airway control. Theoretically, based on animal models, concern has been raised as to whether rigid plate fixation may limit facial growth and development in humans (Resnick, Kinney, & Kawamoto, 1990), though clear evidence that this occurs has not yet been demonstrated (Posnick, Wells, & Pron, 1993). As a result of this concern, however, long segments of plate fixation should be avoided in children and consideration should be given to plate removal following fracture healing (Bartlett & DeLozier, 1992).

Particular care must be taken in the placement of plates and screws in the maxilla to avoid damaging tooth roots and undescended teeth. In some cases, plate and screw placement may not be possible, and mandibular maxillary fixation will need to be maintained in the postoperative period to insure fracture fixation. Fortunately, the period of mandibular maxillary fixation need not be more than 2 to 3 weeks in the pediatric population, as fracture healing is rapid and usually complete during this interval (Gussack, Luterman, Powell, Rodgers, & Ramenofsky, 1987).

Superior Orbital Rim and Roof Fractures

A substantial impact to the superior orbital rim in a younger child, prior to the formation of the frontal si-

nus, may result in superior orbital rim and roof fractures. This same force in an older child or adult is more likely to be transmitted to the frontal sinus and result in a fracture of this structure. The frontal sinus, therefore, acts as a barrier to intracranial injury which the younger child does not have. Fractures of the superior orbital rim and roof should be regarded as cranial fractures in children and the possibility of intracranial injury must be considered. CT scan evaluation is mandatory (see Figure 19–6).

Superior orbital rim fractures may be reduced through existing lacerations or a bicoronal incision. Fixation can be best accomplished with 1.0-mm microplates. Orbital roof fractures may occur without an associated rim fracture, similar to pure orbital floor fractures. Children with nondisplaced orbital roof fractures or superiorly displaced orbital roof fractures are treated expectantly. A child with inferiorly displaced orbital roof fractures risks the development of a late orbital encephalocele and surgical repair is indicated, usually through an intracranial approach (Messinger, Radkowski, Greenwald, & Pensler, 1989).

Nasoethmoid Fractures

Nasoethmoid fractures are complex injuries involving the bones of the nose, medial orbit, and ethmoid sinus. The injury may be part of a Le Fort III fracture or may exist as a distinct entity, though it is most commonly seen in association with other facial fractures. The fractured bones are displaced posteriorly and laterally, resulting in telecanthus of the eyes and a concave nasal dorsum or saddle nose deformity. Periorbital edema and ecchymosis are always present and are usually severe. A CT scan will confirm the presence of the fracture, as well as assess the possibility of cranial injury and other facial fractures (Figure 19–10).

Nasoethmoid fractures are frequently accompanied by an overlying laceration which can serve to expose the fracture during surgical treatment (Figure 19–11). A bicoronal incision is frequently used if lacerations are not present. Alternatively, the H-shaped open sky incision can be utilized, though the potentially noticeable scar is a relative disadvantage (Converse & Hogan, 1970).

The most important aspect in the treatment of nasoethmoid fractures is restoration of the correct intercanthal distance (Markowitz et al., 1991). Identification of the medial canthal tendon is the first step in fracture exposure to avoid inadvertent damage to this structure. The medial canthal tendon is almost always attached to a "central fragment" of bone. The preservation of this attachment is a key aspect in reconstruction. A transnasal wire is placed through drill holes in the central fragment superior and posterior to the lacrimal fossa and tightened to restore intercanthal distance. The bone fragments from the nose and the medial orbit are then

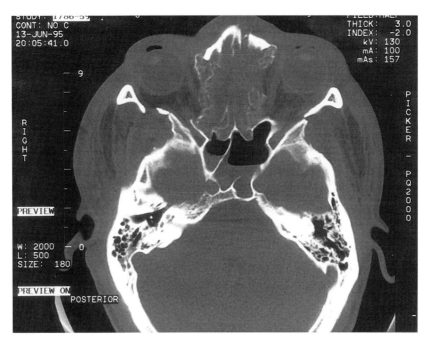

Figure 19-10. Axial CT scan view of a nasoethmoid fracture. Note the posterior displacement of the nasal bones into the ethmoid sinus and the lateral displacement of the medial orbital walls resulting in traumatic telecanthus. This patient also sustained a Le Fort III fracture as demonstrated by the fractures of both frontozygomatic sutures.

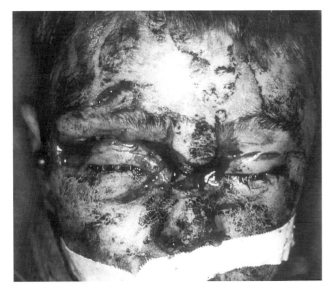

Figure 19-11. Clinical presentation of a Le Fort III fracture. Bilateral periorbital edema and ecchymosis are typically severe. Surgical access to the nasoethmoid area can frequently be obtained via overlying lacerations such as is present in this child.

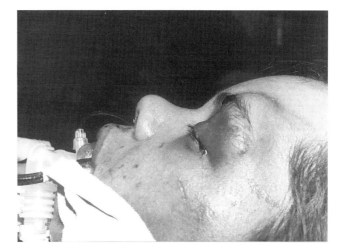

Figure 19-12. Saddle nose deformity seen in conjunction with a nasoethmoid fracture. The posterior displacement of the nasal dorsum results from a loss of both bony and cartilaginous support.

realigned and secured. One-mm microplates have proved to be valuable in the fixation of these fragile pieces of bone.

A persistent saddle nose deformity following fracture reduction occurs secondary to cartilaginous damage including destruction of the septum (Figure 19–12).

This is typically corrected with a dorsal cantilever bone graft (Figure 19–13). The use of onlay bone grafts in the pediatric population, however, is controversial (Bartlett & DeLozier, 1992). A minor contour deformity in the child may remodel over time and a bone graft could cause a secondary growth disturbance. A severe deformity, however, may justify a bone graft to prevent contracture of the soft tissue envelope of nasal skin. In general, bone grafting of the nasal dorsum in nasoethmoid

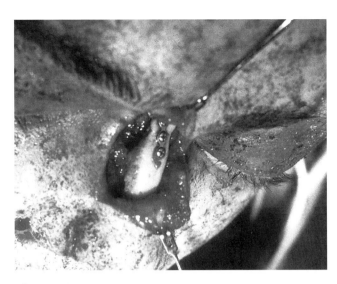

Figure 19-13. Repair of a nasoethmoid fracture with split cranial bone graft reconstruction of the nasal dorsum. The exposure is through an overlying laceration. The use of cranial bone grafts in nasoethmoid fractures in a child is limited to the most severe cases.

fractures should be much less frequent than for the same injury in the adult.

References

Bartlett, S. P., & DeLozier, J. B. (1992). Controversies in the management of pediatric facial fractures. *Clinical Plastic Surgery, 19,* 245–258.

Converse, J. M., & Dingman, R. O. (1977). Facial injuries in children. In J. M. Converse (Ed.), *Reconstructive plastic surgery* (2nd ed., pp. 794–821). Philadelphia: W. B. Saunders.

Converse, J. M., & Hogan, V. M. (1970). Open-sky approach for reduction of naso-orbital fractures. *Plastic and Reconstructive Surgery, 46,* 396–398.

Converse, J. M., & Smith, B. (1957). Enophthalmos and diplopian fracture of the orbital floor. *British Journal of Plastic Surgery, 9,* 265.

Dufresne, C. R., & Manson, P. N. (1990). Pediatric facial trauma. In J. G. McCarthy (Ed.), *Plastic surgery* (pp. 1142–1187). Philadelphia: W. B. Saunders.

Fujino, T., & Makino, K. (1980). Entrapment mechanism and ocular injury in orbital blowout fracture. *Plastic and Reconstructive Surgery, 65,* 571–574.

Grymer, L. F., Gutierrez, C., & Stoksted, P. (1985). Nasal fractures in children: Influence on the development of the nose. *Journal of Laryngology and Otology, 99,* 735–739.

Gussack, G. S., Luterman, A., Powell, R. W., Rodgers, K., & Ramenofsky, M. L. (1987). Pediatric maxillofacial trauma: Unique features in diagnosis and treatment. *Laryngoscope, 97,* 925–930.

Koltai, P. J. (1993). Maxillofacial injuries in children. In J. D. Smith & R. Bumsted (Eds.), *Pediatric facial plastic and reconstructive surgery* (pp. 283–315). New York: Raven Press.

Manson, P. N., Crawley, W. A., Yaremchuk, M. J., Rochman, G. M., Hoopes, J. E., & French, J. H. (1985). Midface fractures: Advantages of immediate extended open reduction and bone grafting. *Plastic and Reconstructive Surgery, 76,* 1–10.

Manson, P. N., Hoopes, J. E., & Su, C. T. (1980). Structural pillars of the facial skeleton: An approach to the management of Le Fort fractures. *Plastic and Reconstructive Surgery, 66,* 54–61.

Markowitz, B. L., Manson, P. N., Sargent, L., Vander Kolk, C. A., Yaremchuk, M., Glassman, D., & Crawley, W. (1991). Management of the medial canthal tendon in nasoethmoid orbital fractures: The importance of the central fragment in classification and treatment. *Plastic and Reconstructive Surgery, 87,* 843–853.

Mermer, R. W., & Orban, R. E. (1995). Repair of orbital floor fractures with absorbable gelatin film. *Journal of Craniomaxillofacial Trauma, 1,* 30–34.

Messinger, A., Radkowski, M. A., Greenwald, M. J., & Pensler, J. M. (1989). Orbital roof fractures in the pediatric population. *Plastic and Reconstructive Surgery, 84,* 213–216.

Posnick, J. C., Wells, M., & Pron, G. E. (1993). Pediatric facial fractures: Evolving patterns of treatment. *Journal of Oral and Maxillofacial Surgery, 51,* 836–844.

Precious, D. S., Delaire, J., & Hoffman, C. D. (1988). The effects of nasomaxillary injury on future facial growth. *Oral Surgery, Oral Medicine, and Oral Pathology, 66,* 525–530.

Putterman, A. M., Stevens, T., & Urist, M. J. (1974). Nonsurgical management of blow-out fractures of the orbital floor. *American Journal of Ophthalmology, 77,* 232–239.

Resnick, J. I., Kinney, B. M., & Kawamoto, H. K. (1990). The effect of rigid internal fixation on cranial growth. *Annals of Plastic Surgery, 25,* 372–374.

Rinehart, G. C., Marsh, J. L., Hemmer, K. M., & Bresna, S. (1989) Internal fixation of malar fractures: An experimental biophysical study. *Plastic and Reconstructive Surgery, 84,* 21–25.

Rowe, N. L. (1968). Fractures of the facial skeleton in children. *Journal of Oral Surgery, 26,* 505–515.

Stucker, F. J., Bryarly, R. C., & Shockley, W. W. (1984). Management of nasal fractures in children. *Archives of Otolaryngology, 110,* 190–192.

Tanaka, N., Uchide, N., Suzuki, K., Tashiro, T., Tomitsuka, K., Kimijima, Y., & Amagasa, T. (1993). Maxillofacial fractures in children. *Journal of Cranio-maxillo-facial Surgery, 21,* 289–293.

Zin, J. E., & Whitaker, L. A. (1983) Membranous versus endochondral bone: Implications for craniofacial reconstruction. *Plastic and Reconstructive Surgery, 72,* 778–784.

20

Pediatric Facial Soft Tissue Trauma

Thomas J. Bitterly, M.D., F.A.C.S.

This chapter describes the assessment and the treatment of pediatric soft tissue trauma. Surprisingly, very little has been specifically written about this topic (Hunter, 1992). It is intended to help the reader become familiar with methods of treating such injuries in both acute and chronic settings. Moreover, it should enable him or her to determine which injuries should be treated by the practitioner and which should be referred to surgeons with particular expertise in the handling of complex soft tissue injuries and reconstruction in children.

INITIAL EXAMINATION

When consulted to evaluate a child with soft tissue injuries of the face, the principles of pediatric advanced trauma life support should be followed. The history should include the mechanism of injury, the time it occurred, the location where the injury occurred, and the overall condition of the patient. Consideration of the above will determine the method and timing of therapeutic intervention.

The mechanism of injury can influence the type of soft tissue injury, wound healing, and the resultant scar. Among these are lacerations from sharp objects, blunt trauma, thermal injuries, bites, gunshot wounds, and abuse. Since the child's head comprises such a large proportion of its body surface area, it is not surprising that it is often involved in pediatric traumatic injuries.

More than 50% of children admitted to pediatric trauma centers have head injuries (Rouse & Eichelberger,

1995). Most common pediatric facial trauma in younger children results from falls (Hunter, 1992). Blunt trauma can result in abrasions, skin contusions, subcutaneous hematomas, lacerations, and facial fractures. The force of the blunt trauma can affect wound healing, especially if it has been significant, such as in a sudden deceleration, which can occur in a motor vehicle accident. In such circumstances, the injury is a crush, which can compromise the vascularity of the tissue resulting in impaired wound healing and resultant scarring. This is important to know, so that the surgeon can reasonably predict the outcome of the soft tissue repair and provide nervous parents with a reasonable prognosis of the outcome of the initial repair, and the potential need for further reconstructive procedures. Furthermore, significant blunt trauma should alert the surgeon to possible significant other injuries such as facial fractures, cervical spine injuries, and closed head injuries.

When examining a laceration, one should practice topographical anticipation. This means that one should suspect potential injury to underlying structures such as nerves, muscles, lacrimal ducts, salivary glands, and the eyes, as well as underlying skeletal and cartilaginous structures, depending on the facial location. One should never overlook the possibility that a laceration may have resulted from either an animal or a human bite. If such an injury is not properly diagnosed and appropriate antibiotic coverage is not given, serious soft tissue infection can ensue, resulting in potential cellulitis, wound infection, abscess, sepsis, hospitalization, and permanent disfigurement from scarring (Ruskin et al., 1993).

Simply suturing a laceration, without thought to the mechanism of injury or possible damage to underlying structures, can result in potential grave harm to the patient. The author has frequently had patients referred to his service by outlying practitioners stating that the reason for the referral was simply for wound closure, insisting that there were no other injuries. Unfortunately the author's experience has been the contrary. This is why a trauma consult is part of the protocol when patients are referred and the mechanism of injury suggests more significant trauma. Aside from the well-being of the patient, the medical-legal aspects of a missed diagnosis need to be considered in the United States of America.

Likewise, the time an injury occurred can influence both perioperative and postoperative management. In general, facial lacerations can be safely closed up to 24 hours from the time of injury because of the excellent vascularity of the face. The greater the time from the injury to the repair, the greater the risk of infection (Lawson, 1982). In cases where there has been a delay in the closure of facial lacerations, it must be explained to the parent(s) that, for the sake of cosmesis, a calculated risk is being taken in closing the laceration and that, despite antibiotic coverage, an infection requiring both drainage of the wound and parenteral antibiotics can occur. This is especially true with bites and heavily contaminated wounds.

The locale where the injury occurred can influence potential antibiotic coverage (Hunter, 1993). A toddler falling and lacerating a forehead on a coffee table may require no antibiotic coverage since the wound is reasonably clean. In contrast, a child thrown from a car into a farm field may need to be treated as a farm injury with broad spectrum antibiotics for gram-positive and gram-negative bacteria, as well as anaerobes. Road wounds heavily contaminated with road dirt should be treated in a similar fashion (Lawson, 1982).

The overall condition of the patient will determine when the soft tissue injuries can be treated. Simple lacerations with no other injuries can be immediately treated. However, the child who is the victim of multiple trauma will obviously need life-threatening injuries treated first. If such patients need to be taken to the OR to treat acute life-threatening injuries or other injuries such as fractures, the surgeon can accompany the patient to the OR, clean and suture any facial lacerations, and later evaluate the patient for underlying fractures or injuries (Lawson, 1982; Walton et al., 1982).

Finally, the eventual outcome of the soft tissue repair may be influenced by many premorbid factors, such as the age of the child; any preexisting medical conditions, such as juvenile diabetes; and medications, such as steroids, which can have a deleterious effect on wound healing.

THE PHYSICAL EXAMINATION

The facial examination includes inspection as well as palpation of the soft tissue and underlying facial bones. The length and configuration of lacerations should be documented. Dirt and other contaminants should be noted. Photographs are the optimal record. They provide an excellent record of the injuries. The treating surgeon may be called upon to testify in a liability suit. In addition, parents sometimes forget the appearance of the original injury. Photographs may help to remind them and potentially protect the surgeon from being sued for malpractice if the parents consider the result to be suboptimal. Finally, photographs are mandatory if one suspects abuse. Bruising should also be noted. It could suggest abuse. Ragged edges with small satellite punctures may suggest a bite. Foreign bodies should be suspected in patients who have struck the windshield or in patients having dirty lacerations embedded with gravel. A retained tooth from a bite should not be overlooked. The motion of the facial musculature should be observed. Lack of movement distal to a laceration can indicate either a contusion or transection of a branch of the facial nerve. The location of the laceration determines whether surgical repair is indicated. Sensation to light touch should be evaluated; however, this may be very difficult to determine in a young child.

Following inspection of the face, light palpation should be done to check for crepitus or step-offs indicating underlying fractures. Foreign bodies sometimes may be palpable. Finally, the oral cavity should be inspected for lacerations.

After the examination has been completed, radiologic studies should be done. These can range from plain radiographs to CT scans. These films should be inspected for fractures as well as foreign bodies.

INITIAL TREATMENT

Following the examination, the first decision that needs to be made is where the actual treatment will take place. This depends on the extent of the laceration and the age of the child. A small, linear facial laceration can usually be treated in the office or the emergency department, even if the child is uncooperative. For more extensive lacerations, where the proper alignment of key structures such as the vermillion border demands a totally cooperative patient, a decision will have to be made as to whether an OR setting is more appropriate. This depends on the maturity of the child and may not simply be age-dependent. The author has seen some older children who are totally uncooperative because of fear and anxiety and toddlers who are totally cooperative.

If the child is going to be treated either in the emergency department or the office, it is imperative that the practitioner gain the child's trust. He should speak directly to the child and in a comforting manner. He should never lie to the child, such as "this won't hurt you" (Hunter, 1992).

After it is determined where the wound will be closed, successful treatment requires a thorough knowledge of the principles of wound healing and Halstead's principles for the handling of tissue. The general phases of wound healing are the inflammatory phase, the proliferative or fibroblastic phase, and the wound contraction or maturation phase. The inflammatory phase is a nonspecific cellular and vascular response that serves to clean the wound of devitalized tissue and particulate matter (Rohrich & Robinson, 1992). If the wound is not properly debrided of all particulate matter, traumatic tattooing and foreign body reactions can result. Copious irrigation as will be described below is needed. The fibroblastic phase consists of epithelialization and the production of granulation tissue and collagen, which provide the framework of the scar. During the maturation phase, the collagen remodels, which provides the wound with tensile strength. This can last 6-18 months (Koopman, 1993). The redness of the wound usually recedes during this phase. The author sometimes describes this as the "red worm phase." This is when parents are usually concerned about the appearance of the wound. Knowledge of this phase permits the surgeon to reassure them that the redness will usually fade. It is for this reason that one should wait at least a year before undertaking a scar revision unless the wound edges are very uneven or there is traumatic tattooing of the wound. Many other factors can affect wound healing. These include nutritional status, premorbid illnesses including diabetes mellitus and inherited disorders such as pseudoxanthomatomata elasticum (Rohrich & Robinson, 1992), medications such as chemotherapeutic agents and steroids, and age. It is generally agreed that children heal more rapidly than adults. However, there is debate as to whether children are more prone to hypertrophic scarring (Farrior & Clark, 1993). Thomas and colleagues (1995) have stated that the causes of hypertrophic scarring are local, resulting from excessive wound tension due to inappropriate wound closure or postoperative wound infection.

When treating a soft tissue injury of the face, the goals should be to close the wound if possible, preserve function, and achieve the best cosmetic result possible. In short, one desires a fine line scar that compromises neither function nor appearance (Rohrich & Robinson, 1992). The eight principles of Halstead for the handling of tissue are best described by Crikelair:

1. Incisions should follow natural skin folds and lines of tension.
2. Tissue should be handled gently with minimal debridement of tissue to insure a clean base.
3. Complete hemostasis.
4. Avoid closing skin edges under tension.
5. Use fine suture, remove early.
6. Avert wound edges.
7. If possible, close wound in patients whose ages are closer to 90 than 9.
8. Allow time for wounds to mature before revising (Crikelair, 1960; Rohrich & Robinson, 1992).

EMERGENCY ROOM OR OFFICE ANESTHESIA

If the surgeon decides to treat the child in either of the above settings, it is imperative that the child be completely comfortable before doing anything, including cleaning and debriding the wound. One common mistake is to start irrigating the wound before anesthetizing the wound. This will guarantee a totally uncooperative child for the remainder of the procedure, resulting in a less than optimal closure and a potentially poor scar.

The author uses either 0.5% or 1% Xylocaine with epinephrine. Epinephrine should not be used in tissue with marginal vascularity (Walton et al., 1982). However, the author has always used this with essentially no resultant tissue loss and improved hemostasis. The addition of bicarbonate buffers the usually acidic local anesthetic, decreasing the pain of injection (Proudfoot, 1995). Some surgeons prefer to use sedation. This is acceptable provided he or she is comfortable with sedation techniques and adequate personnel and equipment are available to monitor the patient. This is usually not the case in most emergency room settings, which is why the author believes that if such a degree of sedation is required to comfortably treat the patient in the emergency room, then the patient is best served by doing the procedure in the OR. Some surgeons use topical solutions to decrease the pain of injection, but the duration of onset may not be for 20 to 60 minutes. Examples are TAC (tetracaine, adrenaline, and cocaine), which can be absorbed and have systemic side effects including hallucinations, seizures, and death; and EMLA (a eutectic mixture of local anesthetics). It cannot be applied to mucous membranes or local wounds or children younger than 1 month (Proudfoot, 1995). The author believes that the use of the above is limited because of the length of time it takes for the drugs to work. In general, the author never uses topical agents or sedation in the emergency room; instead he relies on the method described below (Hunter, 1992). Furthermore, he does not use the once popular lytic "pediatric cocktail" DPT consisting of Demerol, Phenergan, and Thorazine. It is now recognized that it is poorly titrable and can cause seizures, dystonic reactions, and even death at standard doses. It usually does not start to work until the closure is finished and can last up to 19 hours. Therefore it is not recommended for general usage (Proudfoot, 1995).

The author's preferred method is as follows. After examining the child, it is explained to them that the laceration, "cut," or "booboo," will need to be cleaned. Some children will become very upset if they hear that they are going to be sutured. Under such circumstances, the author informs the child that he must clean the wound. The author does not feel that this is lying to the child because closing a wound is actually part of the cleansing process. He then explains to the child that he will need to numb the area so that it does not hurt while he is cleaning it. He also makes it clear that the numbing process is going to hurt for a minute or so. At this point the wound is anesthetized. Usually, a small child will be upset for a few minutes. The author usually leaves the patient for about 5 minutes while he sets up his instruments. He then returns and tests the area to see if it is anesthetized, usually by gently irrigating it. If the wound is numb, he proceeds to clean it. At this point, he shines the operative light into the child's eyes. He then asks the child if he or she wants his eyes covered. The answer is usually yes. At this point the wound is prepped and draped, making sure to provide adequate ventilation and access to and visibility of a parent. The surgeon then proceeds with the closure of the wound. This technique is primarily applicable in toddlers and older children with relatively minor facial wounds. More extensive lacerations should be treated in an OR. Some children may require restraint in a Papoose Board (Olympic Medical Corp., Seattle, Washington).

Once the wound is anesthetized, it should be thoroughly cleaned before preparation and draping. The amount of cleaning and irrigation depends on the wound. Copious irrigation is desirable using a pulsatile stream after the removal of all large pieces of debris. For minimally contaminated wounds, a 35-cc syringe fitted with a 19-gauge needle will generate a pressure of 7 pounds per square inch (Lawson, 1982). More heavily contaminated wounds are best treated with jet lavage (Walton et al., 1982). Bites and heavily contaminated wounds may require several liters or more. Some surgeons prefer to add antibiotics to the irrigant. Ground-in dirt must be mechanically debrided to avoid traumatic tattooing. In addition, debridement can reduce the risk of wound infection 30-fold (Lackmann, 1992). This may require scrubbing with brushes or sharp surgical debridement—in the special cases of road dirt, chemical agents such as Polaximer 188 should be used (Hunter, 1993). The author has used mayonnaise to emulsify the dirt and tar and remove it (Eriksson, 1985). Most hospital kitchens are usually confused by this request, but the author has had excellent results using mayonnaise. This technique can be alternated with lavage until all of the particulate debris is removed. Failure to do so can prolong the inflammatory phase of wound healing, ultimately affecting the scar (Thomas et al., 1995). If scrubbing or emollients such as mayonnaise are not successful in removing the dirt, an 18-gauge needle or toothbrush can be used. In certain circumstances, it is not possible to surgically remove all ground-in dirt by debridement without risking distortion of the tissue and permanent disfigurement. The use of shields and drapes during irrigation and debridement to protect the OR personnel is usually appreciated. Preparation and draping are done after the wound has been cleaned as much as possible. Draping prior to cleaning the wound does not seem to make much sense to the author.

BITES

Mammalian bites account for 1% of all visits to the emergency departments. Fifty percent of the population experiences at least one bite during a lifetime (Kahn & Goldstein, 1993; Ruskin et al., 1993). Although human saliva can contain up to 10×8 bacteria per ml, representing as many as 42 species, *Streptococcus* and *Staphylococcus* are the species most commonly cultured. Also isolated are *Micrococcus, Bacteroides, Neisseria, Eikenella, Spirochetes,* gram-negative organisms, and occasional *Clostridia.* Animal bites are less virulent than human bites. In addition to *Staphylococcus* and *Streptococcus, Pasteurella multocida* is also isolated from canine and feline saliva (Ruskin et al., 1993).

All bites should be covered with antibiotics. A parenteral dose is usually administered in the outpatient setting, followed by oral antibiotics for 4 to 5 days (Kahn & Goldstein, 1993). Longer administration of parenteral antibiotics may be necessary if there has been extensive soft tissue injury. For parenteral use a good choice is ampicillin sodium/sulbactam sodium (Unasyn). The oral equivalent is amoxicillin and clavulanate sodium (Augmentin) (Goldstein, 1992; Kahn & Goldstein, 1993).

Bite wounds can be closed up to 6 to 8 hours after the injury following copious irrigation and judicious debridement. The closure should be done with simple, interrupted, nonabsorbable monofilament suture, avoiding dermal and subcutaneous sutures, which can act as a foreign body and a nidus for infection in bites (Hunter, 1992). Occasionally, a subcuticular suture may be needed for proper alignment of the wound. Puncture wounds should never be closed (Ruskin et al., 1993). When closing bites, the parents should be told that a calculated risk is being taken in closing a facial bite for the sake of cosmesis and that there is still a risk of cellulitis and hospitalization. Failure to recognize bites and treat them appropriately can have disastrous consequences (Ruskin et al., 1993). Finally, precautions against rabies should be taken.

PROPHYLACTIC ANTIBIOTICS

In addition to bites, all traumatic wounds should be considered as contaminated or infected according to the American College of Surgeons Committee on the

Control of Surgical Infections. A wound infection can be caused by the presence of 10×5 bacteria per gram of tissue. Broad-spectrum antibiotics effective against penicillinase-resistant *Staphylococcus* should be used. Early administration before the development of a fibrous coagulum, which can interfere with the delivery of the antibiotic to the wound, is recommended (Bried et al., 1995b). Finally, the surgeon must make sure that patients with both bites and other traumatic facial wounds have been adequately prophylaxed against tetanus.

CLOSURE OF THE FACIAL WOUND

Once the wound has been thoroughly cleaned, it is prepped and draped using sterile technique as one would in the OR. The author believes that surgical masks should be used. The type of closure depends on the wound. In the final analysis, there are really only four ways in which a wound can be closed: (1) primary closure; (2) healing by secondary intention; (3) skin grafting; and (4) flap coverage. Methods of closure should follow the so-called reconstructive ladder, proceeding from the simplest to the more complex (Bried et al., 1995b). This is sometimes described in more colloquial terms as the "KISS principle" which stands for Keep It Simple, Stupid. For simpler wounds, proper closure at the time of initial treatment will yield the best results. More complex wounds involving the loss of tissue may require more complex methods of closure either acutely or on a delayed basis if the wound is heavily contaminated. This chapter deals primarily with initial treatment of facial wounds in the pediatric population and techniques for closure. A detailed description of more advanced methods of reconstruction is beyond the scope of this chapter. General treatment common to all facial wounds will be described first, followed by a discussion of special areas of importance such as the lips, ears, eyes, and nose.

When closing a facial wound, it is important that all anatomic landmarks be properly aligned. In a linear laceration, this is straightforward. One can close the wound by placing a series of sutures that continuously bisect the wound. For stellate lacerations with multiple flaps, provided they are viable, the flaps should be replaced back into their original anatomic position. At the time of the original treatment, it is sometimes not possible to determine if flaps are viable. In this case, the wise course of action is to suture the questionable tissue back into position, with a plan to return and debride the tissue if it proves eventually not to be viable (Figures 20–1 and 20–2).

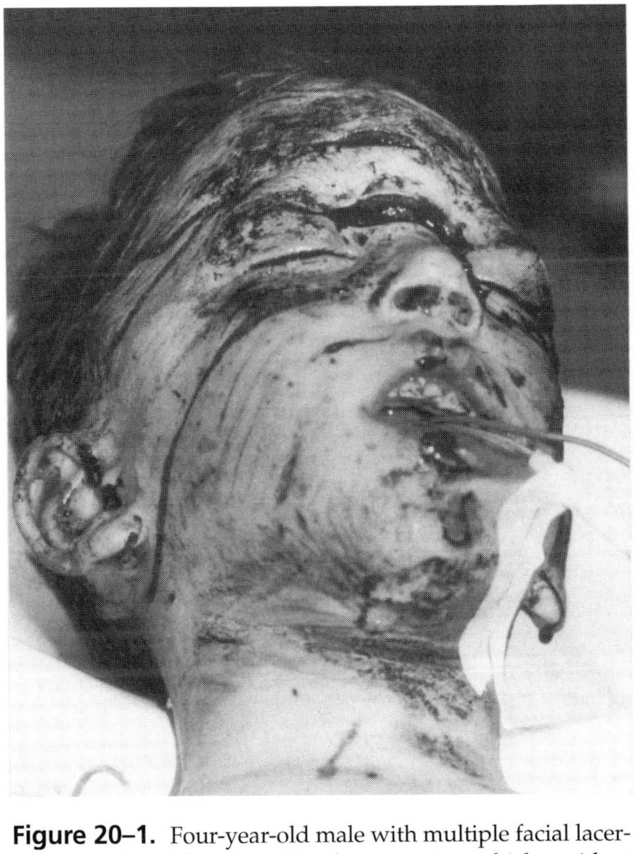

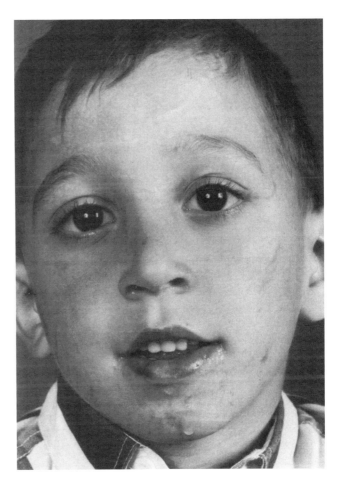

Figure 20–1. Four-year-old male with multiple facial lacerations totalling 30 cm resulting from a motor vehicle accident (MVA). Treated in OR.

Figure 20–2. Same patient shown in Figure 20–1 13 months later.

If there is an avulsion injury with actual loss of tissue, then the tissue should be aligned as best possible. This will help to outline the actual extent of the soft tissue loss (Figures 20–3, 20–4 and 20–5). If the tissue is mobile, local flaps can be used to close the defect. It is imperative that any type of closure does not result in the distortion of surrounding uninjured anatomic structures. For example, one would not close a cheek wound, that could result in an ectropion of the lower eyelid. Most important is the proper alignment of key anatomic structure, such as the vermilion border of the lips, before closing the remainder of the wound. The author firmly believes in what he terms the "key stitch" when closing a wound. If one can place this suture in a position that results in the correct alignment of the tissue, the remainder of the closure falls into place. This may be a trial-and-error process demanding great patience. However, the ultimate reward is a well-closed wound that will result in minimally noticeable scars when healed (Figure 20–6).

Wound edges can be debrided as long as this does not result in distortion of the surrounding tissue and key structures. Borges (1990) notes that "debridement, which in French means cutting loose adhesions and not trimming, frequently could be seen as an ill-advised premature application of fusiform scar revision." Borges is an advocate of minimal use of scar revision techniques at the time of initial closure. In addition, he advocates delayed scar revisions using Z-plasty techniques, so that scars fall within natural skin line. However, many surgeons, including the author, believe that proper handling of the initial closure yields the best results. "If the primary repair is unsatisfactory, the result is always disappointing" (Thomas et al., 1995). In younger children and infants, the surgeon may have to guess where these lines may eventually occur later in life. A wide debridement of tissue for the sake of a linear closure could potentially result in the distortion of surrounding tissue and structures. Sometimes wounds can be allowed to heal secondarily as in shown in Figure 20–7. This 6-year-old child was injured in a motor vehicle accident. She suffered an avulsion injury of her forehead secondary to striking glass. An attempt was made to try immediate tissue expansion (Figure 20–8), a technique described by Sasalo (1987). It was not possible. Therefore, local forehead flaps were elevated, with scoring of the galea to stretch the tissue so that the exposed frontal bone could be covered (Figure 20–9). There was a loss of skin on the subcutaneous tissue/muscle flap covering the exposed bone. The plan was to let the wound granulate and eventually skin graft the open wound. The postoperative treatment was aided by hyperbaric oxygen therapy, which the author feels is a valuable adjunct in promoting vascularity and the development of granulation tissue in wounds. However, it became obvious that the wound was starting to contract and heal by secondary intention (Figure 20–10). Both the child and her parents were

patient, and in the end were rewarded with an excellent flat wound with minimal color mismatch (Figure 20–11).

The type of suture used depends on the surgeon's preference and training. In general, the author prefers a two-layer closure of clean lacerations. Buried dermal absorbable suture such as braided Vicryl (polyglactin 910, Ethicon, Inc., Somerville, NJ) or the newer monofilament poliglecaprone (Monocryl) is placed. This takes tension off the closure, which could otherwise result in a spread scar (Wray, 1983). These are usually placed after permanent monofilament sutures have been placed to properly align the wound or key structures. This is followed by the placement of interrupted 5-0 or 6-0 monofilament sutures. These are usually left in place for 4 to 5 days. Further delay in removal could result in the development of permanent suture marks from the epithelialization of the suture tracts. Exceptions are heavily contaminated wounds, which may need to be closed in one layer or with minimal dermal sutures. In a simple straight laceration, a running subcuticular suture of permanent monofilament can be placed after the dermal sutures (Lackmann, 1992). This lessens the chance of suture marks and can be left in place longer. It further reduces tension on the closure. All suture techniques should result in everted skin edges, which decreases the chance of a depressed scar (Figures 20–12 and 20–13). Inverted or uneven edges result in scars that are more noticeable, because when light strikes them from certain angles, they cast a shadow across the depression, making the scar more noticeable.

SPECIFIC FACIAL ANATOMIC AREAS

The face can be divided into specific anatomic regions, each of which deserves special consideration.

Lips

The key to proper lip closure is the exact alignment of the vermillion border. This can be done by placing a 5-0 or 6-0 monofilament suture through the vermillion on each side of the wound. The suture can be left untied until the underlying sutures are placed. A full-thickness laceration is closed in three layers. The musculature is closed with either 4-0 or 5-0 absorbable suture. The dermis of the white lip is closed in a similar fashion with buried sutures. This takes tension off the closure, which otherwise could result in a widened scar. The skin is closed with 6-0 nonabsorbable monofilament. The red lip and intraoral mucosa is finally closed with a 5-0 braided absorbable suture. These may need to be removed later, but are more comfortable than stiffer absorbable sutures such as surgical gut.

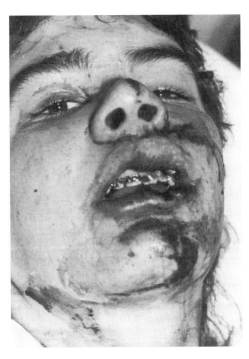

Figure 20–3. A 15-year-old male with multiple lacerations including avulsion of lip secondary to a motorcycle accident.

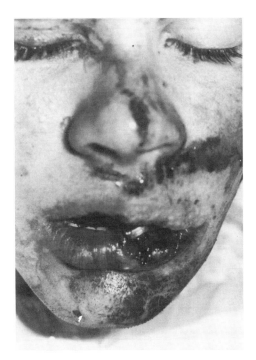

Figure 20–4. Extent of lip laceration and avulsion, in patient shown in 20–3.

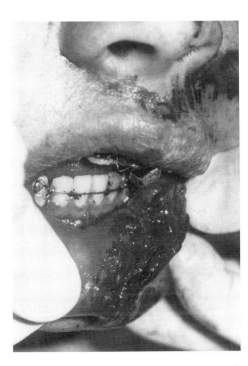

Figure 20–5. Intraoral extent of the lacerations. Vermillion spared.

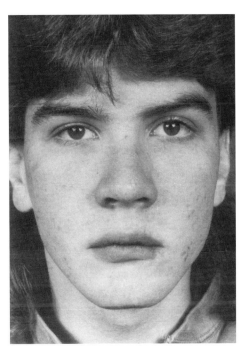

Figure 20–6. Result 1 year later. This cooperative patient was repaired in the emergency room.

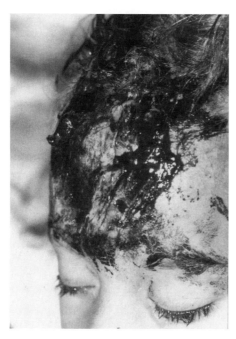

Figure 20–7. Six-year-old female with forehead avulsion and exposed frontal bone secondary to glass lacerations from an MVA.

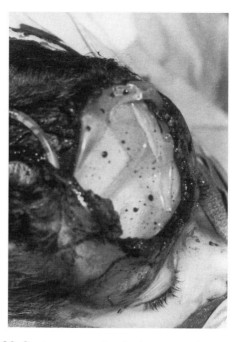

Figure 20–8. Attempt to close by intraoperative immediate tissue expansion in patient shown in Figure 20–7.

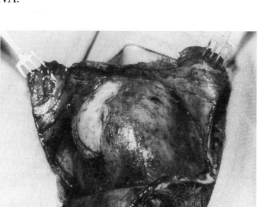

Figure 20–9. Elevation of forehead flaps with galeal scoring.

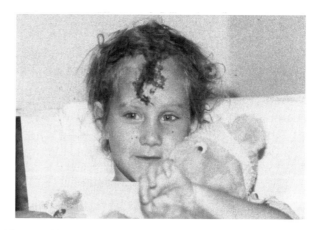

Figure 20–10. Wound healing by secondary intention in conjunction with hyperbaric oxygen therapy.

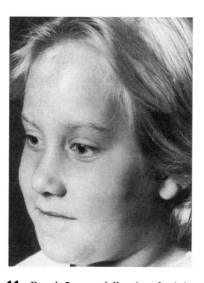

Figure 20–11. Result 2 years following the injury.

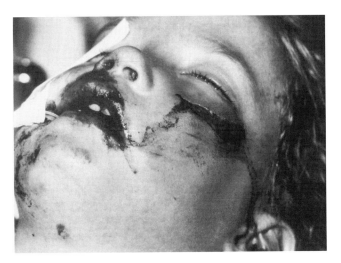

Figure 20–12. Three-year-old female with cheek and lip lacerations secondary to dog bite.

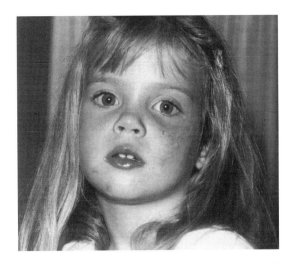

Figure 20–13. Result following wound maturation. Note that eversion of skin edges and proper alignment of vermillion have resulted in barely noticable scars.

If there are complex flap lacerations, the same technique of starting with vermillion alignment should be done first. The flaps should then be sutured back into position. If tissue is missing, then a local tissue rearrangement may be necessary (Figure 20–14). Distortion of anatomic landmarks should be avoided. In the author's experience, it is better to horizontally advance tissue. This results in a vertical scar. Even if it extends into the white lip, the scar is less noticeable (Figure 20–15) than vertical advancement flaps or closure, which can result in a shortening of the height of the lip, distortion of the red lip, and a more noticeable scar which is very difficult to correct later.

Nose

The most difficult nasal lacerations are those involving the alar regions. Full-thickness lacerations into the nasal vestibule can occur. Repair requires precise alignment of the alar rim. The nasal mucosa is closed with absorbable 5-0 suture with the knots in the vestibule. The alar cartilage must be repaired with either absorbable or nonabsorbable suture depending on the surgeon's preference. This is followed by closure of the skin in the manner previously described. Significant tissue loss may require flap closure or grafting techniques, the descriptions of which are beyond the scope of this chapter. Although one would prefer to do these in the acute setting, if there is major tissue contamination or loss, it may be preferable to close as much of the wound as possible to avoid distortion of the surrounding tissues, and return for the definitive flap closure several days later. Proper alignment of tissue is mandatory to avoid nasal stenosis and consequent airway obstruction (Lawson, 1982).

Eyelids

Lacerations of the eyelids demand meticulous attention to detail. The eyelids consist of skin, a muscular layer comprising the orbicularis oculi, levator, and Mueller's muscle, a semirigid tarsal plate, and conjunctiva. All layers must be properly aligned in lacerations of the lids. Prior to any repair, the surgeon must make sure that there has not been any damage to the eye itself or the cornea. In addition, lacerations around the medial canthus could involve the lacrimal system. If any of the above are noted, an ophthalmologist should be consulted.

Simple lacerations or linear lacerations can be directly closed (Figures 20–16, 20–17, and 20–18). In addition to a local anesthetic injected into the wound edges, a topical ophthalmic anesthetic should be applied to the eye and conjunctiva. This will result in a more comfortable and cooperative patient. Unfortunately, younger children may be very frightened; therefore it is in their best interest to repair such injuries in the OR if one is to achieve an anatomic repair. Debridement or ragged edges can be judiciously performed. The closure should be done without tension. Primary closure is possible with up to 25% lid loss (30% in the elderly with lax skin) (Burns, 1994). If there is tension, lateral canthotomy and cantholysis can gain up to 5–8 mm additional length (Mustardé, 1983).

The eyelid should be closed in three layers: conjunctiva and tarsus, muscular layer, and skin. If there is greater than 25% loss of tissue, more complex reconstructive methods are required. Flaps from the lower lid are usually used to reconstruct full-thickness losses of the mobile upper lid, whereas local cheek flaps are used to reconstruct the more static lower lid. Damage to the lacrimal system requires stenting, which is best per-

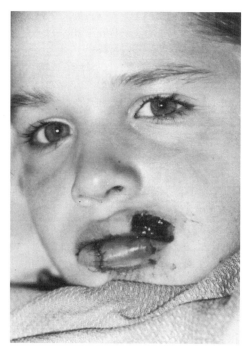

Figure 20–14. Eight-year-old male with lip avulsion injury secondary to dog bite.

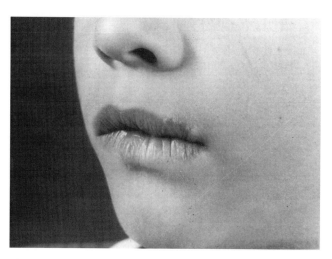

Figure 20–15. Result 2 years later after local advancement flaps.

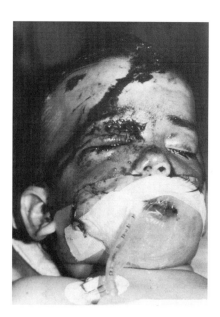

Figure 20–16. Eighteen-month-old male with upper eyelid and multiple facial lacerations secondary to MVA.

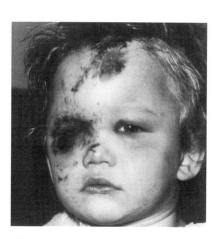

Figure 20–17. Wounds several days after closure.

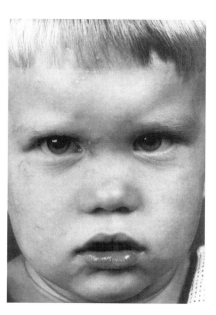

Figure 20–18. Result 3 months later.

formed by an ophthalmologist, unless the surgeon has expertise and training in this area.

Delicate sutures are required for eyelid repair. Usually, 5-0 or 6-0 silk is used to close the skin if there is a possibility of contact of the suture ends with the cornea, to prevent abrasions. The muscle and conjuncti-

va can be closed with fine absorbable suture, taking care to bury knots on the conjunctival closure to again avoid corneal abrasion.

Following repair, patching of the eye after the application of antibiotic ointment is required for 24 to 48 hours.

Ears

Lacerations of the auricle require meticulous alignment of the cartilage. Simple laceration can be closed in layers with absorbable suture to align the cartilage, and the skin closed with 5-0 or 6-0 nonabsorbable monofilament; judicious debridement should be performed. If there are significant abrasions and skin loss with the preservation of perichondrium, split-thickness skin grafting can be performed. Full-thickness losses can be closed with either wedge resections and primary closure or advancement flaps. Significant tissue loss and/or avulsions can be closed with postauricular flaps, which can then be divided at a second stage. Significant loss of the cartilaginous framework requires replacement either from the same or contralateral cartilage. Nearly avulsed ears with a vascular pedicle in the form of a thin flap should be placed back in an anatomic position. Mladick (1978) reports that success can be good because of the excellent vascularity of the ear. In such cases, if venous congestion occurs, the author has used a combination of medicinal leeches and hyperbaric oxygen therapy (Lawson, 1982).

Replacement of totally avulsed ears as composite grafts is not recommended, whereas microvascular replantations have been successful (Snively, 1991).

The ear which is primarily repaired should be dressed with petroleum gauze, coated with antibiotic ointment, and carefully padded and wrapped for 5–7 days. Contaminated wounds or bites should be inspected sooner. Hematoma should be drained and treated with compression dressing to avoid the complication of a cauliflower ear. Trauma and infection can result in perichondritis and significant deformity (Lawson, 1982).

Eyebrows

These should be carefully aligned, and under no circumstances should they be shaved because of the possibility that they will not grow back (Walton et al., 1982).

Cheek Lacerations and Salivary Glands

Lacerations to the cheeks which are either deep or full thickness should alert the practitioner to the possibility of damage to the parotid duct. If this is the case, the duct should be repaired under magnification and the duct stented. Otherwise salivary fistulas can result.

Facial Nerve Branches

If the laceration occurs lateral to the lateral canthus, direct repair with microscopic magnification should be performed within 72 hours. In a heavily contaminated wound or bite, the ends should be identified and tagged for later repair. Small branches medial to the lateral canthus are usually too small to be repaired (Anderson, 1991; Hunter, 1992).

Massive Soft Tissue Trauma

Sometimes the practitioner is faced with massive soft tissue injuries in association with underlying facial fractures. These are usually associated with gunshot wounds. However, there can be unusual circumstances, as the following case illustrates. It also demonstrates many of the points discussed above.

The patient was a 2½-year-old female who stuck her face into a large attic vertical cooling fan. She suffered massive facial injuries, including multiple facial fractures and multiple flap lacerations of the overlying skin (Figure 20–19). A multidisciplinary team approach was used at our tertiary care level I trauma center. After the general surgery trauma team had stabilized the patient, a team consisting of an otolaryngologist, oral surgeon, and plastic surgeon treated the wounds. First, the underlying fractures were reduced using rigid fixation, as well as cranial bone grafting. After this was done, the soft tissue injuries were repaired. This required the careful identification and alignment of the key landmarks, as were discussed above. Avulsed tissue was placed in as anatomic a position as possible. Some of the tissue was of questionable viability and hyperbaric oxygen therapy was initiated (Figure 20–20). The tip of a large left cheek flap did not survive (Figure 20–21). Following debridement, the wound healed secondarily (Figures 20–21 and 20–22). The patient eventually had this defect repaired with tissue expansion. She is currently undergoing repair of her severed facial nerve with a combination of cross-facial nerve grafts and a muscle transfer.

CONCLUSION

Facial soft tissue injuries in children, whether simple or complex, require meticulous attention to detail and expertise. Although any facial scarring can be distressing to a patient, it is especially so for parents. They usually expect their child to be returned to the premorbid state and are often heartbroken when they learn that the scars will be permanent. The author believes that, where possible, a meticulous primary closure at the time of the injury yields the best results. However, under certain conditions, definitive repair may need to be delayed. Successful closure and reconstruction demand a thorough understanding of facial anatomy so that damage to underlying structures is not overlooked. Such attention to detail will result in a better result and happier patients and parents.

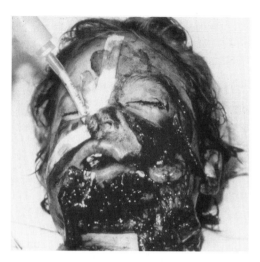

Figure 20–19. Two-year-old female who stuck her face into a large attic fan, with resultant flap lacerations and mandibular fractures.

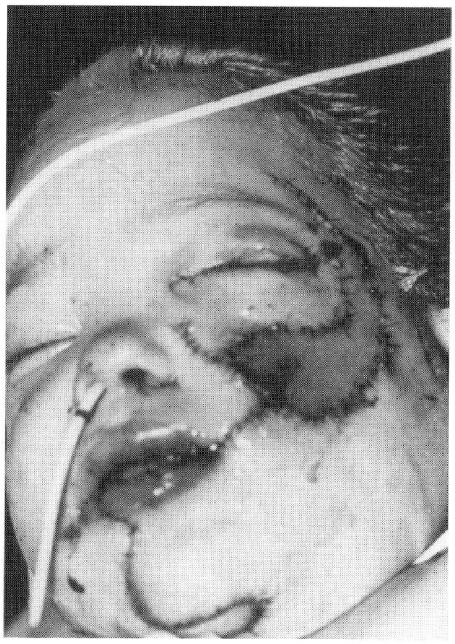

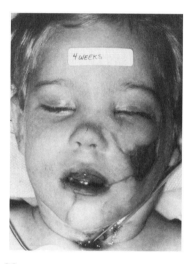

Figure 20–20. Appearance of wounds after open reduction and internal fixation (ORIF) of fractures including bone grafting, and alignment of key structures. Note ischemia of flap.

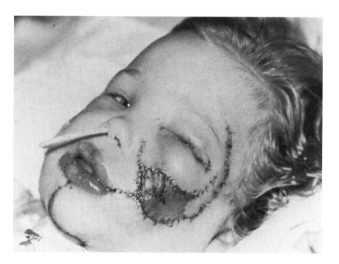

Figure 20–21. Continued flap necrosis, despite hyperbaric oxygen therapy.

Figure 20–22. Four weeks after hyperbaric therapy.

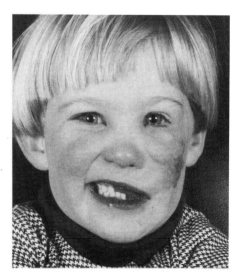

Figure 20–23. Result several months later after allowing the defect to heal secondarily and prior to further reconstructive procedures.

References

Anderson, R. G. (1991). Facial nerve disorders. *Selected Readings in Plastic Surgery (Overview), 6,* 9–10.

Borges, A. F. (1990). Timing of scar revision techniques. *Clinics in Plastic Surgery, 17,* 71–76.

Bried, M. C., Jurkiewicz, M. J., Elias, D. L., & Lintner, T. B. (1995a). Complex wound management: Part I. History and introduction to basic principles of wound management. *Surgical Physician Assistant, 1,* 34–40.

Bried, M. C., Jurkiewicz, M. J., Elias, D. L., & Lintner, T. B. (1995b). Complex wound management: Part II. General principles of wound reconstruction. *Surgical Physician Assistant, 1,* 5.

Burns, A. J. (1994). Eyelid reconstruction. *Selected Readings in Plastic Surgery (Overview), 7,* 1–12.

Crikelair, G. F. (1960). Surgical approach to facial scarring. *JAMA, 172,* 140.

Eriksson, O. (1985, October). Lecture burn symposium. Rochester, NY.

Farrior, R. T., Clark, D.A. (1993). Soft tissue trauma in children. In J. D. Smith & R. Bumstead (Eds.), *Pediatric facial plastic and reconstructive surgery.* New York: Raven Press.

Goldstein, E. J. (1992). Bite wounds and infection. *Clinical Infectious Diseases, 14,* 633–640.

Hunter, J. G. (1992). Pedatric maxillofacial trauma. *Pediatric Clinics of North America, 39,* 1127–1143.

Jelks, G. W., & Smith, B. C. (1990). Reconstruction of the eyelids and associated structures. In J. G. McCarthy (Ed.), *Plastic surgery* (pp. 1685–1688). Philadelphia: W.B. Saunders.

Kahn, R. M., &, Goldstein, E. J. (1993). Common bacterial skin infections. *Postgraduate Medicine, 93,* 175–182.

Key, S. J., Thomas, D. W., & Shepherd, J. P. (1995). The management of soft tissue facial wounds. *British Journal of Oral and Maxillofacial Surgery, 33,* 76–85.

Koopman, C. F. (1993). Wound healing and scar revision in the pediatric patient. In J. D. Smith & R. Bumsted (Eds.), *Pediatric facial plastic and reconstructive surgery* (pp. 317–335). New York: Raven Press.

Lackmann, G. M., Draf, W., Isselstein, G., & Töllner, U. (1992). Surgical treatment of facial dog bite injuries in children. *Journal of Cranio-Maxillo-Facial Surgery, 20,* 81–86.

Lawson, W. (1982). Management of soft tissue injuries of the face. *Otolaryngologic Clinics of North America, 15,* 35–48.

Losken, H. W., & Auchincloss, J. A.(1984). Human bites of the lip. *Clinics in Plastic Surgery, 11,* 773–775.

Mladick, R. A. (1978). Salvage of the ear in acute trauma. *Clinics in Plastic Surgery, 5,* 427–435.

Mustardé, J. C. (1983). Reconstruction of the eyelids. *Annals of Surgery, 11,* 149–169

Polhgeers, A., & Ruddy, R. M. (1995). An update on pediatric trauma. *Emergency Medicine Clinics of North America, 13,* 267–287.

Proudfoot, J. (1995). Analgesia, anesthesia, and conscious sedation. *Emergency Medicine Clinics of North America, 13,* 357–379.

Rohrich, R. J., & Robinson, J. B. (1992). Wound healing and closure, abnormal scars, tattoos, envenomation, and extravasation injuries. *Selected Readings in Plastic Surgery (Overview), 7,* 2–3.

Rosenberg, N. R., Stewart, G. M., Quan, L., & Horton, M. A. (1993). Laceration management. *Pediatric Emergency Care, 9,* 247–250.

Rouse, T. M., & Eichelberger, M. R. (1992). Trends in the management of pediatric trauma. *Surgical Clinics of North America, 72,* 1347–1363.

Ruskin, J. D., Laney, T. J., & Wendt, S. V. (1993). Treatment of mammalian bite wounds of the maxillofacial region. *Journal of Oral Maxillofacial Surgery, 51,* 174–176.

Sasalo, G. H. (1987). Intraoperative sustained limited expansion (ISLE) as an immediate reconstructive technique. *Clinics in Plastic Surgery, 14,* 563–73.

Schafermeyer, R. (1993). Pediatric trauma. *Emergency Medicine Clinics of North America, 11,* 187–201.

Snively, S. L. (1991). Deformities of the external ear and their correction. *Selected Readings in Plastic Surgery (Overview), 6,* 18–21.

Thomas, D. W., O'Neill, I. D., Harding, K. G., & Shepherd, J. P. (1995). Cutaneous wound healing: A current perspective. *Journal of Oral and Maxillofacial Surgery, 53,* 442–447.

Tittle, B. J., & Rohrich, R. J. (1994). Lip, cheek and scalp reconstruction and hair replacement. *Selected Readings in Plastic Surgery, 7,* 5.

Walton, R. L., Hagan, K. F., Parry, S. H., & Deluchi, S. F. (1982). Maxillofacial trauma. *Surgical Clinics of North America, 62,* 73–95.

Wray, R. C. (1983). Force required for wound closure and scar appearance. *Plastic and Reconstructive Surgery, 72,* 380.

21

Pediatric Laryngeal Trauma

Thomas L. Kennedy, M.D., F.A.C.S.

PEDIATRIC LARYNGEAL TRAUMA

Trauma to the larynx is a rare occurrence at any age, and in the pediatric population the type of injury sustained is, in some respects, related to the age of the child (Table 21–1). Laryngeal injury during birth is not infrequent and can result in dislocation of the cricothyroid or cricoarytenoid articulations. Unilateral or bilateral recurrent nerve injury from traumatic forceps delivery may also occur. The infant and young child are exposed to mostly iatrogenic injuries from intubation and laryngeal surgery in early development. Blunt external trauma to the larynx is seen in the teenage or adolescent group and is uncommon in the very young child for anatomical reasons. The higher location in the neck of a child's larynx enables the mandible to protect the larynx from direct blunt trauma. Furthermore, the size of the larynx is much smaller in the child than in the adult, and the cartilaginous framework is more elastic and forgiving. One disadvantage, however, is the greater possibility of endolaryngeal soft tissue injury without a cartilage fracture or the overt signs of laryngeal trauma. This may lead to significant swelling in the airway that may initially go unrecognized by medical personnel. In general, however, internal injuries to the larynx are more commonly seen than external injuries and include iatrogenic, inha-

Table 21–1. Pediatric laryngotracheal trauma.

Age Range	Type of Injury
At birth	Cartilaginous dislocations Recurrent nerve damage
Neonates	Intubation
Infants to early childhood	Intubation Surgery (tracheotomy, benign lesions) Infectious Thermal Chemical
Teenage-Adolescent	Blunt/Penetrating Cricotracheal separation Mechanical Chemical

239

lation, caustic ingestion, nasogastric tubes, and reflux (Table 21–2).

ANATOMICAL CONSIDERATIONS

Before discussing the various causes of laryngeal trauma, certain points concerning anatomy need to be reviewed in order to understand the complex nature of these injuries, and the difficulty that reconstruction sometimes presents. The larynx is composed of ligaments, cartilage, membranes, musculature, vasculature, and an extensive mucosal covering. The important cartilage structures that can be injured are the thyroid, cricoid, and the paired arytenoid cartilages. When these are damaged, the functions of respiration, deglutition, and speech are affected. This is especially true when the cricoid or arytenoid cartilages are injured. When the cricoid is fractured, stenosis of the subglottic space may result. If the arytenoids are damaged, dislocated, or exposed, the healing may lead to glottic incompetence and a permanent dysphonia. Besides the disruption of the cartilage framework, damage to the delicate internal mucosal lining is what makes laryngeal repair so difficult. The loose mucosa with little submucosa, the fragile arytenoids, the precarious blood supply to the cartilage structures, and the constant stretching and movement of the larynx during swallowing and speaking all contribute to the poor wound healing in laryngeal injuries. This, in turn, promotes healing by secondary intention with scarring and stricture formation.

EXTERNAL LARYNGEAL TRAUMA

As commented on earlier, this form of laryngeal injury is unlikely to occur in the small child. In our own series of penetrating and blunt injuries to the larynx, the youngest patient was 15 years of age. This correlates with other studies and is related to the increased size of the adolescent larynx and their more aggressive physical behavior (Kadish, Schunk, & Woodward, 1994). Sport vehicles like motorcycles, snowmobiles, and jet skis have added to the blunt trauma and clothesline injuries,

while sporting events like karate and snowboarding have resulted in direct blows to the head and neck regions. Automobiles and the refusal to wear a lap belt and shoulder harness by young drivers or passengers, is still a major factor in neck and laryngeal injuries. Table 21–3 lists the acute laryngeal injuries that occur in all patients, with the older pediatric patients sustaining soft tissue injuries along with a supraglottic or lateral glottic fracture of the thyroid or cricoid cartilage (Figures 21–1 and 21–2).

Laryngotracheal disruption or avulsion of the trachea from the larynx, a life-threatening blunt injury in a child, is a rare occurrence that results from an anterior horizontal blow low in the neck which forces the larynx and trachea against the spine (Figure 21–3). Most patients with these injuries are young teenagers using recreational vehicles producing the so-called clothesline injury. A tremendous force occurring low in an extended neck results in a pull of the relatively elastic laryngeal structures cephalad, separating them from the more stationary caudad trachea. The younger patient is more likely to sustain this injury because the intercartilaginous membranes are not fully mature, and the laryngeal cartilages are more resistant to crush injuries than the adult larynx. Surgical repair is complicated by recurrent nerve damage.

Penetrating injuries are another form of external laryngeal trauma and are more common than blunt laryngeal trauma in the pediatric age group (Ford, Gardner, & Lynch, 1995). These injuries are associated with accidental trauma and assaults which may involve injury to the esophagus as well. Penetrating injuries to younger children are now occurring with alarming frequency as a result of youths finding unsecured weapons within the home. Attempted suicide by teenage youths is also on the rise and this has resulted in wounds to the neck that cause laryngeal damage. One form of penetrating injury that deserves mention is the emergency tracheotomy in the child. Although a rare event,

Table 21–2. Causes of laryngeal trauma.

External trauma
  Blunt
  Penetrating
  Iatrogenic (tracheotomy, birth delivery injuries)

Internal trauma
  Iatrogenic (intubation, surgery for benign disease, tracheotomy)
  Thermal (inhalation from burns)
  Chemical (reflux, caustic ingestion, etc.)
  Mechanical (nasogastric tubes, foreign bodies, voice abuse, etc.)

Table 21–3. Acute (penetrating and blunt) laryngeal injuries.

Laryngeal soft tissue
  Mucosal edema, hematoma, laceration
  Arytenoid dislocation
  Cricothyroid joint dislocation
  Vocal cord paralysis

Laryngeal fractures
  Supraglottic
  Lateral glottic
  Combined frontal comminuted
  Massive injury with cartilage loss

Laryngeal-Tracheal
  Cricotracheal separation

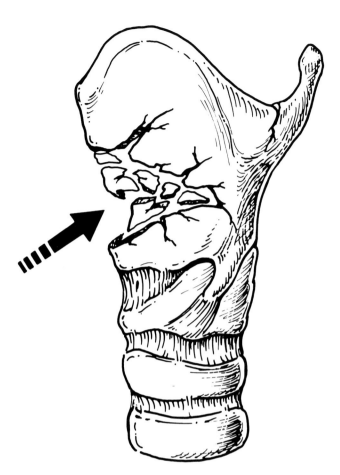

Figure 21–1. Supraglottic fracture.

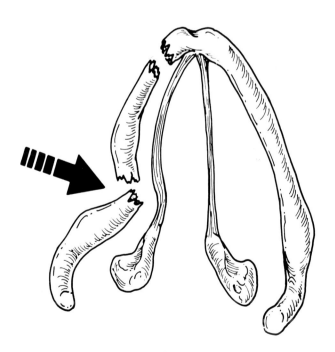

Figure 21–2. Lateral glottic fracture.

an uncontrolled situation may occur and the resultant tracheotomy may lead to cartilage or recurrent nerve injury.

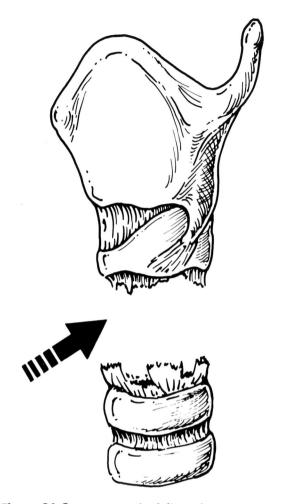

Figure 21–3. Laryngotracheal disruption.

INTERNAL LARYNGEAL TRAUMA

The most common internal or endolaryngeal injury in the pediatric age would have to be attributed to complications from intubation. This, along with the other iatrogenic causes of internal injury, make up the largest category of internal laryngeal trauma (Table 21–2). Intubation injuries can be divided into two kinds: those at the time of intubation and those caused by the duration of intubation. Complications of intubation include pharyngeal and laryngeal lacerations; cricoarytenoid dislocation; glottic and subglottic damage from placement of too large a tube or cuff; and neural injury to the lingual, hypoglossal, or laryngeal nerves. The dislocations and nerve injuries are the most difficult to resolve or repair. The pathophysiology of trauma from prolonged endotracheal intubation is complex and the topic is controversial. It is not the scope of this discussion to deal with this matter, except to state there are many variables that come into play, as listed in Table 21–4. The two factors that remain the most significant are the duration of intubation and the size of the airway. The one exception to this relates to infants who are able to withstand longer periods of intubation. This is, in

Table 21–4. Variables to consider in intubation injury.

Anatomy of the upper respiratory tract (females), narrower internal diameter

Movement between the laryngotracheal complex and the endotracheal tube

Size, shape, and biological properties of the tube

Type of cuff

Cuff pressure

Increased vulnerability of mucosa
   Hypotension
   Infection
   Diabetes
   Steroids

Duration of intubation

part, due to the flexibility of their airways and the cuff-less nature of the endotracheal tubes that are used in this age. Intubation trauma is more likely to occur in an abnormal larynx than in a normal one. For example, it has been found that 12% of the pediatric patients intubated for airway obstruction due to acute laryngotracheitis could not be successfully extubated after 7 days, and two out of three needed a tracheotomy (McEniery et al., 1991). The injuries sustained by long-term intubation are mostly chronic and are listed in Table 21–5.

Surgical removal of laryngeal lesions and tracheotomy are the remaining iatrogenic etiologies of laryngeal injury. In the pediatric group the removal of laryngeal papillomas can lead to scarring of the glottis, most notably at the anterior commissure. Aggressive laryngeal removal of other benign lesions in children can result in irreversible damage, especially if carried out by an inexperienced surgeon. A high-placed tracheotomy, the use of too large a tracheotomy tube, recurrent nerve injury, and improper postoperative tracheotomy care are a few reasons for tracheotomy-related injury to the larynx.

Injuries from caustic ingestion typically are seen in the pediatric population. These are secondary to a variety of household cleaners. The oral cavity, pharynx, and esophagus are usually the most affected. The laryngeal injury results from direct contact by ingestion and regurgitation of the offending agent. The degree of injury depends on the amount of the material ingested and the duration of exposure. Inhalation injury or thermal energy damage secondary to burns is another form of internal laryngeal trauma. Children account for almost half of all burn patients requiring hospital care, and burns in children are the second most common type of fatal trauma (Calhoun et al., 1988). The only initial sign of thermal injury may be redness in the larynx, but it can later lead to airway obstruction when edema results from fluid resuscitation. Another form of internal injury is chemical change as a result of GER with or without the placement of a nasogastric tube. Reflux leads to mucosal inflammation, ulceration, edema, and granulation formation. This problem has recently become more recognized and treated. A nasogastric tube placed in a patient who already has a larynx injury increases the reflux chemical irritation and adds to the production of postcricoid ulceration, infection, and necrosis.

Table 21–5. Chronic laryngeal injury.

Isolated
   Supraglottic
      Epiglottic displacement
      Stenosis
   Glottic
      Webs, stenosis
      Interarytenoid scarring
      Arytenoid dislocation and fixation
      Vocal cord paralysis
   Subglottic
      Stenosis
   Tracheal
      Stenosis
      Tracheoesophageal fistula

Compound
   Supraglottic-glottic stenosis
   Glottic-subglottic stenosis
   Subglottic-tracheal stenosis
   Supraglottic-glottic-subglottic stenosis

ASSESSMENT OF ACUTE INJURY

The diagnosis of external laryngeal injury at birth is sometimes delayed and is suspected when the infant reveals a raspy or breathy cry. Difficulty with feeding and occasional aspiration may be the next presenting symptoms of neural injury. The diagnosis is made by fiberoptic laryngoscopy and treatment is usually observation, since greater than 50% recover with time.

When blunt external trauma occurs in the older child, the major symptoms center around a disruption of phonation, respiration, and deglutition. In minor laryngeal trauma, the quality of the voice may change, the patient may have some pain with swallowing, or there may be some noisy breathing. As the severity of the trauma increases, these symptoms lead to acute signs of impending airway obstruction with stridor, cyanosis, and restlessness. Crepitance or subcutaneous air is always an indication of a ruptured viscus, possibly the hypopharynx, the esophagus, the pulmonary system, or the laryngotracheal complex. If fractures are present, they may be palpated through the neck or there may be anterior cervical flattening with loss of the laryngeal prominence. Laryngoscopy, indirect or fiberoptic, is the initial and most important examination when the patient is first seen. This evaluation will determine the need for further work-up or immediate intervention. CT scanning is the best test for laryngeal cartilaginous fractures. Aerosolized epinephrine may temporarily decrease swelling in children and provide more time to plan treatment. Direct laryngoscopy may be indicated to further define the extent of the damage. At this point it is necessary to determine if emergency exploration is required because of the possibility of airway obstruction. Laryngeal surgery is considered for the following reasons: marked displaced cartilage fractures, cricotracheal separation, significant laryngeal mucosal lacerations, and rapidly increasing subcutaneous emphysema. When exploration is required, a temporary tracheotomy is usually carried out. Even the most severe laryngeal injury can be repaired with good results if acutely done. A delay in diagnosis and treatment leads to local infection and granulation build-up that dramatically alters the reconstruction success rate. This, in turn, can result in chronic stenosis in one or more regions of the larynx.

MANAGEMENT OF LARYNGEAL TRAUMA

The goals of management in laryngotracheal injury for the child are the same as in the adult and include: the establishment of an adequate airway and swallowing mechanism without aspiration, prevention of long-term sequelae, and voice preservation. Restoration of speech, the last objective, is the most important to the patient. As in any other type of surgical repair, the first attempt is the best chance at a successful reconstruction. Delay in treatment, or an inexperienced operator, may result in irreversible damage to the larynx and trachea. There are a variety of repair techniques used in the management of acute and chronic laryngeal injury. The principles behind each procedure remain the same. Take extreme care to realign structures, make sure all internal surfaces are lined by mucosa or skin grafts, and use stents only when support has been lost to injury. Early recognition of an injury with appropriate treatment can prevent permanent scarring and long-term disability.

References

Calhoun, K. H., Deskin, R. W., Garza, C., McCracken, M. M., Nicholas, R. J., Jr., Hokanson, J. A., & Herndon D. N. (1998). Long-term airway sequelae in a pediatric burn population. *Laryngoscope, 98,* 721–725.

Ford, H. R., Gardner, M. J., & Lynch, J. M. (1995). Laryngotracheal disruption from blunt pediatric neck injuries: Impact of early recognition and intervention on outcome. *Journal of Pediatric Surgery 30,* 331–335.

Kadish, H., Schunk, J., & Woodward, G. A. (1994). Blunt pediatric laryngotracheal trauma: Case reports and review of the literature. *American Journal of Emergency Medicine, 12,* 207–211.

McEniery, J., Gillis, J., Kilham, H., & Benjamin, B. (1991). Review of intubation in severe laryngotracheobronchitis. *Pediatrics, 87,* 847–853.

22

Anesthesia for Pediatric Ear, Nose, and Throat Procedures

George Tenedios, M.D., and Jan Schwartz, M.D.

Providing anesthesia care to children is an experience that is generally fun, often challenging, and always anxiety-provoking! The pediatric anesthesiologist must be knowledgeable in the discipline of pediatrics, as well as the practice of anesthesia. The anesthesiologist who prepares the child for surgery must be ever mindful of the often unrecognized stresses experienced by the family unit. Long-lasting behavioral disturbances are observed after poorly prepared children have been subjected to stormy anesthetic inductions (Eckenhoff, 1953; Levy, 1945). By the same token, seemingly comfortable but inadequately prepared parents often describe their child's anesthetic as a terrifying and even horrific event (Schofield & White, 1989; White, 1985). Therefore, during the preanesthetic evaluation of the pediatric surgical patient, the anesthesiologist needs to identify strategies for dealing with the child's and parents' anxiety during the perioperative period. In the perioperative period, the anesthesiologist must also be a "developmental specialist" and be cognizant of age-dependent variations in the child's physiology and maturation. The pediatric specialist must command a particular knowledge of developmental anatomy and physiology, with special clinical awareness of airway growth and development, maturation of the physiological processes responsible for drug metabolism, respiratory drive, and temperature regulation. Furthermore, the pediatric anesthesiologist must be appreciative of how a disease's signs and symptoms are manifested in different pediatric age groups. The pediatric anesthesiologist wears many hats well to ensure the safety of the pediatric patient undergoing a surgical procedure

(Keenan, Shapiro, & Dawson, 1991; Keenan, Shapiro, Kane, & Simpson, 1994).

This chapter considers the anesthetic methods and management of common pediatric ear, nose, and throat (ENT) procedures such as myringotomy tube placement, endoscopy, tonsillectomy, and adenoidectomy. Our discussion will focus on some of the shared and competing concerns of anesthesiologists and otolaryngologists about patient readiness, perioperative pain, and critical management schemes to permit simultaneous access to the child's breathing system. Anesthesia for pediatric ENT procedures is especially challenging and often problematic during surgeries when both specialists share a compromised life-giving airway.

GENERAL PRINCIPLES OF PEDIATRIC ANESTHESIA

Preoperative Evaluation

The preoperative clinical visit of the child, parent, and anesthesiologist helps to establish rapport, as well as to obtain the needed information about the patient from the medical history and physical examination. The preanesthetic care for children is initiated by developing rapport with the child and the parent during a clinical "work-up." A special perioperative staging area that is comfortable and supportive for children is helpful in diminishing the child's fears about impending surgery. This comfortable environment where families will meet with the anesthesiologist can be accomplished with toys, books, or videos. During the preoperative interview, the pediatric anesthesiologist has an opportunity to communicate his or her special commitment to the parents by helping them cope with the real and perceived risks of the anesthesia through a positive attitude toward their child's welfare. If the parent conveys the appearance of being comfortable about leaving the child with the anesthesiologist, then the child will respond appropriately and most likely be able to easily separate from the parents. During the medical interview, the anesthesiologist must establish an age-appropriate alliance with the child. Children intellectually and psychologically respond in developmentally different styles to the prospect of surgery. For example, psychologists have observed that the infant favorably responds to gentle voices and the comfort of holding and rocking. The child of 1 to 3 years of age has more difficulty establishing trust. He or she is less likely to separate from his or her parents, is intellectually less likely to understand the explanations, and easily views the world as a fantasy and is therefore more receptive to stories or songs. The older child of 3 to 6 years of age is literal in his or her thinking. When using the phrase "being put to sleep" the child might grasp images of his or her pet no longer living. Children from 7 to 12 years of age are more concrete in their thinking and cannot think abstractly. For example, they will not be able to distinguish between "a pound of feathers and a pound of rocks." They will demand more explanation and participation in the anesthetic process. Adolescents, like adults, are more likely to be cooperative with the anesthesiologist if clear explanations and assurances are provided (McGraw, 1994).

The preoperative history and physical examination by the anesthesiologist are the mainstays of the perioperative evaluation. Obtaining complete medical history before surgery is important to assess and identify the pediatric patients in whom perioperative respiratory, cardiac, neurologic, metabolic, and coagulopathic compromise is most likely to develop (Table 22–1). The medical history should seek information about allergies (Kerner & Newman, 1993), congenital abnormalities (Foley, Beste, & Farber, 1997), recent exposure to communicable diseases, existing medical conditions, and the current functional level of the major organ systems. A review by Gerber, O'Connor, Adler, and Myer (1996) showed the importance of such questioning. Their conclusion was that pediatric patients younger than 3 years of age with neuromuscular disorders, chromosomal abnormalities, difficulty in breathing, or an upper respiratory tract infection within 4 weeks of surgery were most at risk for perioperative respiratory compromise after undergoing adenotonsillectomy. The preoperative review of old anesthetic records is an important aid in assessing potential airway difficulties, such as difficulty with procurement of the airway, or postextubation stridor or croup. A review of the family history is particu-

larly important for exposing the possibilities of anesthetic-triggered disease such as malignant hyperthermia (Wackym & Blackwell, 1994). The appraisal of medications currently being administered and their potential interaction with the anesthetic administered is important to prevent incompatibilities of drugs.

A thorough physical examination is important to identify the functional activity of the major organ systems such as heart, lungs, kidney, hepatic, and neurological system. The detailed clinical examination should also assess the fluid status of the patient, as well as signs of limited physiologic reserve as revealed with the presence of cyanosis. The observation of loose teeth should be noted to prevent unintentional aspiration. Preoperative laboratory blood tests for general screening of pediatric patients are not generally recommended (Nigam, Ahmed, & Drake-Lee, 1990; Zwack & Derkay, 1997). These recommendations are based on large outcome studies of healthy patients undergoing elective surgical procedures. Routine laboratory tests of coagulation prothrombin time (PT) and activated partial thromboplastin time (PTT) fail to identify otherwise healthy patients who develop excessive postoperative bleeding after ENT surgery (Burk, Miller, Handler, & Cohen, 1992; Close, Kryzer, Nowlin, & Alving, 1994; Livesey, 1993; Wall, Wilimas, & Manco-Johnson, 1993). Similar studies show no measurable improvements in outcome when patients without manifest clinical disease or risk factors are screened with blood tests before elective surgery (Manning, Beste, McBride, & Goldberg, 1987).

A preoperative chest radiograph can be diagnostic of an aspirated foreign body if there is persistent air trapping on an expiratory or lateral film. A lateral neck radiograph may be helpful to diagnose inflamed supraglottic structures such as a retropharyngeal abscess or epiglottitis. The preoperative radiograph is helpful as a comparison in the postoperative period to evaluate the efficacy of the endoscopy as well as development of atelectasis or pneumothorax from the surgical procedure (Redleaf & Fennessy, 1995).

However, a study looking at the benefit of reviewing preoperative chest x-rays to predict postoperative respiratory complications in 355 pediatric patients undergoing tonsillectomy and adenoidectomy found no predictive value in obtaining a routine film (Biavati, Manning, & Phillips, 1977). After the preoperative evaluation the anesthesiologist must summarize and document in the patient's record pertinent findings of the patient's history and physical examination, along with pertinent laboratory findings, and determine the functional capacity and reserve of the patient. Specific potential complications related to the patient's overall health should be noted and an anesthetic plan and technique must be formulated that minimizes the risks and maximizes the benefits for the patient to proceed with the surgery.

Preoperative Medications

The ideal sedation technique is when the child can easily separate from the parent. There are a variety of techniques reported to help a young, anxious child cooperatively participate in the anesthetic process (Table 22–2). Noninjected sedatives and narcotics administered by mouth (Epstein et al., 1996), nasal instillation (Schreuder, Bosenberg, & Murray, 1992), or per rectum (Karl, Keifer, Rosenberger, Larach, & Ruffie, 1992; Zedie, Amory, Wagner, & O'Hara, 1996) have all been demonstrated to be safe and effective.

Many pediatric institutions also gain the confidence and cooperation of young patients through extensive prehospital educational programs or by permitting the patients to be accompanied by parents into the OR or induction area (McCormick & Spargo, 1996). While no single technique is shown to be preferable for all ages, it is very clear that all efforts to alleviate anxiety and limit the incidence of children who are forcibly anesthetized are helpful when evaluated from the perspective of postoperative behavior. As a cautionary note, preoperative sedatives and narcotics should be avoided if there are concerns about further compromising the child's airway.

Using agents to reduce gastric acidity or volume is an unresolved question in children. Sodium citrate is distasteful and most children will refuse to drink it. The

Table 22-1. Examples of medical conditions and possible postoperative complications during ENT procedures.

Coexistent Medical Condition	Common Perioperative Problems
Familial periodic paralysis	Prolonged muscle weakness (Bunting & Allen, 1997)
Renal disease	Respiratory failure after codeine (Talbott, Lynn, Levy, & Zelikovic)
Down syndrome	Postop airway obstruction (Bower & Richmond, 1995; Jacobs, Gray, & Todd, 1995)
Congenital airway disease	Death (Kirse, Tryka, Seibert, & Bower, 1996)
Beckwith Wiedemann syndrome	Airway obstruction (Rimell, Shapiro, Shoemaker, & Kenna, 1995)
Prematurity	Postoperative airway obstruction (McGowan, Kenna, Fleming, & O'Connor, 1992)
Inherited bleeding disorders	Life-threatening hemorrhage (Prinsley, Wood, & Lee, 1993)
Duchenne's muscular dystrophy	Sudden cardiac arrest (Benton & Wolgat, 1993)

Table 22-2. Preoperative sedation medications.

Medication	Site of Administration	Dose
Midazolam (Cray, Dixon, Heard, & Selsby, 1996; Patel & Meakin, 1997)	Oral	0.4–0.75 mg/kg
Ketamine (Cioaca & Canavera, 1996; Sekerci, Donmez, Ates, & Okten, 1996)	Oral	6 mg/kg
Midazolam (Zedie, Amory, Wagner, & O'Hara, 1996)	Intranasal	0.2 mg/kg
Sufentanil (Karl, Keifer, Rosenberger, Larach, & Ruffle, 1992)	Intranasal	2 mcg/kg
Methohexital (Khalil, Flordence, Van den Nieuwenhuyzen, Wu, & Stanley, 1990)	Rectal	25 mg/kg of 1%

new histamine H_2 receptor antagonist, famotidine, given to children by mouth either the evening before or the morning of elective surgery does increase gastric pH; however, it failed to reduce gastric volume (Jahr, Burckhart, Smith, Shapiro, & Cook, 1992). The same observations were made in children administered intravenous ranitidine and metoclopramide in that there was an increase in gastric pH but no decrease in gastric volume (Christensen, Farrow-Gillespie, & Lerman, 1990). The use of antisialagogues such as atropine and glycopyrrolate in children undergoing endoscopy also does not provide significant benefits (Hofley et al., 1995; Randall, Saarnivaaran, Oikkonen, & Lindgren, 1992), as compared to the efficacy shown in adults (Gronnebech, Johansson, Smedebol, & Valentin, 1993) .

Inductions

Many children arrive at the OR already frightened and agitated following separation from their parents. The strange OR environment, the smell of the inhaled gases, and the physical placement of a mask over the nose and mouth may become overwhelming for a youngster. There are numerous approaches to make the child less anxious prior to the initiation of the anesthetic induction (McGraw, 1994). Such strategies include allowing the parents to be present during the induction of anesthesia (Gillerman, Hinkle, Green, & Connell, 1996; Kain, Ferris, Mayes, & Riman, 1996; Kain et al., 1996; Larosa-Nash, Murphy, Wade, & Clasby, 1995), administering sedative premedications (Cray et al., 1996; Warner, Cabaret, & Velling, 1995), and educating the child and parents (Hannalah, 1995).

Induction of anesthesia, the transition from an awake to an unconscious state, may be accomplished by oral administration (Bragg & Miller, 1990; Patel & Meakin, 1997; Warner et al., 1995), intranasal administration (Diaz, 1997), intravenous or intramuscular injection, rectal drug administration (Guidbrand & Mellstrom, 1995; Schrenk et al., 1992), and by inhalation of anesthetic agents (Greenspahn, Hannalah, Wellborn, & Norden, 1995; Johannesen, Floren, & Lindahl, 1995). Intravenous and inhalational inductions are the most common techniques (LeSaint, 1995). The chosen induction technique is generally determined by the child's age (Berry, 1990). When asked, most children (and parents of young or preverbal children) will request an inhalation induction. Anesthesia commences with the child breathing an agent through a mask. An intravenous catheter is inserted after the patient is anesthetized. Despite this generally observed preference of a mask induction among patients and parents, a recent study reviewing 90 children undergoing routine ENT operations indicated the children who underwent inhalational inductions had significantly more postoperative negative psychological outcomes when compared

with children in whom an intravenous catheter was started before anesthesia (Kotiniemi & Ryhanen, 1996).

Intraoperative Management

Once in the OR, the safe administration of anesthesia to children requires meticulous attention to details (Bloch, 1992). General anesthesia for most children undergoing ENT procedures begins with the inhalational induction of anesthetic gases through a clear plastic Guedel face mask placed over the child's nose and mouth. A mixture of nitrous oxide, oxygen, and halothane, a potent, strong-smelling agent, has been the standard since the 1970s. More recently, halothane has been replaced by sevoflurane, a less objectionable-smelling agent that appears to be better tolerated by children (Wark, 1997). After the patient is sufficiently deeply asleep from the inhalational anesthetic, one can place the intravenous cannula. This placement can be a major undertaking in the pediatric age group. In the infant population, veins may be difficult to find due to added tissue and small size. It is important to adequately secure the catheter with tape and an armboard. The intravenous cannula is especially needed for fluid replacement and resuscitation or emergent treatment of a posttonsillectomy hemorrhage.

Patient monitoring guidelines are established by the American Society of Anesthesiologists Committee on Standards. Standard monitoring for routine anesthetics includes the placement of a precordial stethoscope, electrocardiogram, temperature probe, fractional inspired and expired oxygen, end tidal CO_2 monitoring (Badswell, 1992), pulse oximetry, and blood pressure recording (Cass, Crosby, & Holland, 1988; Pearsall, Davison, & Asbury, 1995). The major concern during the sharing of the airway by the otolaryngologist and anesthesiologist is the impedance of oxygen delivery, resulting in hypoxia. Continuous pulse oximetry is the most valuable monitor for assessment of the adequacy of oxygen delivery through detection of oxygen saturation (Goldhill et al., 1990; Mihm & Halperin, 1985; O'Connor & Jones, 1990; Schnapf, 1991). Clinical signs of hypoxemia, such as cyanosis and bradycardia, are late clinical observations. Continuous pulse oximetry enables the anesthesiologist to monitor these hypoxic events earlier and prior to an adverse event such as hypoxic cardiac arrest (Cote, Goldstein, Cote, Hoaglin, & Ryan, 1988; Morray et al., 1993). Blood pressure measurements are more difficult and complicated in children and particularly infants compared to adults, because appropriate cuff sizes and reference values are needed (Menard, 1995; Steiss & Roscher, 1996). In our experience, patients may have falsely elevated blood pressure recording during the anesthetic because of placement of inappropriately sized cuffs. These erroneous measurements lead to treatment errors by administering additional narcotics and increasing inhalational concentration to control the patient's fictional hypertension. This overtreatment may lead to complications of delayed emergence and delays in normal recovery of respiratory activity.

The intubation is accomplished either under deep inhalational agent or by intravenous administration of a neuromuscular agent. The oral RAE (Ring Adair Elwyn) endotracheal tube is preferred for this procedure because its preformed curve angulates away from the operating field. The operating surgeon will place a mouth gag for better exposure prior to the incision. Throughout the surgical procedure, it is important to check for equal breath sounds because the mouth gag may have compressed and displaced the endotracheal tube (Black & Mackersie, 1997; McCoy, Russell, & Webb, 1997).

Postoperative Care

Pain is a common problem after ENT procedures (Toma, Blanshard, Eyman-Lewis, & Bridges, 1995). A recent prospective survey of 167 children aged 1–7 years who had undergone adenoidectomy as a day case revealed the significant impact that this type of surgery has on a child's postoperative course (Kokki & Ahonen, 1997). In this study, 83% of children had pain at home and 17% had moderate or severe pain on a 4-point verbal rating scale. Eighty percent of children required pain medication at home. Consequently, the pediatric patient and their parents are justifiably concerned about the possibility of postoperative pain and the proper and safe relief from such distress. For the patient, the parent, and the healthcare providers, the assessment and treatment of pain in the first 24 hours can be a significant challenge (Bartley & Connew, 1994; Gedaly-Duff & Ziebarth, 1994; Lee & Sharp, 1996; Romsing, Moller-Sonnergaard, Hertel, Lee & Sharp, 1996; Romsing, Moller-Sonnergaard, Hertel, & Rasmussen, 1996; Sutters & Miaskowski, 1997).

A diversity of etiologic factors may contribute to the child's perception of pain (McGrath, 1995). The child's experience of pain may be from the actual physical tissue trauma of the surgical procedure, from progression of the disease process as in a neoplastic growth, and also from the complex interaction of cognitive and emotional developmental behaviors of the child (McGrath & Alpine, 1993). The severity of surgical pain can be related to the surgical technique as seen in patient reports of pain in comparing tonsillectomy performed with a diathermy unit or by ligation technique, (less reportable with diathermy) (Tay, 1996; Weimert, Babyak, & Richter, 1990).

The anesthesiologist controls a large number of pharmacologic agents to relieve pain during otolaryngologic procedures (Majcher, 1992; Yaster, Sola, Pegoli,

& Paidas, 1994). A couple of studies have shown the efficacy of preincisional infiltration of local anesthetics into the peritonsillar pillars prior to tonsillectomy in lessening postoperative pain by blocking nociceptive input (Goldsher et al., 1996; Jebeles, Reilly, Gutierrez, Bradley, & Kissin, 1994). The administration of acetaminophen or ketamine before the operation has been shown to be both safe and effective for alleviating postoperative pain (Murray, Yankelowitz, LeRoux, & Bester, 1987; Romej, Vuepel-Lewis, Merkel, Reynolds, & Quinn, 1996). Ibuprofen is as effective as acetaminophen combined with codeine for postoperative pain control in children after tonsillectomy (St. Charles, Matt, Hamilton, & Katz, 1997). Additionally, the administration of intravenous morphine may be required as a rescue dose in the recovery room period to relieve the child's postoperative discomfort (Mather & Peutrell, 1995). Intraoperatively, the use of steroids injected intravenously has been shown to lessen the postoperative symptoms such as trismus, vomiting, and subsequently more oral intake (April, Callan, Nowak, & Hausdorff, 1996). Even the use of dantrolene has been shown to be effective in the reduction of analgesic requirements after tonsillectomy (Salassa et al., 1988). The use of intraoperative nonsteroidal inflammatory drugs should be used with caution during tonsillectomies because of the observations of increased surgical-site bleeding after the operations (Forrest, Heitlinger, & Revell, 1997; Gallagher, Blauth, & Fornadley, 1995; Judkins, Dray, & Hubbell, 1996; Romsing & Walther-Larsen, 1997; Splinter, Rhine, Roberts, Reid, & MacNeil, 1996). The child who undergoes bilateral myringotomy tube (BMT) procedure will generally require some form of analgesia (Finley, McGrath, Forward, McNeill, & Fitzgerald). The timing of pain medicine administration is especially important for children who are scheduled for brief operations without intravenous catheters. For patients undergoing myringotomy and tube insertion under general anesthesia, the application of 4% lidocaine in antibiotic drops may significantly improve postoperative analgesia (Lawhorn et al., 1996). Oral acetaminophen (15 mg/kg) taken 20 to 40 minutes before BMT surgery assures therapeutic blood levels of the drug after operation. Fifty-four percent of these children will be comfortable in the postanesthesia care unit. Tobias, Lowe, Hersey, Rasmussen, and Werkhaven (1995) further demonstrated in a recent prospective study that the preoperative administration of oral acetaminophen (10 mg/kg) and codeine (1 mg/kg) was significantly more reliable for postoperative pain relief than acetaminophen (15 mg/kg) alone. Watcha and colleagues (1992) compared the postoperative analgesic effects of oral acetaminophen (10 mg/kg) or ketorolac (1 mg/kg) when administered 30 minutes before induction of anesthesia for patients undergoing bilateral myringotomy and concluded that the preoperative administration of oral ketorolac, but not acetaminophen, provided better postoperative pain control. However, there is a concern that the increased cost of ketorolac is not justified for the slight analgesic benefit when compared to acetaminophen (Bean-Lijewski & Stinson, 1997).

The concern with postoperative narcotics for pain control is the documented effect of increasing vomiting, where nonopioid analgesics appear to provide a more satisfactory analgesia and a decreased incidence of vomiting (Kermode, Walker, & Webb, 1995; Matthew & Peutrell, 1995). The incidence of postoperative vomiting after myringotomy is reported to be 2% to 31% and appears to increase with the age of the patient (Markowitz-Spence, Brodsky, Syed, Stanievich, & Volk, 1990; Splinter, Roberts, Rhine, MacNeill, & Komocan, 1995). The incidence of vomiting after tonsillectomy has been reported to be as high as 72% to 25% (Karlsson, Larsson, & Nilsson, 1990; Splinter, Baxter et al., 1995). Recent reports have suggested that the preoperative administration of steroids (Splinter & Roberts, 1996), midazolam (Splinter, MacNeill et al., 1995), ondansetron, or gastrokinetic drug (Ferrari & Donlan, 1992) may be effective in the prevention of nausea and vomiting after tonsillectomy and adenoidectomy. Propofol-based anesthetics as compared to inhalational-based anesthetics have been shown to decrease the incidence of postoperative vomiting in children following tonsillectomy (Barst et al., 1995). Dexamethasone given intraoperatively is also effective in significantly reducing both postoperative pain and vomiting (Catlin & Grimes, 1991; Tom, Templeton, Thompson, & Marsh, 1996). Postoperative nausea and vomiting can be relieved with a variety of antiemetics such as droperidol, metoclopramide, and ondansetron (Lawhorn et al., 1996; Morton et al., 1997; Rose & Martin, 1996). More importantly, prophylactic ondansetron appears more effective than metoclopramide or placebo for the prevention of vomiting after tonsillectomy or adenotonsillectomy (Stene, Seay, Young, Bohnsack, & Bostrom, 1996). Specifically, odanestron administered at 150-μg/kg dose is more effective than the other antiemetics to reduce the incidence of vomiting in posttonsillectomy children (Furst & Rodarte, 1994). However, in a few selective patients, postoperative vomiting may persist despite antiemetic treatment and the avoidance of narcotics. In these particular situations, patients will require hospitalization for intravenous hydration.

SPECIAL ANESTHETIC CONSIDERATIONS

Myringotomy and Insertion of Tympanotomy Tubes

One of the most commonly performed surgical procedures in children is placement of BMTs for recur-

rent otitis media (Bright, Moore, Jeng, Sharkness, & Hamburger, 1993). Patients presenting for myringotomy and tympanotomy are usually healthy. Nevertheless, because ear infections are a commonly diagnosed illness in the pediatric population, the anesthesiologist will encounter a wide spectrum of pediatric patients undergoing surgical placement of myringotomy tubes, with an additional variety of congenital and medical conditions. By far the most common and most controversial coexisting condition in this group of patients is an acute upper respiratory infection (URI) (Van der Walt, 1995).

Children with URIs create a dilemma for the anesthesiologist (Martin, 1994). In 1991, Cohen and Cameron prospectively studied 1,283 children undergoing anesthesia and surgery with a preoperative URI and 20,876 children without URI symptoms (Cohen & Cameron, 1991). Their study discovered that children with a URI were two to seven times more likely to experience respiratory-related adverse events during the intraoperative, recovery room, and postoperative phases of their operative experience. The documented respiratory events included laryngospasm, bronchospasm, stridor, breathholding, and postoperative croup. If a child with a URI required endotracheal intubation, the risk of a respiratory complication increased 11-fold. Their recommendation for children with significant preoperative symptoms of URI is that elective surgery should be postponed for several weeks. Several recent studies have found that children with URI signs and symptoms at the time of surgery or a history of URI in the previous week are at an increased risk of developing transient postoperative hypoxemia (DeSoto, Patel, Soliman, & Hannallah, 1998; Rolf & Cote, 1992). Hypoxemia may not be clinically detected in the OR, and may be first observed in the recovery room after supplemental oxygen has been discontinued (DeSoto et al., Fennelly & Hall, 1990; Levy, Pandit, Lewis, & Tait, 1992). However, the decision to delay BMT surgery in children with acute URI symptoms is controversial (Hinkle, 1989; Jacoby & Hirshman, 1990). While some studies conclude that children with URIs should not be electively anesthetized, one recent retrospective survey of 3,585 patients aged newborn to 20 years undergoing elective surgical procedures reported no significant differences in complication rates between asymptomatic patients (1.61 per 100) and those with URI symptoms (1.64 per 100) (Tait & Knight, 1987a). However, in this study, patients who were asymptomatic but had a recent history of an URI had a significantly higher complication rate (5.31 per 100; $p<.05$) than the asymptomatic patients. There were no significant differences in intraoperative complications between patients managed with and without tracheal intubation, nor was there any association between the type of anesthetic agent used and the development of intraoperative respiratory complications. In fact, patients with chronic infectious nasal discharge can get relief from URI symptoms by the surgical placement of ventilating ear tubes (Tait & Knight, 1987b). Because of the substantial difference of opinion in the literature of managing children with URI symptoms, the anesthesiologist must unavoidably rely on his of her own judgment and skill of what is safe and necessary surgery for the patient. The risk-to-benefit ratio of the surgical procedure must be considered on an individual patient basis. If the patient has significant respiratory symptoms and the surgical procedure is purely elective, then the procedure should be postponed. The more difficult patient scenario is the patient with a nasal discharge, sneezing, and malaise, and no other symptoms. Do the child's symptoms represent a chronic allergic condition or a potentially progressive respiratory illness? What is the degree of risk and benefit for this patient? Pneumonia and pulmonary collapse have been documented as occurring during the anesthetic in the pediatric surgical patient with an existing URI (Campbell, 1990; Williams, Hills, & Goddard, 1992). In today's medical-legal climate, during the postoperative period the anesthesiologist may find it difficult to explain to the parents the child's pneumonic process occurring from the natural course of the preoperative respiratory infection, or secondary to the administration of the anesthetic. The anesthesiologist is preoperatively obliged to inform and discuss with the parent the possible natural sequelae of a respiratory tract allergic or infectious response, and the concerns with administering an anesthetic during this period of illness. The discussion should include the observation of the several previous URI studies mentioned. The parent, anesthesiologist, and surgeon can then make an informed and appropriate plan for the child.

Anesthetic Management

The surgical procedure is generally very short and lasts 5 to 10 minutes in an experienced surgeon's hands. Most anesthesiologists will not place an intravenous catheter for such a short surgical procedure. While this may appear to simplify perioperative care, the anesthesiologist should not minimize the potential anesthetic risks during short surgical procedures. One recent study of 510 children during tympanotomy tube placement reported a 13% incidence of airway obstruction that required interventions including airway manipulation, positive pressure ventilation, and endotracheal intubation (Markowitz-Spence et al., 1990). The decision to forgo vascular access places additional burdens on the practitioner who must be prepared to start an intravenous catheter in the event of an emergency. He must

also insure that the child is adequately hydrated *per os* prior to discharge from the day surgery unit.

Anesthetic Management of the Child Undergoing Tonsillectomy and Adenoidectomy

This section will highlight important considerations when delivering anesthesia for the pediatric patient undergoing tonsillectomy and adenoidectomy. Tonsillectomy and adenoidectomy is one of the most common inpatient surgical procedures in children under 15 years of age (Derkay, 1993).

The clinical assessment of fluid losses and subsequent replacement of intravenous fluid can be difficult for the anesthesiologist. The reason for this is the inability to accurately measure blood loss during the removal of adenoids and tonsils because of the unmeasured blood draining into the stomach. Therefore, many anesthesiologists are encouraged to be liberal with fluid replacement to counteract for the period of preoperative fasting, the blood loss during the procedure, and postoperatively when the patient may be unable to adequately meet fluid requirements because of pain and vomiting. The anesthesiologist should be infusing a hypertonic solution, such as normal saline or Normosol, to prevent the complication of iatrogenic hyponatremia (McRae, Weissburg, & Chang, 1994).

Once the surgical procedure is complete and prior to extubation, an orogastric tube should be gently placed to empty the stomach of any residual blood. Blood in the stomach may be a strong stimulus for postoperative nausea and vomiting. The oral cavity should also be inspected for active bleeding and suctioned for blood and secretions prior to extubation. Any throat packs should be accounted for and removed. Most anesthesiologists extubate the child awake because the patient's protective airway reflexes are intact and airway patency is easier to maintain (Karam, Najm, Kattar, & Raphael, 1995). A few anesthesiologists recommend deep extubation because of the belief that there is less coughing and blood pressure elevation, which may result in increased tonsillar bed bleeding. A recent study did show increased respiratory episodes of desaturation during awake tracheal extubation when compared to extubation during the deeply anesthetized state (Pounder, Blackstock, & Steward, 1991). However, Patel et al. (1991) confirmed no differences between the two styles of extubation in the incidence of airway-related complications such as laryngospasm, croup, sore throat, excessive coughing, and arrhythmias The patient is transported to the recovery room in the lateral position to prevent aspiration of blood. The patient in the recovery room is watched for any bleeding and any signs of airway obstruction. Intravenous fluids are continued for several hours until the patient can adequately take fluids by mouth.

Postoperative Problems

Postoperative bleeding is a most alarming complication after tonsillectomy. Hemorrhage is the most frequent complication of tonsillectomy and is responsible for the majority of posttonsillectomy fatalities. Despite continued efforts to reduce this problem, it remains a persistent risk (Szeremeta, Novelly, & Benninger, 1996). A recent study by Myssiorek and Alvi (1996) reviewed the charts of 1,138 patients who underwent tonsillectomy with or without adenoidectomy and found posttonsillectomy hemorrhage occurred in 36 patients (3%). Postoperative bleeding occurred more often in older patients (69% over age 11 years). The majority of these patients presented after postoperative day one (83%). Other studies have shown that postoperative bleeding occurs earlier, within the first 12 hours, and a smaller number 1 week later (Irani & Berkowitz, 1997; Schroeder, 1995). The patient that presents for reoperation for persistent bleeding creates many potential problems for the anesthesiologist. The patient may be hypovolemic from the blood loss and have cardiac instability on induction of the anesthetic. During the induction, the patient can aspirate residual blood clots in the stomach, leading to pneumonitis. The attempted intubation of the airway may be difficult to visualize because of blood obscuring the trachea. The patient can develop obstruction of the airway from a blood clot, leading to subsequent hypoxia. Therefore, for the safety of the patient, prior to induction the anesthesiologist must be sure of an adequately functioning intravenous catheter, have blood typed and crossed, restore intravascular volume losses, and have the presence of the surgeon with available emergency airway equipment.

ANESTHESIA FOR ENDOSCOPY AND BRONCHOSCOPY

Pediatric Endoscopy and Microsurgery of the Airway

Patients with a variety of congenital and acquired airway or pulmonary problems require laryngoscopy or bronchoscopy. Most of these children present with some degree of respiratory distress manifested by stridor, such as obstruction to normal airflow through the tracheobronchial tree. Pediatric conditions that may present with stridor include tracheal foreign body (Black, Johnson, & Matlack), congential tracheomalacia (Mancuso, 1996), congenital vascular anomalies (Valleta,

Pregarz, Bergama-Andreis, & Boners, 1997), laryngeal trauma (Gold, Gerber, Shott, & Myer, 1997), juvenile papillomatosis (Sakoh et al., 1993), epiglottitis, and bacterial tracheitis (Eckel, Widemann, Domm, & Roth, 1993). Serial airway examinations may be undertaken after tracheotomy (Tom, Miller, Wetmore, Handler, & Potsic, 1993) or tracheobronchial reconstruction (Kamata et al., 1997).

Among all of the procedures in the operating suite, endoscopic procedures require the closest cooperation between the anesthesiologist and the surgeon, whose functional roles of ventilation and examination are often in conflict. This is no place for novices, the meek, or the faint of heart! Techniques of extraordinary permissive hypercapnia (Dries, 1995), intermittent jet ventilation (Baraka, 1996; Chan, Wei, Lau, & Lam, 1990; Donner, Schragh, & Aloy, 1997), or spontaneous stimulated ventilation through extremely narrow endoscopic equipment, demand exquisite attention to details of gas concentrations and delivery and often subtle changes in the patient's cardiorespiratory physiology.

Preoperative Preparation

Procedures during which the airway is shared by the anesthesiologist and surgeon will require a thorough preoperative assessment of the child's most probable surgical pathology. The delivery of anesthetic agents and ventilation of children with suspected epiglottitis, tracheal foreign body, or laryngomalacia may be very different than for confirmation of a vascular ring or right middle lobe pneumonia (Table 22–3)

Preoperative Medications

Preoperative considerations of the surgical condition will influence decisions about premedication. Children with altered mental states, disordered control of ventilation, a history of apnea, or symptoms of airway obstruction are observed to demonstrate impaired or even paradoxical ventilatory depression in the face of hypoxia or hypercarbia (Alexander & Gross, 1988; Arens et al., 1994; Gozal, Arens, Omlin, Jacobs & Keens, 1995; Knill & Gelb, 1978; Liv et al., 1983). These symptoms may be exacerbated by the administration of sedatives or narcotics (Henson & Ward, 1994; Yaster, Nichols, Deshpande, & Wetzel, 1990). Understanding that narcotics, sedatives, and general anesthetics all depress respirations, it may be judicious to limit sedation of patients for whom spontaneous ventilation during surgery will be desirable. By the same token, intraoperative respiratory stimulants (e.g., doxapram) (O'Connor, Levy, & Peacock, 1996; Sun, 1990; Yoshikawa, Yamamoto, Nishimura, & Kawakami, 1987) may be helpful in preserving spontaneous ventilation during airway procedures.

Intraoperative Care

Most patients undergoing endoscopy with a rigid device will require general anesthesia using any of a variety of combinations of inhaled and intravenous agents and local anesthetics, utilizing many ventilation techniques (Table 22–4). Apneic oxygenation or permissive hypoventilation has been used to permit access to the airway for procedures that cannot be accomplished with an endotracheal tube or other artificial airway in the trachea. Severe hypercapnia in children from airway obstruction up to 269 torr is tolerated without long-term cardiac or neurological sequelae as long as arterial oxygen saturation is preserved (Goldstein & Shannon, 1990).

Table 22-3. Ventilation during airway procedures.

Spontaneous ventilation is desirable	
Laryngomalacia[a]	Diagnosis by direct visualization of laryngeal collapses during inspiration.
Tracheal foreign body[b]	Life-threatening total airway obstruction may occur if the foreign body moves deeper into the airway with positive pressure ventilation.[c]
Epiglottitis[d]	In severe cases, the spontaneous movement of air through an inflamed edematous epiglottis may be the only means of identifying the patient's larynx.
Spontaneous ventilation is not necessary	
Lung lavage	
Tracheal reconstruction	
Confirmation of congenital vascular ring	

[a]Baxter, 1994; Hinton, O'Connell, von Besouw, & Wyatt, 1997; Waters, Woo, Mortelliti, & Colton, 1996
[b]Kain & O'Conner, 1994
[c]Woods, 1990
[d]Morgan-Hughes & Wilkinson, 1995; Stehling, 1987

Table 22-4. Ventilation devices used during endoscopic procedures.

Ventilating bronchoscope	Ventilation through a specialized sidearm on the bronchoscope. *Advantages:* Permits excellent visibility for the airway evaluation by the surgeon and continuous uninterrupted spontaneous or controlled ventilation. *Disadvantages:* airway resistance may increase with telescope in place leading to impaired ventilation or hyperinflation of the lungs (Hoeve, Rombout,& Meursing, 1993; Redleaf et al., 1995).
Manual jet ventilation (Gros et al., 1997)	Ventilation accomplished by using high velocity jets of air and oxygen directed from a canula placed in the oral pharynx. Technique does not require endotracheal intubation and is therefore useful during laryngoscopic, but not bronchoscopic, procedures. *Advantages:* Permits controlled ventilation without the placement of a device into the trachea. *Disadvantages:* Does not permit the use of inhaled anesthetic agents and the control of anesthetic depth. Increased incidence of barotrauma. Cannot be used during laser surgery.
Pharyngeal insufflation (Aun, Houghton, So, Van Hasselt, & Oh, 1990; Baxter, 1994)	Spontaneous ventilation of anesthetic agents at high flow rates using a cannula placed in the mouth. *Advantages:* Permits airway surgery free of bulky mechanical devices obstructing access to the airway. *Disadvantages:* High incidence of hypoxia and hypoventilation. Operating suite pollution in excess of OSHA guidelines (Rita, Seleny, & Holinger, 1983; Sorensen, 1987).
Apneic oxygenation (Cohen, Herbert, & Thompson, 1988; Hawkins & Joseph, 1990; Weisberger & Ernhardt, 1996)	The endotracheal tube is removed for the laser procedure. The patient is constantly paralyzed and O_2 saturation is monitored. *Advantages:* Unobstructed view of the airway and no concern for ignition of the endotracheal tube. *Disadvantages:* The surgical time is limited to 2 to 4 minutes and periodic intubation of the airway is required. Hypoventilation can lead to acidosis and arrhythmias.

Pouiseille's Law

Anatomic or equipment-induced obstruction to airflow is observed during many endoscopic procedures. There are two components to this: resistance to laminar flow and turbulence created when air passes through tubes that are partially obstructed. The first component, resistance to laminar airflow, is due to the overall narrow diameter of the pediatric trachea and bronchi. Pouiseille's equation, $R = 8ln/r^4$, describes this relationship. Resistance to the flow of air through a tube is directly related to the viscosity (n) of the air and inversely proportional to the fourth power of its radius (r). Predictably, the smaller pediatric airway will offer more resistance to airflow than the trachea of a larger adult. Hence, airway resistance is normally high in children. The resistance to airflow through a very narrow bronchoscope can be extremely high. In this situation, the addition of helium to the inspired gas mixture is effective in improving ventilation by decreasing inspired air viscosity component of airway resistance (McGee, Wald, & Hinchliffe, 1997).

A graphic representation of laminar and turbulent airflow is seen in the Figure 22–1. Inspired air through an airway flows smoothly (A), until passing though an area of sudden obstruction (B), where eddies of deflected air current are established. These areas of less organized turbulence are less effective sources of ventilation.

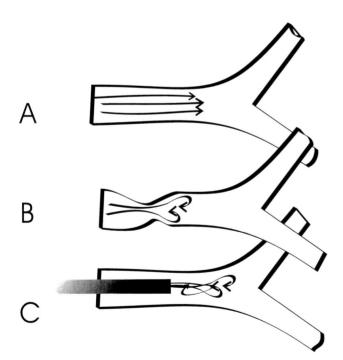

Figure 22–1. Flow characteristics through an obstructed airway: laminar vs. turbulent airflow. **A.** Laminar flow through a normal airway. **B.** Inefficient turbulent airflow passing through an area of tracheal obstruction. **C.** Turbulent flow patterns of gas directed through a narrow ventilating bronchoscope placed in a small child's trachea.

Emergence and Postoperative Care

On completion of the endoscopy, the anesthesiologist must be prepared to reestablish the patient's airway. Before the endoscopist removes the scope from the airway, there needs to be an assessment of the patient's ability to adequately maintain his or her own airway. Should the bronchoscope be removed and the patient satisfactorily masked during the emergence or should an endotracheal tube be placed to guarantee an adequate airway? The nature of the surgical procedure can cause increased airway edema from prolonged instrumentation, and therefore an endotracheal tube with concomitant administration of steroids will be needed for a period of time. Was the induction of the patient difficult with frequent airway obstruction? Was it difficult to maintain an adequate seal with the mask and appropriately to ventilate the patient? This preoperative situation may warrant placement of an endotracheal tube until the patient is alert and able to maintain pharyngeal tone to keep the airway patent. Is the patient's stomach empty of air or gastric contents? Does a suction catheter need to be passed to relieve gastric distension from possible positive pressure mask ventilation? In addition, the endoscopist and bronchoscopy equipment must remain in the OR during the extubation. During emergence one must be concerned about laryngospasm and a plan developed as to how to treat the event. Is the intravenous line still functioning and is it secure? Is there an available endotracheal tube and laryngoscope for reintubation? Are intubating drugs readily available? Postoperative stridor and dyspnea following instrumentation are frequent. The patient should be observed in the OR for a period of time after extubation for the possibility of progressive airway obstruction (Hoeve et al., 1993). The patient may have mild to moderate airway stridor, and may benefit from a trial of racemic epinephrine or steroids. The OR is the best time to treat these events, *not* the time the child is being wheeled down the corridor. The patient should receive oxygen during transport and in the recovery room to guard against unrecognized hypoxia (Brown, Purcell, & Traugott, 1990; Fossum & Knowles, 1995; Xue et al., 1996). After discontinuation of oxygen therapy, the patient should have a confirmed normal oxygen saturation on room air prior to being discharged from the recovery room. The final decision to discharge the patient from the hospital depends on on a number of factors, such as the difficulty of the procedure, whether the patient still has or has the potential for significant airway compromise, and the age of the patient.

LARYNGEAL MICROSURGERY WITH THE LASER

A laser (light amplification by the stimulated emission of radiation) is a device that produces an intense beam of light that can be focused and precisely controlled to coagulate, incise, or vaporize tissue. Laser surgery provides a bloodless field with minimal edema. Lasers are used for excision of a number of airway lesions. There are a number of types of lasers used for specific airway surgery, such as the CO_2, Nd:Yag laser, and the potassium titanyl phosphate (KTP) laser. The CO_2 laser emits infrared light, which is absorbed by the water in the tissue, and is therefore used to excise pathological tissue. A common use of the CO_2 laser is the management of laryngeal papillomatosis. These viral tumors multiply and can cause significant airway compromise. Often, children with laryngeal papillomatosis require multiple surgical procedures throughout childhood to maintain airway patency. The ND:Yag laser is better absorbed by pigmented tissue and is primarily used for treatment of hemangiomas and debulking tumors. The KTP laser is increasingly used in flexible fiberoptic laser systems. The use of a flexible fiberoptic laser provides a means of delivering laser energy into extremely small airways that are unreachable by the common CO_2 techniques (Rimelli et al., 1996).

Anesthetic Management

The anesthetic principles for laser surgery are for the most part similar to the basic considerations during endoscopy. However, laser surgery has inherent hazards related to high-energy ray (Sliney, 1995). During laser airway surgery, risk of fire in the airway is the greatest morbidity factor. The laser beam can ignite the endotracheal tube, the breathing circuit, drapes, oil-based lubricants, and basically any combustible material. One needs to protect and cover the patient's eyes with saline-soaked gauze. OR personnel need to wear specially tinted safety glasses that absorb the spectral energy of potentially stray laser light. Most patients undergoing laser airway surgery need to be immobilized, so that laser rays are intentionally directed to abnormal tissue and do not accidentally strike normal tissue or combustible material. Therefore, most laser surgery procedures are done under general anesthesia with muscle paralysis to ensure no random or stray laser beams. Airway patency can be maintained with an endotracheal tube in place or by a laryngoscope in combination with jet ventilation. If the anesthesiologist should choose the use of an endotracheal tube, he or she must be aware of the potential flammability of the tube. Endotracheal tubes vary in their ignitability and flammability (Fontenot, Bailey, Stiernberg, & Jenicek, 1987; Sosis, Braverman, & Caldarelli, 1996; Wolf & Simpson, 1987). A number of manufacturers make special tubes that will not ignite, such as those made of spiral stainless steel (Fried et al., 1991). However, many of these tubes may have a PVC cuff that is flammable. If one uses a tube with a cuff, it is encouraged to inflate the tube with saline to which a small amount of methyl-

ene blue has been added. The saline acts as a heat sink to absorb the laser energy and lessens the chance of ignition; the colored saline will be an indicator of a possible cuff perforation from an inadvertent laser beam. One can cover such tubes with metal foil in an overlapping fashion to lessen the chance for ignition (Sosis & Braverman, 1993; Sosis et al., 1996; Sosi & Dillon, 1990). However, covered tubes and specially designed tubes can catch fire in the presence of oxygen. Polyvinyl tubes and silicon tubes can ignite when pulsed by a laser beam, and specially shielded laser tubes and red rubber endotracheal tubes will ignite in an atmosphere of 30% oxygen in helium when the laser is used in the continuous mode (Ossoff, 1989). The fractional concentration of oxygen delivered in the airway should be minimized to reduce the maintenance combustion. The concentration of air to oxygen should be maximally 30%, as long as adequate oxygenation is insured by measurements from the continuous use of pulse oximetry. Nitrous oxide should not be used because it can support combustion (Wolf & Simpson, 1987). It is safe to use helium in place of air because it has a higher thermal conductivity, which could delay the ignition time of an endotracheal tube. However, helium oxygen mixture has only proven safe with the CO_2 laser; the use of KTP laser helium did not delay the ignition times at various oxygen concentrations (Al Haddad & Brenner, 1994). The treatment of fire in the airway is to stop the source of oxygen, douse the fire with sterile water or saline, remove the tube, and subsequently ventilate with oxygen. Another endotracheal tube and a bronchoscope should be available to reestablish and examine the injured airway. If the airway damage is severe, the patient may need a prolonged course of mechanical ventilation. Steroids or antibiotics may be necessary. If the damage to the airway is severe, the surgeon may have to perform an emergent tracheostomy. Airway fires have been reported without the use of lasers. There are a number of case reports of endotracheal tube fires from an electrocautery during tracheostomy and during electrodissection of tonsils (Keller, Elliott, & Hubbell, 1992; Le Clair, Gartner, & Halma, 1990; Lew, Mittleman, & Murray, 1991; Marsh & Riley, 1992; Simpson & Wolf, 1986).

Other hazards irrespective of fire in the airway during laser surgery are inadvertent injury to normal tissue, smoke inhalation, and particulate debris aspirated in the airway.

References:

Alexander, C. M., & Gross, J. B. (1988). Sedative doses of midazolam depress hypoxic ventilatory responses in humans. *Anesthesia and Analgesia, 67*(4), 377–382.

Al Haddad, S., & Brenner, J. (1994). Helium and lower oxygen concentration do not prolong tracheal tube ignition time during potassium titanyl phosphate laser use. *Anesthesiology, 80*(4), 936–938.

April, M. M., Callan, N. D., Nowak, D. M., & Hausdorff, M. A. (1996). The effect of intravenous dexamethasone in pediatric adenotonsillectomy. *Archives of Otolaryngology—Head and Neck Surgery, 122*(2), 117–120

Arens, R., Gozal, D., Omlin, K. J., Livingston, F. R., Liu, J., Keens, T. G., & Ward, S. L. (1994). Hypoxic and hypercapnic ventilatory responses in Prader-Willi syndrome. *Journal of Applied Physiology. 77*(5), 2224–2230.

Aun, C. S., Houghton, I. T., So, H. Y., Van Hasselt, C. A., & Oh, T. E. (1990). Tubeless anaesthesia for microlaryngeal surgery. *Anaesthesia and Intensive Care, 18*(4), 497–503.

Badgwell, J. M. (1992). Respiratory gas monitoring in the pediatric patient. *International Anesthesiology Clinics, 30*(3), 131–146.

Baraka, A. (1996). Oxygen enrichment of entrained room air during venturi jet ventilation of children undergoing bronchoscopy. *Paediatric Anaesthesia, 6*(5), 383–385.

Barst, S. M., Markowitz, A., Yossefy, Y., Abramson, A., Lebowitz, P. , & Bienkowsk, R. S. (1995). Propofol reduces the incidence of vomiting after tonsillectomy in children. *Paediatric Anaesthesia, 5*(4), 249–252.

Bartley, J. R., & Connew, A. M. (1995). Parental attitudes and postoperative problems related to paediatric day stay tonsillectomy. *New Zealand Medical Journal, 107*(989), 451–452.

Baxter, M. R. (1994). Congenital laryngomalacia. [Review]. *Canadian Journal of Anaesthesia, 41*(4), 332–339.

Bean-Lijewski, J. D., & Stinson, J. C. (1997). Acetaminophen or ketorolac for post myringotomy pain in children? A prospective, double-blinded comparison. *Paediatric Anaesthesia, 7*(2), 131–137.

Benton, N. C., & Wolgat, R. A. (1993). Sudden cardiac arrest during adenotonsillectomy in a patient with subclinical Duchenne's muscular dystrophy. *Ear, Nose, and Throat Journal, 72*(2), 130–131.

Berry, F. A. (1990). *Anesthetic management of difficult routine pediatric patients* (2nd ed., p. 37). London: Churchill Livingston.

Biavati, M. J., Manning, S. C., & Phillips, D. L. (1997). Predictive factors for respiratory complications after tonsillectomy and adenoidectomy in children. *Archives of Otolaryngology—Head and Neck Surgery, 123*(5), 517-521.

Black, A. E., & Mackersie, A. M. (1991). Accidental bronchial intubation with RAE tubes. *Anaesthesia, 46*(1), 42–43.

Black, R. E., Johnson, D. G., & Matlak, M. E (1994). Bronchoscopic removal of aspirated foreign bodies in children. *Journal of Pediatric Surgery, 29*(5), 682–684.

Bloch, E. C. (1992). Update on anesthesia management for infants and children. *Surgical Clinics of North America, 72*(6), 1207–1221.

Bower, C. M., & Richmond, D. (1995). Tonsillectomy and adenoidectomy in patients with Down syndrome. *International Journal of Pediatric Otorhinolaryngology, 33*(2), 141-148.

Bragg, C. I., & Miller, B. R. (1990). Oral ketamine facilitates induction in a combative mentally retarded patient. *Journal of Clinical Anesthesia, 2*(2), 121-122.

Bright, R. A., Moore, R. M, Jr., Jeng, L. L., Sharkness, C. M., Hamburger, S. E., & Hamilton, P. M. (1988). The prevalence of tympanostomy tubes in children in the United States, 1988. *American Journal of Public Health, 3*(7), 1026-1028.

Brown, L. T., Purcell, G. J., & Traugott, F. M. (1990). Hypoxaemia during postoperative recovery using continuous pulse oximetry. *Anethesia and Intensive Care, 18*(4), 509–516.

Bunting, H. E., & Allen, R. W. (1997). Prolonged muscle weakness following emergency tonsillectomy in a patient with familial periodic paralysis and infectious mononucleosis. *Paediatric Anaesthesia, 7*(2), 171–175.

Burk, C. D., Miller, L., Handler, S. D., & Cohen, A. R. (1992). Preoperative history and coagulation screening in children undergoing tonsillectomy. *Pediatrics, 89*(4, Pt. 2), 691–695.

Campbell, N. N. (1990). Respiratory tract infection and anaesthesia. Haemophilus influenzae pneumonia that developed under anaesthesia. *Anaesthesia, 45*(7), 561–562.

Cass, N. M., Crosby, W. M., & Holland, R. B. (1988). Minimal monitoring standards. *Anaesthesia and Intensive Care, 16*(1), 110–113.

Catlin, F. I., & Grimes, W. J. (1991). The effect of steroid therapy on recovery from tonsillectomy in children. *Archives of Otolaryngology—Head and Neck Surgery. 117*(6), 649–652.

Chan, A. S., Wei, W. I., Lau, W. F., & Lam, K. H. (1990). Modified jet ventilation during total laryngectomy: A prospective study using pulse oximetry and a pressure regulator. *Anaesthesia and Intensive Care, 18*(4), 504–508.

Christensen, S., Farrow-Gillespie, A., & Lerman, J. (1990). Effects of ranitidine and metoclopramide on gastric fluid pH and volume in children. *British Journal of Anaesthesia, 65*(4), 456–460.

Cioaca, R., & Canavea, I. (1996). Oral transmucosal ketamine: An effective premedication in children. *Paediatric Anaesthesia, 6*(5), 361–365.

Close, H. L., Kryzer, T. C., Nowlin, J. H., & Alving, B. M. (1994). Hemostatic assessment of patients before tonsillectomy: A prospective study. *Otolaryngology—Head and Neck Surgery, 111*(6), 733-738.

Cohen, M. M., & Cameron, C. B. (1991). Should you cancel the operation when a child has an upper respiratory tract infection? *Anesthesia and Analgesia, 72*(3), 282–288.

Cohen, S. R., Herbert, W. I., & Thompson, J. W. (1988). Anesthesia management of microlaryngeal laser surgery in children: Apneic technique anesthesia. *Laryngoscope, 98*(3), 347–348.

Cote, C. J., Goldstein, E. A., Cote, M. A., Hoaglin, D. C., & Ryan, J. F. (1988). A single-blind study of pulse oximetry in children. *Anesthesiology, 68*(2), 184–188.

Cray, S. H., Dixon, J. L., Heard, C. M, & Selsby, D. S. (1996). Oral midazolam premedication for paediatric day case patients. *Paediatric Anaesthesia, 6*(4), 265–270.

Derkay, C. S. (1993). Pediatric otolaryngology procedures in the United States: 1977–1987. *International Journal of Pediatric Otorhinolaryngology, 25*(1/3), 1–12.

DeSoto, H., Patel, R. I., Soliman, I. E., & Hannallah, R. S. (1988). Changes in oxygen saturation following general anesthesia in children with upper respiratory infection signs and symptoms undergoing otolaryngological procedures. *Anesthesiology, 68*(2), 276–279.

Diaz, J. H. (1997). Intranasal ketamine preinduction of paediatric outpatients. *Paediatric Anaesthesia, 7*(4), 273-278.

Dries, D. J. (1995). Permissive hypercapnia. [Review]. *Journal of Trauma, 39*(5), 984–969.

Eckel, H. E., Widemann, B., Damm, M., & Roth, B. (1993). Airway endoscopy in the diagnosis and treatment of bacterial tracheitis in children. *International Journal of Pediatric Otorhinolaryngology, 27*(2), 147–157.

Eckenhoff, J. E. (1953). Relationship of anesthesia to postoperative personality changes in children. *American Journal of Disabilities in Children, 86*, 587–591.

Epstein, R. H., Mendel, H. G., Witkowski, T. A., Waters, R., Guarniari, K. M., Marr, A. T., & Lessin, J. B. (1996). The safety and efficacy of oral transmucosal fentanyl citrate for preoperative sedation in young children. *Anesthesia and Analgesia, 83*(6), 1200–1205.

Fennelly, M. E., & Hall, G. M. (1990). Anaesthesia and upper respiratory tract infections—a non-existent hazard? *British Journal of Anaesthesia, 64*(5), 535–536.

Ferrari, L. R., & Donlon, J. V. (1992). Metoclopramide reduces the incidence of vomiting after tonsillectomy in children. *Anesthesia and Analgesia, 75*(3), 351–354.

Finley, G. A., McGrath, P. J., Forward, S. P., McNeill, G., & Fitzgerald, P. (1996). Parents' management of children's pain following "minor" surgery. *Pain, 64*(1), 838-847.

Foley, P. J., Beste, D. J., & Farber, N. E. (1997). Massive blood loss during tonsillectomy in a child with congenital venous malformation. *Paediatric Anaesthesia, 7*(3), 243–246.

Fontenot, R., Jr., Bailey, B. J., Stiernberg, C. M., & Jenicek, J. A. (1987). Endotracheal tube safety during laser surgery. *Laryngoscope, 97*(8, Pt. 1), 919–921.

Forrest, J. B., Heitlinger, E. L., & Revell, S. (1997). Ketorolac for postoperative pain management in children. *Drug Safety, 16*(5), 309–329.

Fossum, S. R., & Knowles, R. (1995). Perioperative oxygen saturation levels of pediatric patients. *Journal of Post Anesthesia Nursing, 10*(6), 313–319.

Fried, M. P., Mallampati, S. R., Liu, F. C., Kaplan, S., Caminear, D. S., & Samonte, B. R. (1991). Laser resistant stainless steel endotracheal tube: Experimental and clinical evaluation. *Lasers in Surgery and Medicine, 11*(3), 301–306.

Furst, S. R., & Rodarte, A. (1994). Prophylactic antiemetic treatment with ondansetron in children undergoing tonsillectomy. *Anesthesiology, 81*(4), 799–803.

Gallagher, J. E., Blauth, J., & Fornadley, J. A. (1995). Perioperative ketorolac tromethamine and postoperative hemorrhage in cases of tonsillectomy and adenoidectomy. *Laryngoscope, 105*(6), 606–609.

Gedaly-Duff, V., & Ziebarth, D. (1994). Mothers' management of adenoid-tonsillectomy pain in 4- to 8-year-olds: A preliminary study. *Pain, 57*(3), 293–299.

Gerber, M. E., O'Connor, D. M., Adler, E., & Myer, C. M., III. (1996). Selected risk factors in pediatric adenotonsillectomy. *Archives of Otolaryngology—Head and Neck Surgery, 122*(8), 811–814.

Gillerman, R. G., Hinkle, A. J., Green, H. M., Cornell, L., & Dodge, C. P. (1996). Parental presence plus oral midazolam decreases frequency of 5% halothane inductions in children. *Journal of Clinical Anesthesia, 8*(6), 480–485.

Gold, S. M., Gerber, M. E., Shott, S. R., & Myer, C. M., III. (1997). Blunt laryngotracheal trauma in children. *Archives of Otolaryngology—Head and Neck Surgery, 123*(1), 83–87.

Goldhill, D. R., Hill, A. J., Whitburn, R. H., Feneck, R. O., George, P. J., & Keeling, P. (1990). Carboxyhaemoglobin concentrations, pulse oximetry and arterial blood-gas tensions during jet ventilation for Nd-YAG laser bronchoscopy. *British Journal of Anaesthesia, 65*(6), 749–753.

Goldsher, M., Podoshin, L., Fradis, M., Malatskey, S., Gerstel, R., Vaida, S., & Gaitini, L. (1995). Effects of peritonsillar infiltration on post-tonsillectomy pain. A double-blind study. *Annals of Otology, Rhinology and Laryngology, 105*(11), 868–870.

Goldstein, B., Shannon, D. C., & Todres, I. D. (1990). Supercarbia in children: clinical course and outcome. *Critical Care Medicine, 18*(2), 166–168.

Gozal, D., Arens, R., Omlin, K. J., Jacobs, R. A., & Keens, T. G. (1995). Peripheral chemoreceptor function in children with myelomeningocele and Arnold-Chiari malformation type 2. *Chest, 108*(2), 425–431.

Grasl, M. C., Donner, A., Schragl, E., & Aloy, A. (1997). Tubeless laryngotracheal surgery in infants and children via jet ventilation laryngoscope. *Laryngoscope, 107*(2), 277–281.

Greenspun, J. C., Hannallah, R. S., Welborn, L. G., & Norden, J. M. (1995). Comparison of sevoflurane and halothane anesthesia in children undergoing outpatient ear, nose, and throat surgery. *Journal of Clinical Anesthesia, 7*(5), 398–402.

Gronnebech, H., Johansson, G., Smedebol, M., & Valentin, N. (1993). Glycopyrrolate vs. atropine during anaesthesia for laryngoscopy and bronchoscopy. *Acta Anaesthesiologica Scandinavica, 37*(5), 454–457.

Guldbrand, P., & Mellstrom, A. (1995). Rectal versus intramuscular morphine-scopolamine as premedication in children. *Acta Anaesthesiologica Scandinavica, 39*(2), 224–227.

Hannallah, R. S. (1995). Pediatric ambulatory anesthesia: role of parents. *Journal of Clinical Anesthesia, 7*(7), 597-599.

Hawkins, D. B., & Joseph, M. M. (1990). Avoiding a wrapped endotracheal tube in laser laryngeal surgery: Experiences with apneic anesthesia and metal laser-flex. *Laryngoscope. 100*(12), 1283–1287.

Henson, L. C., & Ward, D. S. (1994). Effects of anaesthetics and sedatives on the control of breathing. [Review]. *Annals of the Academy of Medicine, Singapore, 23*(6, Suppl.), 125–129.

Hinkle, A. J. (1989). What wisdom is there in administering elective general anesthesia to children with active upper respiratory tract infection? *Anesthesia and Analgesia, 68*(3), 414–415.

Hinton, A. E., O'Connell, J. M., van Besouw, J. P., & Wyatt, M. E. (1997). Neonatal and paediatric fibre-optic laryngoscopy and bronchoscopy using the laryngeal mask airway. *Journal of Laryngology and Otology, 111*(4), 349–353.

Hoeve, L. J., Rombout, J., & Meursing, A. E. (1993). Complications of rigid laryngo-bronchoscopy in children. *International Journal of Pediatric Otorhinolaryngology, 26*(1), 47–56.

Hofley, M. A., Hofley, P. M., Keon, T. P., Gallagher, P. R., Poon, C., & Liacouras, C. A. (1995). A placebo-controlled trial using intravenous atropine as an adjunct to conscious sedation in pediatric esophagogastroduodenoscopy. *Gastrointestinal Endoscopy, 42*(5), 457–460.

Irani, D. B., & Berkowitz, R. G. (1997). Management of secondary hemorrhage following pediatric adenotonsillectomy. *International Journal of Pediatric Otorhinolaryngology, 40*(2/3), 115–124.

Jacobs, I. N., Gray, R. F., & Todd, N. W. (1996). Upper airway obstruction in children with Down syndrome. *Archives of Otolaryngology—Head and Neck Surgery, 122*(9), 945–950.

Jacoby, D. B., & Hirshman, C. A. (1991). General anesthesia in patients with viral respiratory infections: an unsound sleep? *Anesthesiology, 74*(6), 969–972.

Jahr, J. S., Burckart, G., Smith, S. S., Shapiro, J., & Cook D. R. (1991). Effects of famotidine on gastric pH and residual volume in pediatric surgery. *Acta Anaesthesiologica Scandinavica, 35*(5), 457–460.

Jebeles, J. A., Reilly, J. S., Gutierrez, J. F., Bradley, E. L , Jr., & Kissin, I. (1991).The effect of pre-incisional infiltration of tonsils with bupivacaine on the pain following tonsillectomy under general anesthesia. *Pain, 47*(3), 305–308.

Johannesson, G. P., Floren, M., & Lindahl, S. G. (1995). Sevoflurane for ENT-surgery in children. A comparison with halothane. *Acta Anaesthesiologica Scandinavica, 39*(4), 546–550.

Judkins, J. H., Dray, T. G., & Hubbell, R. N. (1996). Intraoperative ketorolac and posttonsillectomy bleeding. *Archives of Otolaryngology—Head and Neck Surgery, 122*(9), 937–940.

Kain, Z. N., Ferris, C. A., Mayes, L. C., & Rimar, S. (1996). Parental presence during induction of anaesthesia: Practice differences between the United States and Great Britain. *Paediatric Anaesthesia, 6*(3), 187–193.

Kain, Z. N., Mayes, L. C., Caramico, L. A., Silver, D., Spieker, M., Nygren, M. M., Anderson, G., & Rimar, S. (1996). Parental presence during induction of anesthesia. A randomized controlled trial. *Anesthesiology, 84*(5), 1060–1067.

Kain, Z. N., O'Connor, T. Z., & Berde, C. B. (1994). Management of tracheobronchial and esophageal foreign bodies in children: A survey study. *Journal of Clinical Anesthesia. 6*(1), 28–32.

Kamata, S., Usui, N., Ishikawa, S., Kitayama, Y., Sawai, T., Okuyama, H., Fukui, Y., & Okada, A. (1997). Experience in tracheobronchial reconstruction with a costal cartilage graft for congenital tracheal stenosis. *Journal of Pediatric Surgery, 32*(1), 54–57.

Karam, R., Najm, J. C., Kattar, M., & Raphael, N. (1995). Respiratory complications in children emerging from halothane anesthesia—awake vs. deep extubation. *Middle East Journal of Anesthesiology, 13*(2), 221–229.

Karl, H. W., Keifer, A. T., Rosenberger, J. L., Larach, M. G., & Ruffle, J. M. (1992). Comparison of the safety and efficacy of intranasal midazolam or sufentanil for preinduction of anesthesia in pediatric patients. *Anesthesiology, 76*(2), 209–215.

Karlsson, E., Larsson, L. E., & Nilsson, K. (1990). Postanaesthetic nausea in children. *Acta Anaesthesiologica Scandinavica, 34*(7), 515–518.

Keenan, R. L., Shapiro, J. H., & Dawson, K. (1991). Frequency of anesthetic cardiac arrests in infants: effect of pediatric anesthesiologist. *Journal of Clinical Anesthesia, 3*(6), 433–437.

Keenan, R. L., Shapiro, J. H., Kane, F. R., & Simpson, P. M. (1994). Bradycardia during anesthesia in infants. An epidemiologic study. *Anesthesiology, 80*(5), 969–971.

Keller, C., Elliott, W., & Hubbell, R. N. Endotracheal tube safety during electrodissection tonsillectomy. *Archives of Otolaryngology—Head and Neck Surgery, 118*(6), 643–645.

Kermode, J., Walker, S., & Webb, I. (1995). Postoperative vomiting in children. *Anaesthesia and Intensive Care, 23*(2), 196–199.

Kerner, M. M., & Newman, A. (1983). Diagnosis and management of latex allergy in surgical patients. *American Journal of Otolaryngology, 14*(6), 440–443.

Khalil, S. N., Florence, F. B., Van den Nieuwenhuyzen, M. C., Wu, A. H., & Stanley, T. H. (1990). Rectal methohexital: Concentration and length of the rectal catheters. *Anesthesia and Analgesia, 70*(6), 645–649.

Kirse, D. J., Tryka, A. F., Seibert, R. W., & Bower, C. M. (1996). Mortality following adenotonsillectomy in a patient with Williams-Campbe syndrome. *Archives of Otolaryngology—Head and Neck Surgery, 122*(9), 1007–1110.

Knill, R. L., & Gelb, A. W. (1978). Ventilatory responses to hypoxia and hypercapnia during halothane sedation and anesthesia in man. *Anesthesiology, 49*(4), 244–251.

Kokki, H., & Ahonen, R. (1997). Pain and activity disturbance after paediatric day case adenoidectomy. *Paediatric Anaesthesia, 7*(3), 227–231.

Kotiniemi, L. H., & Ryhanen, P. T. (1996). Behavioural changes and children's memories after intravenous, inhalation and rectal induction of anaesthesia. *Paediatric Anaesthesia. 6*(3), 201–207.

Larosa-Nash, P. A., Murphy, J. M., Wade, L. A., & Clasby, L. L. (1995). Implementing a parent-present induction program. *AORN Journal, 61*(3), 526–531.

Lawhorn, C. D., Bower, C., Brown, R. E., Jr., Schmitz, M. L., Kymer, P. J., Stoner, J., Vollers, J. M., & Shirey, R. (1996). Ondansetron decreases postoperative vomiting in pediatric patients undergoing tonsillectomy and adenoidectomy. *International Journal of Pediatric Otorhinolaryngology, 36*(2), 99–108.

Lawhorn, C. D., Bower, C. M., Brown, R. E., Jr., Schmitz, M. L., Kymer, P. J., Volpe, P., & Shirey, R. (1996). Topical lidocaine for postoperative analgesia following myringotomy and tube placement. *International Journal of Pediatric Otorhinolaryngology, 35*(1), 19–24.

Le Clair, J., Gartner, S., & Halma, G. (1990). Endotracheal tube cuff ignited by electrocautery during tracheostomy. *AANA Journal, 58*(4), 259–261.

Lee, W. C., & Sharp, J. F. (1996). Complications of paediatric tonsillectomy post-discharge. *Journal of Laryngology and Otology, 110*(2), 136–140.

LeSaint, P. W., & Hemmen, M. S. (1995). Pediatric anesthesia. *Seminars in Perioperative Nursing, 4*(2), 117–119.

Levy, D. M. (1945). Psychic trauma of operations in children. *American Journal of Disabilities in Children, 69*, 7–25.

Levy, L., Pandit, U. A., Randel, G. I., Lewis, I. H., & Tait, A. R. (1992). Upper respiratory tract infections and general anaesthesia in children: Peri-operative complications and oxygen saturation. *Anaesthesia, 47*(8), 678–682.

Lew, E. O., Mittleman, R. E., & Murray, D. (1991). Endotracheal tube ignition by electrocautery during tracheostomy: Case report with autopsy findings. *Journal of Forensic Sciences, 36*(5), 1586–1589.

Liu, L. M., Cote, C. J., Goudsouzian, N. G., Ryan, J. F., Firestone, S., Dedrick, D. F., Liu, P. L., & Todres, I. D. (1983). Life-threatening apnea in infants recovering from anesthesia. *Anesthesiology, 59*(6), 506–510.

Livesey, J. R. (1993). Are haematological tests warranted prior to tonsillectomy? *Journal of Laryngology and Otology, 107*(3), 205–207.

Majcher, T. A., & Means, L. J. (1992). Pain management in children. *Seminars in Pediatric Surgery, 1*(1), 55–64.

Mancuso, R. F. (1996) Stridor in neonates. *Pediatric Clinics of North America, 43*(6), 1339–1356.

Manning, S. C., Beste, D., McBride, T., & Goldberg, A. (1987). An assessment of preoperative coagulation screening for tonsillectomy and adenoidectomy. *International Journal of Pediatric Otorhinolaryngology, 13*(3), 237–244.

Markowitz-Spence, L., Brodsky, L., Syed, N., Stankievich, J., & Volk, M. (1990). Anesthetic complications of tympanotomy tube placement in children. *Archives of Otolaryngology—Head and Neck Surgery, 116*(7), 809–712.

Marsh, B., & Riley, R. H. (1992). Double-lumen tube fire during tracheostomy. [Letter]. *Anesthesiology, 76*(3), 480–481.

Martin, L. D. (1994). Anesthetic implications of an upper respiratory infection in children. *Pediatric Clinics of North America, 41*(1), 121–130.

Mather, S. J., & Peutrell, J. M. (1995). Postoperative morphine requirements, nausea and vomiting following anaesthesia for tonsillectomy. Comparison of intravenous morphine and non-opioid analgesic techniques. *Paediatric Anaesthesia, 5*(3), 185–188.

McCormick, A. S., & Spargo, P. M. (1996). Parents in the anaesthetic room: A questionnaire survey of departments of anaesthesia. *Paediatric Anaesthesia, 6*(3), 183–186.

McCoy, E. P., Russell, W. J., & Webb, R. K. (1997). Accidental bronchial intubation. An analysis of AIMS incident reports from 1988 to 1994 inclusive. *Anaesthesia, 52*(1), 24–31.

McGee, D. L., Wald, D. A., & Hinchliffe, S. (1997). Helium-oxygen therapy in the emergency department. [Review]. *Journal of Emergency Medicine, 15*(3), 291–296.

McGowan, F. X., Kenna, M. A., Fleming, J. A., & O'Connor, T. (1992). Adenotonsillectomy for upper airway obstruction carries increased risk in children with a history of prematurity. *Pediatric Pulmonology, 13*(4), 222–226.

McGrath, P. A. (1995). Pain in the pediatric patient: practical aspects of assessment. *Pediatric Annals, 24*(3), 126–133, 137–138.

McGrath, P. J., & McAlpine, L. (1993). Psychologic perspectives on pediatric pain. *Journal of Pediatrics, 122*(5, Pt. 2), S2–S8.

McGraw, T. (1994). Preparing children for the operating room: psychological issues. *Canadian Journal of Anaesthesia, 41*(11), 1094–1103.

McRae, R. G., Weissburg, A. J., & Chang, K. W. (1994). Iatrogenic hyponatremia: A cause of death following pediatric tonsillectomy. *International Journal of Pediatric Otorhinolaryngology, 30*(3), 227–232.

Menard, S. W. (1995). Preoperative assessment of the infant, child, and adolescent. *Seminars in Perioperative Nursing, 4*(2), 88–91.

Mihm, F. G., & Halperin, B. D. (1985). Noninvasive detection of profound arterial desaturations using a pulse oximetry device. *Anesthesiology, 62*(1), 85–87.

Morgan-Hughes, J. O., & Wilkinson, K. A. (1995). Anaesthesia in epiglottitis. *Anaesthesia and Intensive Care, 23*(4), 519.

Morray, J. P., Geiduschek, J. M., Caplan, R. A., Posner, K. L., Gild, W. M., & Cheney, F. W. (1993). A comparison of pediatric and adult anesthesia closed malpractice claims. *Anesthesiology, 78*(3), 461–467.

Morton, N. S., Camu, F., Dorman, T., Knudsen, K. E., Kvalsvik, O., Nellgard, P., Saint-Maurice, C. P., Wilhelm, W., & Cohen, L. A. (1997). Ondansetron reduces nausea and vomiting after paediatric adenotonsillectomy. *Paediatric Anaesthesia, 7*(1), 37–45.

Murray, W. B., Yankelowitz, S. M., le Roux, M., & Bester, H. F. (1987). Prevention of post-tonsillectomy pain with analgesic doses of ketamine. *South African Medical Journal, 72*(12), 839–842.

Myssiorek, D., & Alvi, A. (1996). Post-tonsillectomy hemorrhage: an assessment of risk factors. *International Journal of Pediatric Otorhinolaryngology, 37*(1), 35–43.

Nigam, A., Ahmed, K., & Drake-Lee, A. B. (1990). The value of pre-operative estimation of haemoglobin in children undergoing tonsillectomy. *Clinical Otolaryngology, 15*(6), 549–551.

O'Connor, B., Levy, D. M., & Peacock, J. E. (1996). The influence of alfentanil pre-treatment on ventilatory effects of doxapram following induction of anaesthesia with propofol. *Acta Anaesthesiologica Scandinavica, 40*(2), 156–159.

O'Connor, K. W., & Jones, S. (1990). Oxygen desaturation is common and clinically underappreciated during elective endoscopic procedures. *Gastrointestinal Endoscopy, 36*(3, Suppl), S2–S4.

Ossoff, R. H. (1989). Laser safety in otolaryngology—head and neck surgery: anesthetic and educational considerations for laryngeal surgery. *Laryngoscope, 99*(8, Pt. 2, Suppl. 48), 1–26.

Patel, D., & Meakin, G. (1997). Oral midazolam compared with diazepam-droperidol and trimeprazine as premedicants in children. *Paediatric Anaesthesia, 7*(4), 287–293.

Patel, R. I., Hannallah, R. S., Norden, J., Casey, W. F., & Verghese, S. T. (1991). Emergence airway complications in children: A comparison of tracheal extubation in awake and deeply anesthetized patients. *Anesthesia and Analgesia, 73*(3), 266–270.

Pearsall, F. J., Davidson, J. A., & Asbury, A. J. (1995). Attitudes to the Association of Anaesthetists recommendations for standards of monitoring during anaesthesia and recovery. *Anaesthesia, 50*(7), 649–653.

Pounder, D. R., Blackstock, D., & Steward, D. J. (1992). Tracheal extubation in children: Halothane versus isoflurane, anesthetized versus awake. *Anesthesiology, 74*(4), 653–655.

Prinsley, P., Wood, M., & Lee, C. A (1993). Adenotonsillectomy in patients with inherited bleeding disorders. *Clinical Otolaryngology, 18*(3), 206–208.

Randell, T., Saarnivaara, L., Oikkonen, M., & Lindgren, L. (1991). Oral atropine enhances the risk for acid aspiration in children. *Acta Anaesthesiologica Scandinavica, 35*(7), 651–653.

Redleaf, M. I., & Fennessy, J. J. (1995). Pneumomediastinum after rigid bronchoscopy. *Annals of Otology, Rhinology and Laryngology, 104*(12), 955–956.

Rimell, F. L., Shapiro, A. M., Mitskavich, M. T., Modreck, P., Post, J. C., & Maisel, R. H. (1996). Pediatric fiberoptic laser rigid bronchoscopy. *Otolaryngology—Head and Neck Surgery, 114*(3), 413–417.

Rimell, F. L., Shapiro, A. M., Shoemaker, D. L., & Kenna, M. A. (1995). Head and neck manifestations of Beckwith Wiedemann syndrome. *Otolaryngology—Head and Neck Surgery, 113*(3), 262–265.

Rita, L., Seleny, F., & Holinger, L. D. (1983). Anesthetic management and gas scavenging for laser surgery of infant subglottic stenosis. *Anesthesiology, 58*(2), 191–193.

Rolf, N., & Cote, C. J. (1992). Frequency and severity of desaturation events during general anesthesia in children with and without upper respiratory infections. *Journal of Clinical Anesthesia, 4*(3), 200–203.

Romej, M., Voepel-Lewis, T., Merkel, S. I., Reynolds, P. I., & Quinn, P. (1996). Effect of preemptive acetaminophen on postoperative pain scores and oral fluid intake in pediatric tonsillectomy patients. *AANA Journal, 64*(6), 535–540.

Romsing, J., Moller-Sonnergaard, J., Hertel, S., & Rasmussen, M. (1996). Postoperative pain in children: Comparison between ratings of children and nurses. *Journal of Pain and Symptom Management, 11*(1), 42–46.

Romsing, J., & Walther-Larsen, S. (1997). Peri-operative use of nonsteroidal anti-inflammatory drugs in children: Analgesic efficacy and bleeding. *Anaesthesia, 52*(7), 673–683.

Rose, J. B., & Martin, T. M. (1996). Post-tonsillectomy vomiting. Ondansetron or metoclopramide during paediatric tonsillectomy: Are two doses better than one? *Paediatric Anaesthesia, 6*(1), 39–44.

Sakoh, T., Fukuda, H., Sasaki, S., Sakaguchi, R., Shiotani, A., Kawaida, M., & Kanzaki, J. (1993). Laryngomicrosurgery with carbon dioxide laser for laryngeal papillomatosis: Application of a two-stage operation. *Auris, Nasus, Larynx, 20*(3), 223–229.

Salassa, J. R., Seaman, S. L., Ruff, T., Lenis, A., Bellens, E. E., & Brown, A. K. (1988). Oral dantrolene sodium for tonsillectomy pain: A double-blind study. *Otolaryngology—Head and Neck Surgery, 98*(1), 26–33.

Schnapf, B. M. (1991). Oxygen desaturation during fiberoptic bronchoscopy in pediatric patients. *Chest, 99*(3), 591–594.

Schofield, N. M., & White, J. B. (1989). Interrelations among children, parents, premedication, and anaesthetists in paediatric day stay surgery. *British Medical Journal, 299*(6712), 1371–1375.

Schreuder, M., Bosenberg, A. T., & Murray, W. B. (1992). Anaesthesia without tears. *South African Medical Journal, 81*(6), 317–318.

Schroeder, W. A., Jr. (1995). Post tonsillectomy hemorrhage: A ten-year retrospective study. *Missouri Medicine, 92*(9), 592–595.

Sekerci, C., Donmez, A., Ates, Y., & Okten, F. (1996). Oral ketamine premedication in children (placebo controlled double-blind study. *European Journal of Anaesthesiology. 13*(6), 606–611.

Simpson, J. I., & Wolf, G. L. (1986). Endotracheal tube fire ignited by pharyngeal electrocautery. *Anesthesiology, 65*(1), 76–77.

Sliney D. H. (1996). Laser safety. [Review]. (Laser Microwave Division, U.S. Army Environmental Hygiene Agency, Aberdeen Proving Ground, Maryland 21010-5422, USA). *Lasers in Surgery and Medicine, 16*(3), 215–225.

Sorensen, B. H., & Thomsen, A. (1987). Bronchoscopy and nitrous oxide pollution. *European Journal of Anaesthesiology, 4*(4), 281–285.

Sosis, M. B., & Braverman, B. (1996). Evaluation of foil coverings for protecting plastic endotracheal tubes from the potassium-titanyl-phosphate laser. *Anesthesia and Analgesia, 77*(3), 589–591.

Sosis, M. B., Braverman, B., & Caldarelli, D. D. (1996). Evaluation of a new laser-resistant fabric and copper foil-wrapped endotracheal tube. *Laryngoscope, 106*(7), 842–844.

Sosis, M., & Dillon, F. (1990). What is the safest foil tape for endotracheal tube protection during Nd-YAG laser surgery? A comparative study. *Anesthesiology, 72*(3), 553–555.

Splinter, W. M., Baxter, M. R., Gould, H. M., Hall, L. E., MacNeill, H. B., Roberts, D. J., & Komocar, L. (1995). Oral ondansetron decreases vomiting after tonsillectomy in children. *Canadian Journal of Anaesthesia, 42*(4), 277–280.

Splinter, W. M., MacNeil, H. B., Menard, E. A., Rhine, E. J., Roberts, D. J., & Gould, M. H. (1995). Midazolam reduces vomiting after tonsillectomy in children. *Canadian Journal of Anaesthesia, 42*(3), 201–203.

Splinter, W. M., Rhine, E. J., Roberts, D. W., Reid, C. W., & MacNeill, H. B. (1996). Preoperative ketorolac increases bleeding after tonsillectomy in children. *Canadian Journal of Anaesthesia, 43*(6), 560–563.

Splinter, W. M., & Roberts, D. J. (1996). Dexamethasone decreases vomiting by children after tonsillectomy. *Anesthesia and Analgesia, 83*(5), 913–916.

Splinter, W. M., Roberts, D. J., Rhine, E. J., MacNeill, H. B., & Komocar, L. (1996). Nitrous oxide does not increase vomiting in children after myringotomy. *Canadian Journal of Anaesthesia, 42*(4), 274–276.

St. Charles, C. S., Matt, B. H., Hamilton, M. M., & Katz, B. P. (1997). A comparison of ibuprofen versus acetaminophen with codeine in the young tonsillectomy patient. *Otolaryngology—Head and Neck Surgery, 117*(1), 76–82.

Stehling, L. C. (1987). Special pediatric airway problems. *Contemporary Anesthesia Practice, 9*, 97–113.

Steiss, J. O., & Rascher, W. (1996). Automated blood pressure measurement in children. *Zeitschrift für Kardiologie, 85*(Suppl 3), 81–84.

Stene, F. N., Seay, R. E., Young, L. A., Bohnsack, L. E. & Bostrom, B. C. (1996). Prospective, randomized, double-blind, placebo-controlled comparison of metoclopramide and ondansetron for prevention of posttonsillectomy or adenotonsillectomy emesis. *Journal of Clinical Anesthesia, 8*(7), 540–544.

Sun, K. O. (1990). Doxapram in tubeless anaesthesia for microlaryngeal surgery. *Anaesthesia and Intensive Care, 18*(4), 497–503.

Sutters, K. A., & Miaskowski, C. (1997). Inadequate pain management and associated morbidity in children at home after tonsillectomy. *Journal of Pediatric Nursing, 12*(3), 178–185.

Szeremeta, W., Novelly, N. J., & Benninger, M. (1996). Postoperative bleeding in tonsillectomy patients. *Ear, Nose, and Throat Journal, 75*(6), 373–376.

Tait, A. R., & Knight, P. R. (1987a). The effects of general anesthesia on upper respiratory tract infections in children. *Anesthesiology, 67*(6), 930–935.

Tait, A, R., & Knight, P. R. (1987b). Intraoperative respiratory complications in patients with upper respiratory tract infections. *Canadian Journal of Anaesthesia, 34*(3, Pt. 1). 300–303.

Talbott, G. A., Lynn, A. M., Levy, F. H., & Zelikovic, I. (1997). Respiratory arrest precipitated by codeine in a child with chronic renal failure. *Clinical Pediatrics, 36*(3), 171–173.

Tay, H. L. (1996). Post-tonsillectomy pain with selective diathermy haemostasis. *Journal of Laryngology and Otology, 110*(5), 446–448.

Tobias, J. D., Lowe, S., Hersey, S., Rasmussen, G. E., & Werkhaven, J. (1995). Analgesia after bilateral myringotomy and placement of pressure equalization tubes in children: acetaminophen versus acetaminophen with codeine. *Anesthesia and Analgesia, 81*(3), 496–500.

Tom, L. W., Miller, L., Wetmore, R. F., Handler, S. D., & Potsic, W. P (1993). Endoscopic assessment in children with tracheotomies. *Archives of Otolaryngology—Head and Neck Surgery, 119*(3), 321–324.

Tom, L. W., Templeton, J. J., Thompson, M. E., & Marsh, R. R. (1996). Dexamethasone in adenotonsillectomy. *International Journal of Pediatric Otorhinolaryngology, 37*(2), 115–120.

Toma A. G., Blanshard J., Eynon-Lewis, N., & Bridger M. W. Post-tonsillectomy pain: the first ten days. *Journal of Laryngology and Otology. 109*(10), 963–964.

Valletta, E. A., Pregarz, M., Bergamo-Andreis, I. A., & Boner, A. L. (1997). Tracheoesophageal compression due to congenital vascular anomalies (vascular rings). *Pediatric Pulmonology, 24*(2), 93–105.

Van der Walt, J. (1995). Anaesthesia in children with viral respiratory tract infections. [Review]. *Paediatric Anaesthesia, 5*(4), 257–262.

Wackym, P. A., & Blackwell, K. E. (1994). Malignant hyperthermia in the otology patient: the UCLA experience. *American Journal of Otology, 15*(3), 371–375.

Wall, J. E., Wilimas, J. A., & Manco-Johnson, M. J. (1993). Preoperative coagulation screening in children. *Pediatrics, 92*(1), 186.

Wark, H. (1997). Is there still a place for halothane in pediatric anesthesia? [Editorial]. *Pediatric Anesthesia, 7*, 359–361.

Warner, D. L., Cabaret, J., & Velling, D. (1995). Ketamine plus midazolam, a most effective paediatric oral premedicant. *Paediatric Anesthesia, 5*(5), 293–295.

Watcha, M. F., Ramirez-Ruiz, M., White, P. F., Jones, M. B., Lagueruela, R. G., & Terkonda, R. P. (1992). Perioperative effects of oral ketorolac and acetaminophen in children undergoing bilateral myringotomy. *Canadian Journal of Anaesthesia. 39*(7), 649–654.

Waters, K. A., Woo, P., Mortelliti, A. J., & Colton, R. (1996). Assessment of the infant airway with videorecorded flexible laryngoscopy and the objective analysis of vocal fold abduction. *Otolaryngology—Head and Neck Surgery, 114*(4), 554–561.

Weimert, T. A., Babyak, J. W., & Richter, H. J. (1990). Electrodissection tonsillectomy. *Archives of Otolaryngology—Head and Neck Surgery, 116*(2), 186–188.

Weisberger, E. C., & Emhardt, J. D. (1996). Apneic anesthesia with intermittent ventilation for microsurgery of the upper airway. *Laryngoscope, 106*(9, Pt. 1), 1099–1102.

While, A. (1985). Personal view. *British Medical Journal, 291*, 343.

Williams, O. A., Hills, R., & Goddard, J. M. (1992). Pulmonary collapse during anaesthesia in children with respiratory tract symptoms. *Anaesthesia, 47*(5), 411–413.

Wolf, G. L., & Simpson, J. I. (1987). Flammability of endotracheal tubes in oxygen and nitrous oxide enriched atmosphere. *Anesthesiology, 67*(2), 236–239.

Woods, M. W. (1990). Anesthetic management of difficult and routine pediatric patients. In F. Berry (Ed.), *Pediatric endoscopy* (2nd ed., chap. 7, p. 218). London: Churchill Livingstone Inc.

Xue, F. S., Huang, Y. G., Luo, L. K., Deng, X. M., Liao, X., Tong, S. Y., & Liu, Q. H (1996). Observation of early postoperative hypoxaemia in children undergoing elective plastic surgery. *Paediatric Anaesthesia, 6*(1), 21–28.

Yaster, M., Nichols, D. G., Deshpande, J. K., & Wetzel, R. C (1990). Midazolam-fentanyl intravenous sedation in children: Case report of respiratory arrest. *Pediatrics, 86*(3), 463–467.

Yaster, M., Sola, J. E., Pegoli, W., Jr., & Paidas, C. N. (1994). The night after surgery. Postoperative management of the pediatric outpatient—surgical and anesthetic aspects. *Pediatric Clinics of North America, 41*(1), 199–220.

Yoshikawa, T.,Yamamoto, H., Nishimura, M., & Kawakami, Y. (1987). Doxapram on blunted respiratory chemosensitivity to hypoxia in hypoxemic, chronic obstructive pulmonary disease. *Japanese Journal of Medicine, 26*(2), 194–202.

Zedie, N., Amory, D. W., Wagner, B. K., & O'Hara, D. A. (1996). Comparison of intranasal midazolam and sufentanil premedication in pediatric outpatients. *Clinical Pharmacology and Therapeutics, 59*(3), 341–348.

Zwack, G. C., & Derkay, C. S. (1997). The utility of preoperative hemostatic assessment in adenotonsillectomy. *International Journal of Pediatric Otorhinolaryngology, 39*(1), 67–76.

I

Index

Esophageal disease *(continued)*
  Barrett's esophagus, 27, 28, 29
  carcinoma, squamous cell, 36, 151
  congenital disorders, 40–42
  cysts, congenital, 41–42
  diverticulum, 42
  esophagitis
    differentiated from GER, 28–29, 31
    endoscopy, 28–29, 31
  foregut duplication, congenital, 41–42
  GER (gastroesophageal reflux)
    antireflux barrier, 25–26
    associated disorders, 27
    barium studies, 28, 29
    Barrett's esophagus, 27, 28, 29
    congenital disorders, 5, 6
    diagnosis, 28–30
    esophageal defense, 26–27
    exacerbation, diet, 30
    fundoplication, 32
    gastric emptying, 26
    hiatus hernia, 26, 37
    LES (lower esophageal sphincter) incompetence, 26
    pathology, 27
    pathophysiology, 25–27
    refluxate, 26
    surgery, 6, 32
    symptoms, 27–28
    treatment, 30–32
  heartburn, 27
  hiatus hernia
    congenital, 37
    GER (gastroesophageal reflux), 26, 37
    pathophysiology, 36–37
    treatment, 37
  stenosis, congenital, 41
  strictures, corrosive, 34–36, 35
    acid injury, 35
    alkaline injury, 34
    damage, degrees of (staging), 35
    self-bougienage, 36
    treatment, 35–36
  TEF (tracheoesophageal fistula), 37–40, 42
    anastomotic leak, 40
    diagnosis, 39
    pathogenesis, 38
    surgery, 39–40
    and tracheotomy, 107
  webs, 41
Esophagitis
  differentiated from GER, 28–29, 31
  endoscopy, 28–29, 31
Esophagogram, barium, 41, 42, 98
Esophagoscopy, 28–29, 98
Exostosis, 164

F

Feeding
  gastrostomy tube, 56
  suprahyoid lesions, 56
Fever, 121, 122, 132
  spiking, 120

Fistulae
  branchial, 50
  cervicoauricular, 51
  retropharyngeal, 116
  salivary, 235
  TEF (tracheoesophageal fistula), 37–40, 42, 107
Fluoroscopy, choking accidents, 19, 20
Fracture. *See* Trauma
Francisella tularensis, 121
Fundoplication, 98
Fusobacterium sp, 62, 112

G

GABHS (group A beta-hemolytic streptococcus), 78–80, 112, 121
  assessment, 80
  carrier state, 79–80
  pathogenesis, 79
  treatment, 80
Gardner syndrome, 153, 165
Gastropexy, 98
Gastrostomy, 40, 41
  tube feeding, 56
Gaucher disease, 120
GER (gastroesophageal reflux), 174, 179
  antireflux barrier, 25–26
  associated disorders, 27
  barium studies, 28, 29, 98
  Barrett's esophagus, 27, 28, 29
  congenital disorders, 5, 6
  differential diagnosis, 28–30
  esophageal defense, 26–27
  exacerbation, diet, 30
  fundoplication, 32
  gastric emptying, 26
  hiatus hernia, 26, 37
  infectious, 98
  LES (lower esophageal sphincter) incompetence, 26
  pathology, 27
  pathophysiology, 25–27
  pH monitoring, 41, 98
  refluxate, 26
  silent, 98
  surgery, 6, 32
  and surgery, 6, 40
  symptoms, 27–28
  treatment, 30–32
Gibson, William S.
  chapter by, 1–8
Glomerulonephritis, 78, 79
Gonorrhea, 82–83
Granuloma, 182
  eosinophilic, 135
  and giant cell lesions, 166
  vocal fold, 98
Granulomatous disease, chronic, 120
Grave's disease, 156
Gynecomastia, 31

H

Haemophilus haemolytica, 112
Haemophilus influenzae, 96, 97, 111